Psychosomatic Energetics Textbook

REIMAR BANIS

Psychosomatic Energetics Textbook

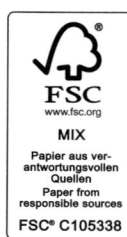

Bibliographical Information Of the German National Library
the German National Library has registered this publication in the German National Bibliography; detailed bibliographical data can be accessed on the Internet via:
HTTP://clnb.d-nb.de.

Author's Address
Dr. Reimar Banis
c/o IGPSE (International Society For Psychosomatic Energetics)
Dörflistrasse 4
CH-6056 Kägiswil
SWITZERLAND

© 2017 Reimar Banis
Translation: David Fogg
Coverdesign, Typesetting, Printing, Production and Layout: BoD – Books on Demand
ISBN: 978-3-7431-8271-4

Illustrations: © Dr. R. Banis and by the named artists below illustrations/photos
Printed in Germany

Also available as e-book

Important information: like any science, medicine is subject to constant development. Research and clinical experience expand our knowledge, especially as regards treatment. To the extent that this book mentions a dosage or an application, the textbook may indeed be assured that authors, editors and publisher have taken great efforts to ensure that this information corresponds to the state of knowledge at the time of publication. However, as regards information concerning dosage instructions and types of applications, the publisher can accept no responsibility with respect to content. It is the responsibility of every user, by careful reading of the package insert and possibly after consulting a specialist, to determine whether the dosage recommendation or the information regarding contraindications deviates from the information in this book. This kind of scrutiny is particularly important when it comes to seldom-used preparations or those which have recently come onto the market. Every dosage or application is at the user's own risk. The authors and the publisher encourage all users to notify them of any inaccuracies that may come to their attention.

Protected product names (brand names ®) are not always clearly labeled as such; therefore, the lack of such information should not be taken to mean that the product is not protected.

All parts of this work are protected by copyright. Any use thereof outside the narrow limits of copyright law and without the specific permission of the publisher is inadmissible and a punishable offense. This applies particularly to duplication, translation, microfilming or storage and processing in electronic systems.

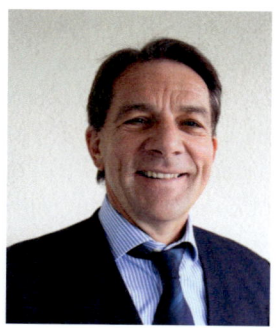

Dr. Reimar Banis

Born 1951 in West Berlin, grew up in the Ruhr valley, alternative service in hospital, after graduation from high school, attended the all-day German Naturopathic School (DH) in Bochum for two years. Passed the naturopathic examination in 1976, then studied human medicine in Heidelberg. Doctorate under Prof. Maria Blohmke (social medicine), dissertation title *Thermoregulation Diagnostics and Focal Diseases,* magna cum laude. 1984 American State Exam (ECFMG). Worked as assistant physician at the internal-medicine ICU in one of Germany's largest rheumatism clinics (University of Hanover).

Since 1985 established physician in general medicine with continuing-education warrant in naturopathic medicine, over a decade as panel doctor with practices in Achern (southern Baden), Stuttgart, Plochingen. Private practices in Ostfildern, Bregenz and Wallerfangen. Intensive collaboration with H.W. Schimmel, developer of the Vegatest. Collaborated in research on electroacupuncture and computerized segment electrography with Prof. G. Heim, Heidelberg University. Seminar activity around the world, and development of Psychosomatic Energetics. Reimar Banis is married to a Swiss woman, lives in the vicinity of Lucerne with three children: Jana, Frederik and David.

Preface

The Psychosomatic Energetics Textbook (PSE) is meant as an aid and reference work for therapists while in training to become "Certified Energy Therapists", but also to be useful later in daily clinical practice. At this point, after more than 15 years, over 600 therapists in German-speaking countries and 50 in North America have been trained, and Psychosomatic Energetics – originally developed from the precursor Vegatest method of H.W. Schimmel – is well on the way to becoming one of the standard methods of modern complementary medicine.

For those interested in the method, this textbook provides a good overview of the possibilities and limits of the method, but it cannot replace practical training. To the uninitiated, energy tests might seem easy to perform, but they are very sensitive and require intensive training in order to obtain good results.

With standardization, PSE aspires to a high level of quality, and this textbook makes an important contribution thereto.

The textbook contains the entire training material for PSE and I'm very grateful that my colleague Dr. Birgitt Holschuh-Lorang, head of PSE training, has looked it over and authorized it.

The textbook is now 16 years old. First published in 1997 by CO'med Verlag in Sulzbach, a thoroughly revised version was published in 2003 in three editions by VAK Verlag in Hinterzarten. In 2013, the textbook again needed to be completely rewritten and brought up to date. It now contains all the studies and scientific research on PSE, as well as an overview of the therapeutic options for a number of different disease pictures. Each procedure is illustrated by means of specific pertinent cases. Because PSE provides a glimpse into the characterological deep structure by which human feelings and actions are subconsciously pre-formed, PSE also makes possible a kind of psychotherapeutic life-counseling, the possibilities of which are likewise thoroughly presented.

Since PSE is active in a relatively unexplored region of the human organism, a certain degree of theoretical underpinning was necessary to indicate what PSE is capable of. The model developed here of the psychosomatic and subtle-energy mesenchymal mode of action should be regarded as provisional; nevertheless, it has a high reality content, since it is based upon decades of clinical experience. It is intended to help therapists to arrive at correct decisions in each case, and also to be able to explain to patients the healing principle of subtle-energy harmonization.

Hergiswil/Switzerland, August 2014
Dr. Reimar Banis

Table of Contents

Part 1
Basics 17

1. Introduction 19
   1.1 How is Psychosomatic Energetics applied in practice? 23
   1.2 Psychosomatic Energetics vs. Orthodox Medicine – just a placebo? . . . 25
   1.3 Healing with Energy Medicine 30
   1.4 The relationship of subtle energy to the mesenchyme,
        soma and Psyche 35

2. The History of Psychosomatic Energetics 39
   2.1 EAV and Vegatest 41
   2.2 The discovery of the conflicts 43
   2.3 Conflict size 48
   2.4 Chakras as conflict storage 54
   2.5 The Central Conflict 57
   2.6 The four character types 58
   2.7 The REBA® Test Device 60

Part 2
Psychosomatic Energetics 63

3. The Subtle Energy Field 65
   3.1 Testing the patient's energy field 65
   3.2 The four energy levels 67
        3.2.1 The Vital Level 68
        3.2.2 The Emotional Level 69
        3.2.3 The Mental Level 72
        3.2.4 The Causal Level 73
   3.3 Life energy and well-being 75
   3.4 Life energy with respect to circulation and pain states 76

4. The Seven Chakras..79
   4.1 Preliminary remarks vis-à-vis "Chakra".....................79
       4.1.1 Hormones, nerve plexus and stem cells................81
       4.1.2 Chakras as psychosomatic control points..............82
       4.1.3 Archetypal significance of Chakras...................83
       4.1.4 PSE and Chakras......................................84
       4.1.5 A lifelong journey through the seven Chakras.........86
   4.2 Definition of the seven Chakras............................89
       4.2.1 First Chakra...89
       4.2.2 Second Chakra..90
       4.2.3 Third Chakra...91
       4.2.4 Fourth Chakra..93
       4.2.5 Fifth Chakra...94
       4.2.6 Sixth Chakra...95
       4.2.7 Seventh Chakra.......................................96
   4.3 Chakra interrelatedness: high/low coupling.................98

5. The 28 Emotional Conflicts of PSE.............................101
   5.1 Example of conflict origin and healing....................101
   5.2 Conflict formation due to emotional repression
       and energetic relocation..................................102
   5.3 Conflict storage and activation...........................106
   5.4 Conflict uncoupling.......................................110
   5.5 Conflict consequences.....................................112
   5.6 Uncovering the 28 unconscious emotional conflicts.........116
       5.6.1 First Chakra conflicts..............................120
       5.6.2 Second Chakra conflicts.............................121
       5.6.3 Third Chakra conflicts..............................123
       5.6.4 Fourth Chakra conflicts.............................124
       5.6.5 Fifth Chakra conflicts..............................126
       5.6.6 Sixth Chakra conflicts..............................127
       5.6.7 Seventh Chakra conflicts............................129

6. The Four Character Types.....................................133
   6.1 Basic laws of PSE characterology..........................136

	6.2	When to talk about character type and when not to	138
	6.3	PSE diagnosis of the four character types	139
	6.4	Description of the four character types	142
		6.4.1 Melancholic	142
		6.4.2 Sanguinic	145
		6.4.3 Choleric	148
		6.4.4 Phlegmatic	150
	6.5	Tips for practical character diagnostics	152
	6.6	Emotional growth in characterology	154
	6.7	Partnership	156
	6.8	Child rearing	158
	6.9	Getting to know the character types	159
	6.10	Does character type trigger specific disease susceptibilities?	161
	6.11	Basic aspects of Central Conflict treatment	162
7.	Character type and Karma		163
	7.1	Reincarnation and depth psychology	164
		7.1.1 Evidence for and against reincarnation	166
		7.1.2 Consequences of former lives and mixed therapeutic experiences	167
		7.1.3 Psychoenergetic dissolution of karmic conflicts	168
	7.2	Reincarnation and PSE – a new transpersonal approach	169
	7.3	Karmic conflicts in PSE	170
8.	The Acute Agents		173
	8.1	Anxiety	173
	8.2	Nervous tension and overexcitement	174
		8.2.1 Autonomic misregulation	174
9.	Geopathy and Electrosmog		177
	9.1	Definition, physical proof and studies	177
	9.2	Diagnosing geopathies	179
	9.3	Medications, relocation reaction, monitoring bedsite cleansing	182
	9.4	Conclusions concerning the topic of geo-radiation	183

9.5	Reliably detecting electrosmog	184
9.6	Just how harmful is electrosmog?	185

10. The Organ Test Kit 187
    10.1 Mesenchymal stress 189
    10.2 Darkfield microscopy 190
    10.3 Acidum lacticum ampoules 193
    10.4 The Organ Test Kit 194
    10.5 Functional organ disorders 197
        10.5.1 Intestinal dysbiosis 197
        10.5.2 Bile duct dysfunction 204
        10.5.3 Pancreatic functional disorder 206
    10.6 Chronic foci 207
        10.6.1 Chronic sinusitis 207
        10.6.2 Dental foci 209
        10.6.3 Chronic tonsillitis 210
        10.6.4 Chronic appendicitis 211
        10.6.5 Pelvic foci (ovaries/uterus/prostate) 212
    10.7 Filtering 213
        10.7.1 Filtering with organ ampoules 214
    10.8 Therapy conclusion 215

Part 3
Clinical practice 217

11. Using Psychosomatic Energetics Correctly 219
    11.1 Test site prerequisites 219
    11.2 Patient prerequisites 220
    11.3 Tester prerequisites 220
    11.4 Step one – patient questioning and examination ... 223
    11.5 Step two – testing the energy levels 224
    11.6 Step three – testing geopathy, Chakras and conflicts ... 227
        11.6.1 Acute agents and masked anxiety disease 229
        11.6.2 Remedy test 231
        11.6.3 Organ Test Kit 232

		11.6.4	Testing other medications	232
	11.7	Step four – conflict size		235
		11.7.1	Therapy recommendation	237
		11.7.2	Testing with the Basic Test Kit	241
		11.7.3	The course of therapy	242
		11.7.4	Chavita plus agent	245
	11.8	Step five – explaining the test procedure to the patient		245
	11.9	Step six – interpreting the test results		248
	11.10	Step seven – discussing character		252
	11.11	Step eight – relationship topics		254
	11.12	Step nine – karmic interpretation of the Central Conflict		255
		11.12.1	Patient resistance and therapist conflicts	257
12.	Useful Information about Energy Testing			261
	12.1	Disturbance due to external influences		262
	12.2	Disturbances due to unconscious mental stress and doubt		263
	12.3	Pitfalls of mental testing and training good testers		268
	12.4	Testers should be more energetically healthy than their patients		269
	12.5	Testing children		270
	12.6	Testing animals		272
13.	Psychosomatic Energetics in Everyday Practice			275
	13.1	Anxiety, AIDS, addiction		275
	13.2	Emotional ailments – Central Conflict dissolution		279
	13.3	Psychiatric ailments		282
	13.4	Venous and arterial circulatory disorders		285
	13.5	Cardiovascular diseases		287
	13.6	Allergies		290
	13.7	Hormonal disorders		294
	13.8	Adjuvant therapy in malignancy cases		294
	13.9	Neurological diseases		296
	13.10	Rheumatological diseases		297
	13.11	Emotionally/physically conditioned ailments		299
	13.12	Spiritual crises		301
	13.13	Limits to PSE		302

13.14 Successful practice management. 304
13.15 The testing process 306
       13.15.1 A testing sequence. 307

Part 4
PSE Therapist training – Studies – Case studies – PSE's accomplishments. . 311

14. Training. 313
    14.1 Studying the basic works 313
    14.2 Training program in detail 314

15. Studies 319
    15.1 Clinical study at a general practice in Bregenz (Austria). 319
    15.2 Mathematical modeling 321
    15.3 Clinical study at a general practice in Saarlouis (Germany). 321
    15.4 PSE as a complementary diagnostic and therapeutic procedure
         in a neurological practice. 323
    15.5 Adjuvant homeopathy (drops) for juvenile behavioral disorders
         (Jupident study) 323
    15.6 The Butterfly Project (Schmetterlings-Projekt)
         with Austrian grade-school students 323
    15.7 Butterfly Project (Schmetterlings-Projekt) .325
    15.8 Burnout syndrome and exhaustion states –
         results of a clinical investigation (2007-2009) 326
    15.9 My "Butterfly Project" (Schmetterlings-Projekt) in a Children's
         Village in Vorarlberg (Austria) – positive experiences with PSE 326
    15.10 Chronic pain: tissue's cry for energy flow –
         clinical practice experience with PSE since 1998 326
    15.11 How stable are healing successes? Long-term study results
         of applying Psychosomatic Energetics 327
    15.12 Multicentric clinical study of Psychosomatic Energetics. 327

16. What PSE is capable of 329
    16.1 The effects of energy deficiency 330
    16.2 Therapeutic results 331

	16.3	Therapists' experiences....................................334
	16.4	Special qualities of Psychosomatic Energetics – an overview 336

Part 5
Appendices... 341

17.	List of the 28 Conflict Themes 343
	17.9 Conflict Theme 9......................................346

18.	Character Type Questionnaire..................................355

19.	Useful Addresses 359

20.	Bibliography 363

Part 1
Basics

1   Introduction

This manual deals with the complementary-medicine method known as Psychosomatic Energetics (PSE), which the author developed in the mid-90s in his naturopathic general practice. As a textbook, it is oriented exclusively towards therapists, and presents the essential knowledge and insights of the method. It contains the learning material for the training course toward becoming a "Certified Energy Therapist", a multiyear PSE-specific extra-occupational supplementary course with written and oral exams as well as obligatory continuing education. This training is authorized by the International Society for Psychosomatic Energetics [IGPSE: Internationale Gesellschaft für Psychosomatische Energetik; website: www.ipse.ch) and is carried out by a team of physicians and naturopathic practitioners.

Along with the multi-volume PSE readers, this manual is meant to serve as a practical reference work when questions arise in daily practice. In order to make this easier, it contains an index as well as an easily understandable copiously illustrated introduction to testing. It also includes many useful case histories as well as a rich variety of answers to frequently asked questions. I hope it will turn out to be a valuable enrichment of each reader's daily practice.

Fortunately, Psychosomatic Energetics has quickly established itself as a new standard procedure in modern complementary medicine. In the opinion of many colleagues, this is attributable primarily to two characteristics of the method: the logical simplicity of its practical application and its high therapeutic efficiency. Meanwhile, in a great many clinical studies, the success rate for common mainstream medicine disease pictures is over 80%, in which more than 1200 patients from the entire range of mainstream medicine diseases have been treated. Many important questions in daily practice can only be answered at this high level of quality and confidence with PSE. In more than a few practices led by experienced therapists, this has now led to Psychosomatic Energetics becoming the primary procedure of choice.

Experience has shown that, with Psychosomatic Energetics, one can practice holistic medicine in the truest sense of the word, which leads for many disease pictures to psychological and somatic improvement or healing. The elimination of conflicts resolves psychoenergetic blocks, so that life energy can once again flow at full strength. A disrupted metabolic system is able to renormalize, amazingly often leading to emotional regeneration as well as physical healing processes. Thus, with PSE, one treats both body and soul – i.e. psychosomatically in the best sense of the word. Amazingly, this often even succeeds nonverbally, so that the method can be used successfully with children and animals, as well as with patients with a negative attitude towards psychotherapy. On the other hand, Psychosomatic Energetics is fundamentally open to the application of adjuvant therapies, such that psychotherapy, hypnosis or other procedures can be performed.

Psychosomatic Energetics is based on two fundamental theses. The first thesis is also one of the fundamentals of Indian Yoga and traditional Chinese energy theory, which says that the quality of the subtle energy field reliably reflects a person's subjective feeling of health, and moreover is crucially related to health and illness – comparable, say, to the relationship between software (energy) and hardware (matter) in a computer. A person with a lot of subtle energy therefore feels fresh, lively and is usually healthy, whereas sick people tend to have low energy and feel tired and listless. The healing principles of Yoga and acupuncture developed from these observations, which are also the basis of Psychosomatic Energetics.

The second fundamental thesis of the method is based on the presence of emotional conflicts in the energy field. Shamans and spiritual healers have long been able to visualize these "demons" and regard them as important causes of disease. Unlike the current conceptual model of modern psychotherapy, PSE can show that emotional conflicts by no means represent purely emotional processes, but rather are permanently stored in the energy field and act there as "energy thieves"(cf. **Fig. 1.1**). For example, if a patient suffering from depression feels tired, his low energy is based on a *Rage* conflict which constantly siphons off energy and which can be viewed energetically as the cause of the patient's depression. With the REBA® Test Device, one can measure the energy stored up in the conflict and thereby determine its size, which is an enormous advantage – vis-à-vis techniques which operate entirely on the mental level – not only for the determination of the clinical picture, but also for monitoring the course of treatment.

Psychosomatic Energetics uses a kind of **quick or focal psychotherapy** in which the conflict contents are briefly summarized in a short phrase. The patient is then asked if there's anything he wants to say about it or if anything occurs to him. In practically all cases, patients recognize that the testable conflict theme addresses the current emotional topic. Many people feel quite relieved to be accepted and correctly understood in the depths of their being. The results of this quick psychotherapy have since come to be regarded as scientifically valid. In particular, the quick response of the conflict contents turns out in many cases to be especially beneficial. The patient maintains his individuality and sovereignty because no regression is performed, and the mental self-healing powers are optimally stimulated.

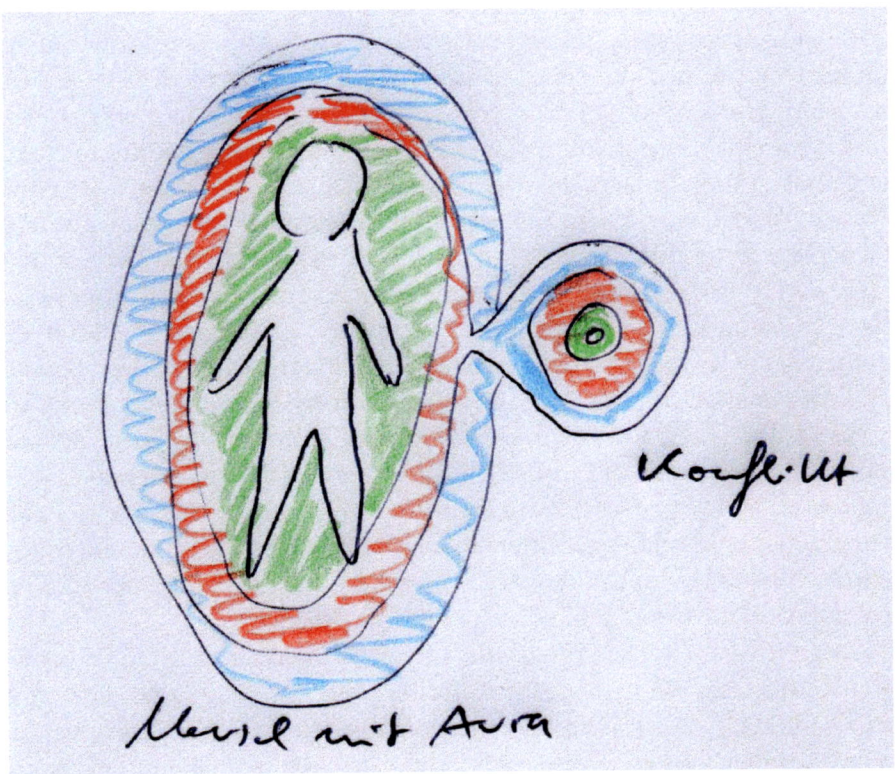

Fig. 1.1 – *Aura levels showing a conflict connected to the Aura via an energetic umbilical cord and feeding vampirically from it (sketch by the author).*

The discussion of the individual **character type**, based on testing of the Central Conflict, leads to particularly profound life counseling sessions. Patients thereby learn about the otherwise subconscious "stage directions" which influence their life scripts and relationships with others. Awareness of the script often enables breakthroughs in personality development, especially when the Central Conflict is dissolved at the same time. Afterwards, people seem more authentic, are more clearly able to express their needs and are better at demarcating boundaries; they put a stop to self-damaging behavioral patterns and once again look optimistically into the future. In the social give-and-take, the theory of character types has proven to be particularly beneficial in the areas of child rearing and choice of partner.

In Psychosomatic Energetics, **energetic conflict resolution** has turned out to be the key healing element, since ultimately the method also works wordlessly. One is thus dealing here with a special form of psychotherapy which is more closely related to modern energy medicine (such as psychokinesiology or Bach Flowers therapy) and humanistic somatic psychotherapy (biodynamic psychology) than, say, to traditional psychoanalysis. The essential point in Psychosomatic Energetics is that, for the first time in the history of medicine, it seems to be possible to portray one's inner emotional "demons" energetically and most precisely by means of resonance over a few months' time.

We now have amassed clinical practice experience from many thousands of patients who have come to us with a great variety of disease pictures, from simply feeling bad all the way to severe chronic ailments. With this treasure trove of experiences, therefore, this manual can offer quite solid instructions in procedures and techniques which have led to success in the majority of cases. Nevertheless, since it is a living method, new experiences and insights are added every day, which makes standing still impossible and which lead to constant improvement. To this extent, Psychosomatic Energetics represents a continuous learning process to which many colleagues, fortunately, constantly contribute. So the method is always being improved and expanded, and every reader is invited to join in this process.

Moreover, I hope that this manual will "infect" as many therapists as possible with the same enthusiasm with which it was written. Because PSE is not just a method with excellent results which is easy to use, but also often an outright adventure for the therapist, which ever and again leads to new stimulating insights. I also hope that this book will impart to my colleagues valuable ideas and information. But above all I hope to stimulate them, as they work with character types, to take on the important role of life counselor, whose comfort and advice is so sorely needed by so many suffering people. The PSE toolkit, which reaches deep into the mental and spiritual realm, makes it possible to impart brand-new insights to many people, which then enable them to reconcile themselves with their destiny and to recognize the truly significant life tasks which each person has, namely to get to know themselves at a very deep level and thereby fully develop their individuality.

1.1 How is Psychosomatic Energetics applied in practice?

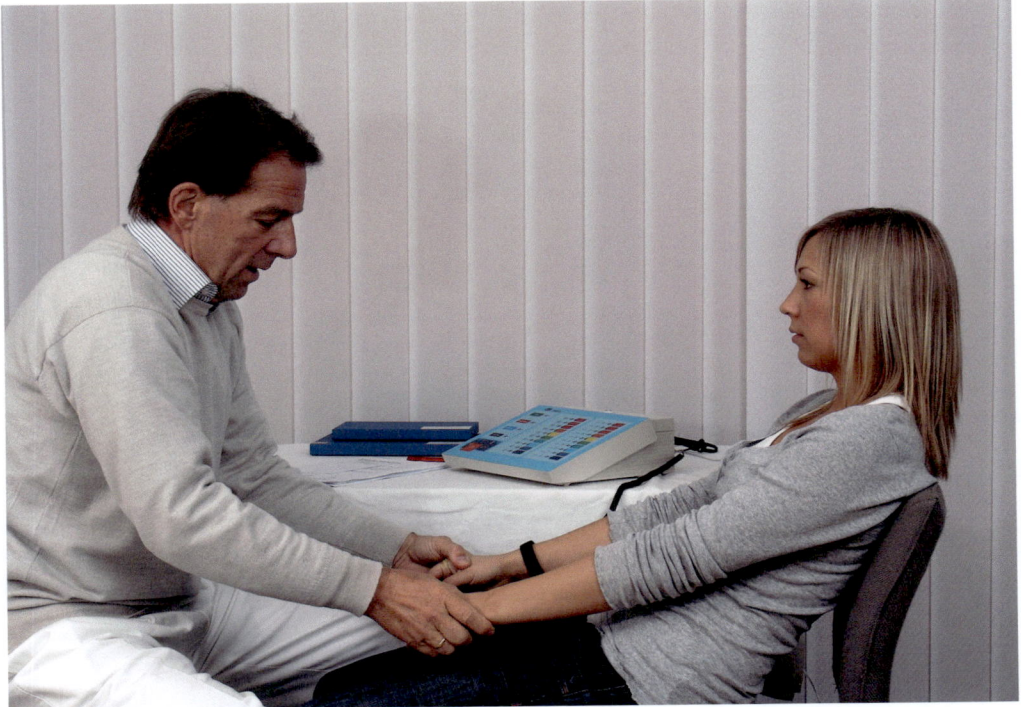

Fig. 1.2 Kinesiological arm-length test with the REBA® Test Device.

In order to give the reader an initial impression of the daily routine with PSE, I would like to describe briefly (in greater detail later on) what a therapist actually does when using PSE. The first step measures the charge on the four subtle-energy levels Vital, Emotional, Mental and Causal using a test device called the REBA® Test Device (Fig. 1.2). The more energy the patient's organism has, the more it can be stressed by the device's vibrations, until finally it exhibits a test reaction. This means, for example in the case of a kinesiological arm-length test, that the position of the patient's parallel arms will become unequal (Fig. 1.3). Other testing procedures can also be used, e.g. a shifting of the pulse wave in the reflex auriculocardial (RAC) test, or an electroacupuncture test device indicating a different value at a measurement point.

> There is a training film available for ESP trainees which presents the rule-consistent use of PSE. Every Basic Seminar participant gets a copy of the DVD so that the testing steps can be calmly learned and rehearsed at home.

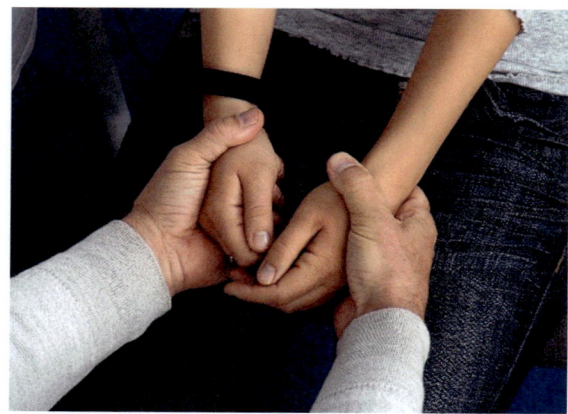

Fig. 1.3 – *Differing arm positions in the kinesiological arm-length test (positive test reaction).*

In the second step, the therapist uses small test tubes filled with homeopathic compound remedies. This is done to find out why the patient has too little energy – i.e. where the energy blocks are located. The test tubes are placed in the test honeycomb one after another to determine when the patient exhibits a reaction to the test. Experience has shown that, at a particular energy block – whether disturbed energy center (Chakra), subconscious conflict, geo-radiation or functional organ disorder – one of the test tubes will respond. Like a sore spot on the skin which hurts when touched, the organism reacts to the subtle vibrational signals of a particular test tube because it also contains the same vibrations.

In the third step, the size of an energy block – i.e. how much energy is taken away from the patient – is determined with the aid of the REBA® Test Device. The duration of therapy can be derived from the conflict size. The final testing step then checks whether the therapy will benefit the patient energetically. Placing the test tube in the pelvic region (Yin zone) simulates taking the agent. Next, the energy levels are retested; if they are noticeably improved or even normal (100%), it may be assumed that the medication in the test tube will be the right healing agent, and so the tested healing agent is prescribed for the patient.

After a few months, the patient is retested with the question now being whether the old energy blocks have disappeared and whether any new ones have surfaced. Case studies of more than 1000 patients have shown that, as a rule, there are good results after 2 to 3 sessions. Thus, PSE is not a fast-acting therapy, but rather takes a great deal of time – which the Psyche evidently needs in order to get reoriented. For this reason, all attempts to accelerate PSE have failed.

1.2   Psychosomatic Energetics vs. Orthodox Medicine – just a placebo?

Modern scientifically-oriented medicine (also known as "mainstream medicine") is known to cover only a portion of the area which makes people sick and for which it can then offer appropriate therapies. One can only estimate how large the region is which mainstream medicine does cover. Based on my decades of experience as a practicing naturopathic physician (going after medical school into a multi-year full-time DH-technical college for training as a naturopath, I've been comprehensively trained in and have a good overview of both areas), it might be 30% or less. Now of course mainstream medicine is constantly improving and discovering new possibilities such as immune-system modulators in cases of inflamed rheumatism, yet this only marginally changes the lack of knowledge, i.e. the incapacity of mainstream medicine will remain pretty much the same for quite some time.

Because mainstream medicine is unaware of large regions which make people sick – for example disturbed intestinal flora or nocturnal geo-radiation stress, as well as disorders on the subtle-energy level – these areas are obviously not treated. However, Psychosomatic Energetics (PSE) knows about these problems and can offer good solutions – it works as a supplement (complement) to mainstream medicine. With this as background, PSE's time has come when the usual mainstream medicine procedures have come to a dead end. However, one first needs a solid mainstream-medicine diagnosis which is then used as the basis for the application of PSE.

PSE complements mainstream medicine without competing with it, since mainstream-medicine diagnostic procedures have their legitimacy and are often indispensable. I'm not just paying lip service here, I also use it in clinical practice, such as when I strongly urge a patient who has not undergone a mainstream-medicine examination to get an examination (cancer checkup, lab tests, x-rays etc.) or therapy (hypertension therapy etc.) as quickly as possible, if the patient has come in for PSE testing, or maybe have it done afterwards.

One tiresome topic is the placebo accusation, since mainstream medicine refuses to acknowledge any possible diagnostic or therapeutic gaps. Instead of learning from alternative or complementary medicine, one mainstream-medicine journal article asserts that: "placebo effects probably account for part or all of the effectiveness of alternative and complementary medicine. Since the administration of […] creates an illusory state of affairs, it needs to be […] checked as to whether or not the deliberate administration of a placebo might not represent […] a deception of the patient." [29] Readers of the *Deutsches Ärzteblatt* [German Medical Journal] thereupon wrote angry letters to the editor, indignant at the above quote by Breidert and Hofbauer, insinuating that they would be guilty of fraud under the law if they were to perform homeopathy (as do about 80% of all established German physicians!). In their response, the authors quickly backpedaled, saying that they "had not even considered professional disbarment for practitioners of alternative and complementary medicine; they were merely concerned that physicians be more aware of the placebo effect."

Ultimately, this confrontation hinges upon what is medically correct and sensible. Anyone who is not convinced of the efficacy of homeopathy will understandably be convinced that the administration of a homeopathic agent constitutes a kind of fraud. However, upon closer inspection, the situation is much less drastic than it sounds at first, because categorical statements of this sort – what is 100% right and what is false, what really works and what does not – are impossible to make from a scientific standpoint: no one can say with absolute certainty that homeopathy is ineffective

- because there are plenty of positive studies concerning homeopathy,
- but above all because, for scientific-theoretic considerations, such dogmatic statements are fundamentally impossible to make in the first place.

The basic idea of the scientific theoretician Karl Popper [109] that one should view science as an "unfinished construction site" (to use a visual metaphor) remains to this day the gold standard of scientific thinking. On principle, serious science may and must not make any final and definitive statements, but rather can only work with probabilities which are subject to constant change. Obviously, critics can nevertheless call into question particular scientifically disputed diagnostic and therapeutic procedures, but they should in all fairness also admit to the proponents that they might under certain circumstances turn out to be right after all. Ultimately, present-day science is something that the scientists of 100 or 200 years ago would largely have found to be absurd and false; one might recall the hostility of his colleagues around 1850 when Semmelweis proposed that unhygienic conditions caused childbed fever. In like manner, it seems thinkable that future research will someday confirm the effectiveness of homeopathy.

> **Note**
> Nobel prize winner Luc Montagnier surprised his colleagues during a scientific conference in 2010 with the statement that aqueous solutions which contained the DNA of pathogenic bacteria and viruses (including HIV) "are capable of emitting low-frequency radio waves which then cause the surrounding water molecules to group themselves into "nanostructures". These water molecules could then in turn emit radio waves. Montagnier showed that water maintained these characteristics when the original solution was massively diluted, even up to the point where the original DNA had in fact vanished. In this manner, water could store the "memory" of substances with which it had been in contact – and physicians could make use of these omissions in order to detect disease.
> Source: www.theaustralian.com/news/health-science/Nobel-Lorient-gives-homeopathy-a-boost/story-e6frg8ys – 122 588 777 2305

Like other complementary-medicine procedures, homeopathy is controversial primarily because it simply has not yet been sufficiently investigated in its fundamentals nor its therapeutic efficacy. One reason that the situation is so unsatisfactory is because no one in the universities believes in such procedures; that which from the outset is believed to be nonsense will not be considered to be worth investigating in the first place. Besides, it is well known that busying oneself with homeopathic topics does not exactly further one's scientific career. The topic is disreputable, i.e. whoever researches such topics should, to be considered a serious scientist, at least demonstrate that homeopathy has little to no effect. So this is indeed what comes out of many studies, but it needs to be said that there are nevertheless a nontrivial number of positive study results (more on this later).

From a business standpoint, when it comes to the serious clinical studies that need to be done, we are talking about expensive material outlays which can run to much more than $3 million, which busts the limited budget of many naturopathic enterprises. In addition, one needs a suitable personnel and economic environment in order to sensibly carry out studies of this sort in the first place – which, considering the global dominance of mainstream medicine in universities and hospitals, turns out, as we all know, to be quite difficult. Any medical outsider faces difficult initial conditions from the very beginning – or is not able to have his therapeutic method rationally examined at all.

Hence, when it comes to scientific investigations of alternative and mainstream medicine, a double standard is employed: those who attack alternative medicine, as can be seen in the quote from the German medical journal, are ultimately merely expressing thereby their strong belief in the current scientific status quo. If one considers contemporary mainstream medicine to be the "true and only church", then anything that deviates from this is basically heretical. One believes exclusively in mainstream medicine and is therefore completely convinced of its correctness.

However, since serious homeopathic research already exists also, which numerous successfully concluded clinical studies and even positive meta-studies demonstrate (mostly carried out in private clinics and special homeopathic departments), there are definitely serious indications that homeopathy is indeed effective.

But the stridency of the confrontation is fueled by other matters. Viewed superficially, it is initially a matter of medical worldviews and current political, business and societal positions – i.e. with objective arguments. But behind these one finds intensely emotional motives such as personal pride, ambition and the like at work. Thus, anyone who is attacked by others will feel personally injured. No wonder, therefore, that the confrontations can at times take a subjective and passionate turn.

For instance, experience has shown that anyone who takes alternative medicine to task in respected medical journals, such as I cited at the beginning of this section, can count on a rapid climb up the academic career ladder. That which seems to be permeated by noble scientific conviction, striving altruistically to discover the truth, is in reality driven by numerous societal and personal motives. In this context, it is worth noting the empty cash registers of the health insurance firms, which understandably makes the intensity of the struggle to legally carve out as big a piece as possible from the shrinking pie of membership fees ever harder and at times more ruthless. To this extent, the article in the German medical journal is an expression of the predominant political and economic *Zeitgeist*.

That the bitter confrontation between mainstream and alternative medicine frequently takes the form of ideological trench warfare can also be seen among the alternative medicine practitioners. Like their opponents, they too often behave subjectively and even polemically. For instance, the question as to whether vaccination is medically correct and sensible, or the radical assertion that, in the cold light of day, the entire field of mainstream medicine is nothing but a corrupt collection of Mafia-type interest groups. Since I myself am not against vaccinations and am in many areas a staunch mainstream medicine practitioner who does not doubt the importance of large regions of mainstream medicine, I do not wish here to expound any further on this topic. Such types of extreme accusations simply highlight the passion with which these religious wars are fought – since ultimately they are nothing more than personal convictions, i.e. ideologies, crashing against each other.

At this point, it should be pointed out that there is often a great deal of ignorance with respect to the actual significance of placebos. Mostly their healing power is assessed to be much greater than it really is, particularly with reference to placebo medications. In cold reality, placebo medications are much less effective than most people think. As a physician with more than 30 years of professional experience – and unlike many critics of alternative medicine who enjoy steady employment in hospitals and universities – it was an existential necessity for me to earn money in my work. I needed to have a full waiting room, but I knew empirically that a placebo-based approach would quickly empty it out, because patients know very well what helps them and what doesn't.

My clinical practice experience agrees with investigations by Peter C. Gotzsche, Director of the Nordic Cochrane Centre Rigshospitalet in Copenhagen, and his colleague Asbjorn Hrobjartsson. In the largest meta-study which has so far been done on the topic of "efficacy of placebos as medications", they found out that placebos are, amazingly, barely or not at all effective. Gotzsche wrote: "In those cases where the clinical results were measured on a binary scale (i.e. improvement/no improvement) we were unable to determine any placebo effect whatever. For this reason, our investigation refutes the claim that the exclusive administration of placebos to patients can result in strong clinical effects." [67]

My own clinical experience agrees completely with the study results of the two Danish researchers. In those rare cases in which I prescribed only placebos, absolutely nothing happened. On the other hand, PSE homeopathic compound agents, used in my practice and those of my colleagues, have achieved positive therapeutic effects of over 80%. Placebo effects, on the other hand, come up at the most to 49%, and for medication-based therapy the response rate, as mentioned, is significantly lower or nearly zero.

1.3   Healing with Energy Medicine

In this Psychosomatic Energetics Textbook [8], I describe the oldest, yet also most comprehensive, healing system known: **treatment of the subtle body**. By subtle body (ind. "Aura") is meant a field that is not perceptible by the normal senses, one which extends out beyond the boundaries of the physical body and, according to ancient Gnostic tradition, is said to be identical with life energy. More detailed clarification will follow in later chapters. Remnants of this knowledge can be found to this day among Siberian shamans, Eskimos and some American Indian tribes. It has long been known that disturbance of the energy body is the primary cause of illness and emotional problems. People lose their *joie de vivre*, their ability to communicate and their bodily harmony if the free flow of life energy is inhibited.

As a general practitioner, I'm expected to heal not only as quickly and gently as possible, but also and above all causally and durably. According to everything that I have learned, this seems to be possible to do with Psychosomatic Energetics – i.e. with the method that I developed over the course of several years. After having examined and treated hundreds of patients using Psychosomatic Energetics, I can say with full conviction that energy-body disturbances are behind most illnesses and interpersonal problems! Even when such disturbances are not the sole cause, they are nevertheless often crucially involved in the appearance or continuation of the problem in question.

Naturally, one might ask oneself why the disturbed energy body plays so big a role. Unfortunately, I cannot give a satisfactory answer in a strictly scientific sense. Evidently, our organism requires free-flowing life energy in order to "function" in a healthy manner and in harmony with its environment. To patients, I like to compare the energy body with a computer's operating system. This is of course just a hypothesis which needs to be more precisely investigated scientifically. I leave the exploration of this topic to the future, and limit myself here to that which I have learned as a practicing physician: when it comes to healing, to trust, above all, sound common sense, my five senses and experience. Proceeding from this pragmatic attitude, I am able to say that the method simply works!

I illustrate the **healing process with an image** for my patients: the patient represents a plant which needs water and light in order to live. Just as a plant gets disturbed and sick if placed in darkness and not watered, so does the patient with respect to life energy. Like the Psyche itself, every one of our body's cells needs enough life energy to stay healthy. Many patients ask: "Doctor, can you make me healthy again?" But the healing process does not essentially depend on me, which is why the question is, at bottom, wrongly put. It is not I, the therapist, who is the actual healer; the patient's self-healing powers effect the cure. This modesty is not merely a pose on my part, but rather my deepest conviction. The therapist is (to stay with the image) simply the good gardener who keeps the plant supplied with light and water; "Mother Nature" does the actual healing.

There is yet another rule that can be derived from the plant image, namely that a plant which is too damaged can no longer be or become healthy. That sounds obvious and yet also sobering. It is thus sometimes a necessary and often painful realization for the patient, to accept the cruel truth that the disease process is too advanced and that not very much more can be done. One thus needs to begin dissolving the energy blocks as soon as possible, or otherwise the self-healing powers will be overwhelmed. In these late stages, one needs more powerful "weapons" in the form, say, of the much-maligned yet often indispensable "repair medicine" of strong chemical medications etc. Energy medicine thus hits its limits in cases of advanced disease processes. Also, many diseases have causes other than energy deficiency, such as infections. One must then proceed causally and fight the pathogen – which of course succeeds much better with a good energy system. Therefore, harmonization of the energy body often represents a very sensible adjuvant therapy. In many British hospitals, spiritual healers are welcome co-therapists, who harmonize the patient's energy field and thereby stimulate the self-healing powers.

Another important viewpoint has to do with the holistic effect of life energy, which influences both body and mind. Harmonic and free-flowing life energy is the most important basis for physical/psychological harmony. We feel good emotionally, are motivated and interested in the world, desire fulfillment and want to do something meaningful when life energy flows freely; we are likewise, as a rule, physically healthy and remain so when life energy flows harmonically. The old Latin saying *mens sana in corpore sano* (a sound mind (lives) in a sound body) needs to be extended as follows: "a sound mind in a sound body – thanks to healthful life energy". **Naming my method "Psychosomatic Energetics"** is based on this context; it unites the three parts or dimensions of man namely Psyche (mind/soul/spirit), Soma (body) and Energy (spiritlike life energy). "Energy check", "Psychoenergetics" and "energy therapy" are often used synonymously. Many patients call the Psychosomatic Energetics testing system an "energy check". The specially trained therapist who conducts it is called a "Certified Energy Therapist".

Because life energy influences the whole person, all healing methods which begin with life energy are holistically oriented toward body and mind – and with that, I would like to talk about the heart and core of Psychosomatic Energetics: it has to do with **bringing out into the light the unconscious conflicts** which can be considered to be the most important causes of energy efficiency. There are of course other causes, but the conflicts are our worst "energy thieves". Every person has such conflicts, which is why I can correctly call them "our" energy thieves. Of course these conflicts are not constantly stealing huge amounts of energy from us, but instead often just tiny bits, such that we normally are hardly aware of their existence. To make matters worse, these conflicts are hard to uncover because they almost always settle into nonverbal and therefore completely unconscious regions.

Most people don't feel their conflicts at all, even though they are to some degree weakened and, over the longer-term, made sick by them – since, sooner or later, conflicts always make one more susceptible to disease, cause subliminal disturbances and very often trigger illnesses. With the aid of Psychosomatic Energetics, we can thus do extremely valuable preventive work by harmonizing people at a very deep level and getting them re-centered. In this manner, many illnesses disappear, and even if they are not always completely eliminated, at least some important impediments to therapy have been moved out of the way so that other healing methods can only then really do their work. Resolving conflicts therefore represents an extremely worthwhile therapeutic goal, one whose profound effect is not matched by any other procedural method.

There is an even deeper significance which reaches deep into human and spiritual realms, and that is the therapeutic activity centering on the largest of the conflicts, the so-called **"Central Conflict"**. The Central Conflict plays a key role in shaping our character and behavior, since it represents the largest psychic "shadow" that we have, since that which, on the psychic level, is the darkest and most suppressed, at the same time influences us most strongly. So if we lead an unhappy and externally determined life, the Central Conflict is often the actual cause. One is reminded of a marionette jiggling with no willpower of its own at the end of its strings. Of course, the Central Conflict shows its destructive nature not just through its often subtle manipulation of behavior, it is also quite directly experienced through illnesses.

Since time immemorial, **healing and self-knowledge** have been viewed as kindred processes. According to this, those who know themselves are expected to grow spiritually and become healthier. In principle, this proposition is a good idea for many health disorders (it goes without saying: not for all of them) as people attempt to figure out their own share of the responsibility for their plight. But the search for self-knowledge has a big catch in clinical practice: the conflicts are usually unconscious and, moreover, bringing the conflict into consciousness represents a problem in itself. Basically, it's the age-old and all too well known problem that many people really do know what's good for them and what they should be doing, but they can't do it for some reason or another. The root of the problem is the unconscious conflicts by means of which one engages in a kind of self-sabotage.

This is the point at which **Psychosomatic Energetics differs substantially from other methods**. According to psychoanalysis, the first step toward healing should be to becoming aware of the conflict – but most patients do not lose their conflicts even though they have been made aware of them. On the contrary, many a physician gets the impression that conflicts even grow and become stronger if they are dealt with intensively. It often does not function exactly like that if one sticks firmly to the good intentions, but mostly it stays at the level of mere wishes, to be implemented after New Year's or some other significant date, only to fade afterwards into oblivion.

Other psychological methods strengthen patients' egos (positive thinking, supportive psychotherapy etc.) or reinforce their positive actions (behavioral therapy). But just as dirt is not really eliminated by painting over it, conflicts do not disappear merely through words of positive encouragement. Still other methods try to clear up the familial environment (family therapy) or guide the deep unconscious onto the right track (hypnosis, meditation). This all sounds very rational and at first inspires both therapists and patients, but it very rarely has any lasting effects. In fact, it can get even worse, because although people might feel healthy after many kinds of therapy, their conflicts have by no means disappeared, and they continue to tick on like a time bomb deep underground.

If you consider them in the context of the biblical passage "By their fruits shall ye know them", then many therapeutic procedures are overwhelmed when it comes to healing large conflicts, and they often fail. I speak from many years of experience with countless patients who have tried out everything possible before coming to me. Looking back, there is nothing that really helped them very much. It is my experience that many well-known therapies suffer from an inability to completely recognize the conflict, to say nothing of properly healing it. Exceptions are strongly transformative therapies with a deep spiritual orientation which correspond to what is designated in the Bible as "purification" or "purging", and in modern terms as "deep personality transformation". In such cases (which are hard to set up voluntarily and which therefore have no general therapeutic value) people undergo change in the core of their being, appearing afterwards as transformed persons. As I said, however, that is seldom the case.

Another small group is made up of people who have worked a great deal on themselves and their unconscious problems. By the way, contrary to popular opinion, this kind of work on one's own personality by no means inevitably entails costly and prolonged psychotherapy, only the courage to face up to one's dark side and overcome it. Naturally, the aid of an experienced therapist can help a lot, not only because one needs some reassurance every now and then, but also because it's good to have someone who will help to get through the jungle of the unconscious. However, I would once again like to emphasize that the current omnipresent glorification of psychotherapy and many similar forms of therapy seems to be excessive and mostly unwarranted.

Therefore, many methods seem to me unable to deal with a conflict because they do not recognize it and certainly do not eliminate it energetically. I can explain what happens – or better yet: what doesn't happen – with an example: no one is surprised when a syphilis sufferer stays sick if the spirochetes are not killed off; only the proper medication can cure the disease. This seems precisely to be the problem in the case of a conflict: it *must* be dissolved energetically for it to disappear and be permanently cured. The tremendous and durable cures which therapists who work with Psychosomatic Energetics experience every day in their clinical practice speak volumes for the correctness of this approach.

> **Therefore, the First Law of PSE is that conflicts must be energetically dissolved in order for the associated energy blocks to disappear, the emotional distortions to cease and life energy to flow freely once again.**

Psychosomatic Energetics thereby becomes an indispensable therapeutic tool, because basically every patient benefits from this kind of procedure. In many cases, the self-healing powers are so strong that healing begins as soon as Psychosomatic Energetics is applied. Occasionally, one might also need other methods, namely when the self-healing powers are no longer sufficient because the disease is already too far advanced. This applies not only to physical illnesses, but also to emotional and social disorders. (I will return to this in the therapy section.)

I would also like to call attention to the important point that many healing techniques have a stronger and quicker effect when Psychosomatic Energetics is used as an adjuvant. This applies to massage, chiropractic and neural therapy on up to psychotherapy. Patients are more relaxed, emotionally more open and react more easily once the energy blocks have been eliminated. Psychotherapists more quickly get "to the point" and patients more easily recognize the negative patterns because they once more can feel that which is good and life-affirming in themselves. In the case of social disruptions, people are either more willing to compromise when a beneficial solution is possible, or on the other hand more vigorous and uncompromising when dealing with self-destructive processes. Thus, students will usually drop their provocative and uncooperative behavior once their conflicts have been eliminated. Contrariwise, a battered wife will more forcefully put an end to her degrading situation.

1.4   The relationship of subtle energy to the mesenchyme, soma and Psyche

We do not yet have a sound model that can properly represent the relationships

- between the coarse body (Soma) and the mental control function (Psyche) – i.e. the two areas of human existence known as yet to traditional medicine –
- as well as two unknown regions, the archaic metabolism, the isotonic primordial sea in which all body cells swim (mesenchyme) as well as subtle energy.

Yet such a model is necessary in order to be able to properly practice complementary medicine. Many people will no doubt register with astonishment that a model of this type actually does exist, although nearly always as experience-based intuition. This kind of model arises automatically over decades of practical experience along the lines of: "As a therapist I know that this or that technique works and that it will have this or that effect." This kind of causally linked experiential knowledge is a kind of model that can not only be applied intuitively, but also put into words – which I have done in what follows. The following model is based on experience from various therapeutic levels, and it is enough so that one can work with it immediately in clinical practice, even if one has not had decades of experience oneself.

The organism as a whole is like a pyramid standing on a broad foundation, with only the upper region visible (Fig. 1.4). The upper region corresponds to that of the individual body cells and all materially detectable body components which can be detected and measured objectively by science-based medicine. As a tree whose root system is invisibly embedded in the ground, and which is essential to the life of the tree, the subtle-energy and mesenchyme regions are likewise crucial to the life of the organism. It's just that they are not visible and therefore not real from the viewpoint of regular science-based medicine.

In complementary medicine, we can influence the non-visible parts of the organism, i.e. the functional metabolism of the mesenchyme (intracellular connective tissue) as well as subtle energy, the latter being slotted in ahead of the mesenchymal level. So, when one harmonizes subtle energy, one thereby automatically affects the mesenchymal level as well. The mesenchymal level is also referred to as "hyperacidity, clogging, premature aging, poisoning"; alkaline vegetarian diets, physical activity outdoors in the fresh air, fasting, therapies involving light, baths (freshwater, seawater, Kneipp baths etc.) are used to try to influence it. The subtle-energy level is treated with homeopathy, acupuncture, energy transmission through laying on of hands, PSE etc.

The health of the mesenchymal level is recognizable by a refreshed appearance, dynamism and vitality, normal body odor, normal bowel movements, elastic skin turgor (the fasting specialist F.X. Mayr checked this by pinching the skin on the temples next to the eyes) as well as a normal blood picture in darkfield microscopy. On the other hand, illness at this level is shown by fatigue, poor appearance, bad body odor, constipation or diarrhea, creased and dry skin turgor at the temples, as well as a poor blood picture in darkfield microscopy.

Basically, health at the subtle-energy level is like the mesenchymal level, but with the addition of mental/energetic characteristics such as good mood, resilience, the joy of discovery, ability to empathize, self-confidence as well as a hospitable and welcoming attitude and healthy logical thoughts and deeds. Illness at the subtle-energy level is precisely characterized by the opposite negative characteristics such as bad mood, irritability, reduced resilience and the like.

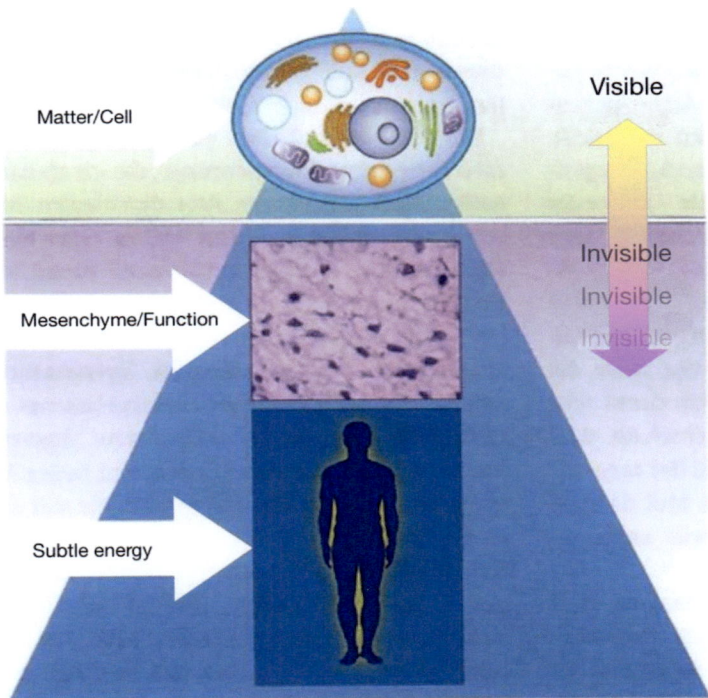

Fig. 1.4 *– From the viewpoint of PSE, the regions of the organism can be likened to a pyramid, of which only the upper (material) tip is visible. Only the tip is detectable by the objective methods of scientific orthodox medicine (cellular level). On the other hand, the other two regions – which exert a much more comprehensive and broader effect on the organism and have more to do with functional regions (archaic organizational structures) and subtle life-energy fields – are indiscernible and can only be revealed via indirect methods such as PSE, darkfield microscopy etc.*

Health at the subtle-energy level can be determined by PSE (REBA® Test Device), and very likely also by a diagnosis in the context of Traditional Chinese Medicine (TCM) with pulse and tongue diagnosis (I assume that this is possible, but I have no comparisons). Good PSE treatment normalizes the subtle-energy level and thereby also improves the mesenchymal level up to a point.

In short, good energy-medicine treatment spares one possible cleansing, unclogging and detoxification measures, and promotes health in the entire organism. One exception to this is blockage at the mesenchymal level, which can be detected using the PSE Organ Test Kit – for example chronic inflammation, chronic sinusitis or functional disorders such as disrupted biliary drainage or intestinal flora dysbioses. Even the best PSE sometimes cannot eliminate these, so that in these cases one must first eliminate the causative mesenchymal disturbance, possibly by healing a chronic sinusitis or surgical removal of chronically inflamed tonsils. This same logic also applies at the cellular level, in which very advanced processes overwhelm the organism's self-healing powers, and mainstream medical procedures are again called for.

2 The History of Psychosomatic Energetics

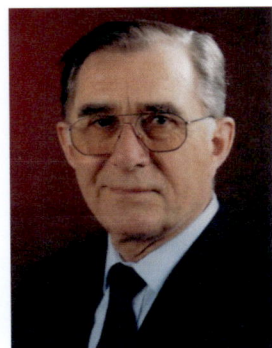

Fig. 2.1 – Dr. Helmut W. Schimmel (MD and DDS), developer of the Vegatest.

I first presented Psychosomatic Energetics in the fall of 1997 at the Baden-Baden Medical Week, the largest alternative-medicine physician's congress in the world. At the end of my presentation on "Psychoenergetic deep structure and its therapy – the new energetic model", my friend and colleague, the physician and dentist Dr. Helmut W. Schimmel (cf. **Fig. 2.1**) – whom I will be talking about later – made me a lovely compliment at the entranceway: "That's a very bold thing you just presented! You are venturing very far forward with it." Schimmel had seen at once that PSE enables us to look deep into the depths of the human soul, and that it takes courage to face the repressed and mainly uncomfortable truths found there.

A year later, the first edition of my book *Psychosomatic Energetics* was published, the REBA° Test Device for measuring energy levels was introduced, and the emotional and chakra remedies came onto the market. Now, more than 15 books about PSE have been published in German, English, Italian and Russian. In just a few years, the method has become established, in more than 20 countries among thousands of therapists, as a valuable alternative-medicine standard method. The nicest compliment I have received as inaugurator of the method I have heard time and again in various different forms, namely my colleagues saying that they can no longer even conceive of working without this method.

PSE came about over several decades through numerous developmental leaps which I underwent as a practicing naturopathic physician, from its unclear beginnings to the very clear methodology which PSE now offers. Because all of this plays out in a dark and sparsely researched area, the complicated developmental process is understandable. I would like to say at the outset that I, as an established general practitioner, did not at first intend to bestow a new method on my colleagues. PSE kind of developed through the back door; looking back, I see that, in my daily medical practice, I evolved a process, the course of which I did not consciously intend or guide – at the end of which there emerged PSE, like a puzzle which finally came together as a whole.

In Fig. 2.2, the various influences which shaped PSE are presented. From this variegated mixture of influences it's not very hard to see that the method is "neither fish nor fowl" so to speak: it deals with homeopathy, acupuncture and Bach Flowers, but also with psychotherapy, shamanism and ancient characterology. It unites East and West, ancient Eastern and Western medicine and psychology. It regards body, soul and subtle energy as a unity which can only be viewed as healthful and life-promoting in the harmonious interplay of all components. At the same time, PSE views crises and conflicts as opportunities for growth, and thus does not promote a sterile image of man oriented exclusively toward positive feelings, a smooth line and a health-aware lifestyle, but rather is aware of the human chasms which are the price of our free will, yet also a chance to grow beyond them.

PSE makes it possible to determine a person's character type by means of an energy test taking only a few minutes, rather than a depth-psychological analysis lasting years. How is this possible? I think it's because psychological reality and energetic reality say much the same thing, and this permits drawing the corresponding conclusions. Thus, PSE is based upon clear and explicit rules which are historically portrayed by various diagnostic and therapeutic systems, which PSE integrates by means of its systematics. Therefore, a complex method such as Psychosomatic Energetics (PSE) is easier to understand if one knows its historical roots. This is why I would next like to describe its history, treating each influence chronologically, out of which the qualities and possibilities of PSE should become clear.

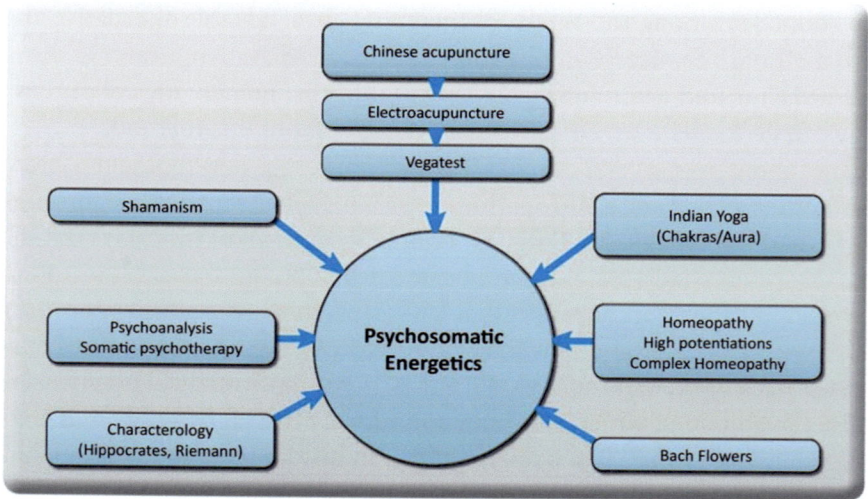

Fig. 2.2 – *The most significant influences which have played a role in the development of PSE.*

2.1 EAV and Vegatest

As a young naturopath in 1976, I learned Bioelectronic Functional Diagnostics (BFD), a further development of Dr. Reinhard Voll's Electroacupuncture (EAV), which in turn was an extension of Chinese acupuncture. The internist Voll (**cf. Fig. 2.3**) had discovered after World War II that the capacitive resistance at acupuncture points changed depending upon disease and disturbance. This change, moreover, could not be reproduced by machine, even if it might subjectively seem to do so by the tester. The EAV tester unknowingly applies a different pressure, which then results in altered test readings. One can take this opportunity to grasp the idea that practically all energy medicine tests such as EAV, RAC pulse diagnosis, kinesiology, one-hand dowsing etc. are based on the same principle, namely a modified muscle play on the part of the tester (I will get into this complex topic in greater detail later on). Because the remedy test deals with subjective phenomena, one should basically not speak in terms of (objective) **measurement**, but rather of (subjectively tinted) **testing**.

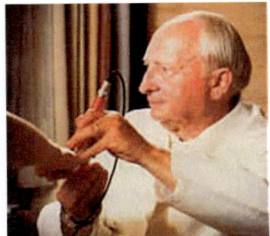

Fig. 2.3 – Dr. Reinhard Voll. (with the kind permission of the International Medical Society for Acupuncture per Voll)

Voll discovered the so-called **"remedy test"** quite by accident: one of his patients happened to have his heart medicine on his person and, against expectation, exhibited normal EAV readings at the points of the Heart meridian. At first, Voll searched irritatedly for the cause of this incorrect test value, since it did not correspond to the patient's clinical state, who continued to have cardiac complaints. At some point, the patient discovered the medicine in his coat pocket and took it out, whereupon the EAV values returned to the expected low readings. So, they had been artificially boosted by the presence of the heart medicine and energetically compensated – a legitimate phenomenon whose significance Voll recognized at once, and which thereupon made possible manifold diagnostic and therapeutic statements, which Voll gradually discovered over time.

By the way, in the 1960s, the inventor of kinesiology, George Goodheart, also discovered the remedy test, which means that it is a universal principle which works for both allopathic and homeopathic medicines and which leads to changes in energy-medicine test results.

> • Note
> The principle of the remedy test is that
> everything responds positively
> • which is energetically similar to a disease or disturbance or
> • which therapeutically changes the energy system.

So the remedy test can thus be used both diagnostically and therapeutically (more on this later). The remedy test plays a large role in PSE, because with its help, one can detect disturbances in the energy centers (Chakras), certain unconscious conflicts, important functional organ disorders or geopathic stresses.

As a young naturopath around 1975, I was looking for a reliable diagnostic technique that would agree with clinical findings and which was also therapeutically reliable, by enabling one to precisely test out what kind of medication was needed. EAV and BFD and the Vegatest method derived from them completely fulfilled my expectations along these lines. I need to qualify that by adding that certain diseases can be so well masked that they are not energetically testable; this includes early and middle phase tumors, mechanical disorders such as a nuclear prolaps etc. certain other diseases such as essential hypertonia are difficult or impossible to test energetically, i.e. blood pressure must be examined in the usual manner and treated correspondingly. In addition, every form of energetic testing has certain sources of failure, so that energy tests should always come into play only after one cannot get any further with standard, scientifically-based methods.

> • Digression
> Voll used the hypothalamus measurement point as a reference at the end of every EAV session. After having tested out hundreds of acupuncture points and dozens of nosodes and homeopathic agents, at the end the hypothalamus measurement point had to be normalized. I knew Voll personally and I'm certain that he never suspected that the hypothalamus measuring point in fact reflected the energetic compensation of the emotional system; Voll still belong to a generation for which all emotional content was to be rejected – and yet, compensating the emotional system was probably the crucial factor in the success of EAV in the first place. Since EAV worked predominantly with nosodes, which primarily affect the emotional system, one realizes that what is actually going on here is in fact emotional conflict therapy. But because the therapy seldom has long-term effects – which I

was able to demonstrate in numerous patients who had previously been treated with EAV – there was a constant need to find new nosodes via further testing with which to continue therapy.

Despite these limitations, my nearly four decades of accumulated experience tell me that energy tests are indispensable for answering important questions:

- Is there a focal process (chronic inflammatory processes such as chronic sinusitis, which stress the entire organism)? Are there functional organ disorders such as intestinal flora dysbiosis? (These questions can now be answered with the PSE Organ Test Kit, which builds on the Vegatest method testing principle.)
- Is there any Geo radiation stress present? Electrosmog?

In my large southern German general practice of the 80s and 90s, besides the Vegatest method, I used numerous other diagnostic procedures such as segment electrography (SEG), thermoregulation diagnostics (TRD) and darkfield microscopy before the Vegatest examination, which supplied additional valuable information. Since testing always has a subjective component, and additional information can guide testing in a new direction, this procedure has well proven itself. Darkfield microscopy in particular has turned out to be very helpful with PSE, covering as it does the area of mesenchymal diagnostics.

2.2   The discovery of the conflicts

Before I developed PSE, I worked for many years with the **Bach Flowers** of the British homeopath Dr. Edward Bach. 30-40% of patients respond very well to Bach Flowers, but the rest hardly at all, unfortunately – not a very good yield if one wants to have a successful practice. A further downside was that there was no end to the therapy: for years and years, I was forced to test out ever new Bach Flowers for the same patients over and over again. I had a similar experience with homeopathic LM high potentiations, which I repertorized and tested out. The positive effects seldom lasted very long, more frequent being a "revolving door effect" – a typical sign of an inadequate therapy. My patients would feel better for a few weeks, and then relapse. Numerous colleges have confirmed this, such that there is probably a general validity here: from the standpoint of PSE, one sees that enduring healing of the emotional body cannot be achieved either with single-remedy homeopathy or Bach Flower essences, because the underlying conflict is not eliminated.

> **• Homeopathy**
> Homeopathy uses the unpotentiated, homeopathically as yet untreated basic tincture – usually an approximately 1:10 dilution of an initial substance – as the first step of the subsequent potentiation (succussion or "dynamization" per Hahnemann). Customary are the decimal potentiations (1:10 dilution, designated as D1, D2 etc.), the centesimal potentiations (1:100, designated as C1, C2 etc.) and the LM potentiations (diluted 1:50,000). However, the crucial point with homeopathy is not the degree of dilution (which the materialistically oriented critics frequently make fun of due to the extreme sounding dilution levels), but rather the information transfer and reinforcement via the potentiation process. Homeopathy can be thought of as information medicine. By comparison: in the process of information transfer, it doesn't matter whether you give a person one or a thousand copies of the same article to read, but rather whether the information is received at all.

Over time, I used increasingly higher homeopathic potentiations and made the astonishing discovery that this did not eliminate the revolving-door effect; only the time intervals between changes or inversions became longer. But I had not yet found the crucial key for long-term healing. Then "chance" came to my aid: a number of tests on myself and on patients in rapid sequence kept pointing to the same homeopathics and potentiation levels. This data collection seemed to be concealing a law or regularity corresponding to the unknown X factor – the secret reason why healing was impermanent.

Energy level	Vital	Emotional	Mental	Causal
Specific potency	DI-C400	C400-800	–	LM16-LM18

Fig. 2.4 *– Energy levels related to the homeopathic potentiation of the emotional remedies.*

As time passed, I collected multiple tests on the same patients using various homeopathics that were strikingly similar to each other. Like a bouquet of wildflowers from the same meadow, these homeopathics evidently represented different aspects of the X factor. This group of homeopathic agents turned up with reliable regularity for certain patients, responding as **compound remedies** in the energy test. Another thing these homeopathic complexes had in common were the similar mental and mood symptoms such as "violent temper" in the case of *Hepar sulfuris*, "angry rage" for lycopodium, "destructive impulses" for tarantula and "irritable, irascible, annoyed" for sulfur – all of them symptoms of repressed anger or rage. Evidently, these homeopathics reflected the various emotional facets of a fundamental emotion; in the case of the complex described above, a feeling of destructive anger and repressed rage. By the way, this complex corresponds to what I later designated as "Emotional Remedy 9".

> **• Homeopathy and PSE**
> Homeopathic agents administered to healthy persons eventually give rise to medication pictures such as are gathered together in review manuals such as Kent, Boerricke etc. Normally, one compares the patient's symptoms with those in a review manual, but they can also be tested out energetically instead (which seems more reliable to me). In this context, striking symptoms such as mental and mood indications are particularly valuable. Clinical practice experience has shown that classical homeopathy hardly ever uses single remedies which, say, are contained in the single remedies of the emotional remedies with which the Central Conflict is treated. Thus, classical homeopathy and PSE each have a completely different thrust and address different areas, specifically: classical homeopathy affects the entire organism and PSE only the conflict. For that reason, one often sees no medication pictures in PSE because the conflict completely absorbs the homeopathic signals, thereby preventing reactions of that sort.

So it was possible that repressed feelings were the true cause of the revolving-door effect. In this manner, I intended to take on the proof that I was able to treat the repressed rage with a mixture of all of 4 of the aforementioned homeopathics, leading to a stable emotional state and long-term healing. Unfortunately, the first attempt with this homeopathic mixture did not function in the hoped-for manner. There had to be something still missing. I found that the answer to the riddle was that it had to do with the overall mood: the right potentiation level was the crucial key to success. It was just necessary to have the four homeopathics administered at different **potentiation levels** in order to succeed. (**cf. Fig. 2.4**):

- D 21 corresponds to the basic tincture and functions as a universal key in that it latently contains all potentiation levels (from the lowest to the highest). Music has the concept of a key's tonic chord, which is conveyed by this potentiation level. The D 21 agent and the emotional remedy complex is the most important, dominating agent.
- C 400-800 acts on the lower Emotional Level (corresponding to the conflict's emotional charge).
- LM 16 acts on the lower and middle Causal Levels (where the conflict has its instinctive automatic anchor point).
- LM 18 acts on the upper Causal Level (corresponding to the deeply-rooted basic beliefs of psychokinesiology; action is similar to LM 16, but more profound).

There seems to be generally valid law that underlies this discovery: homeopathic potentiation levels and be compared to different frequencies. As in a radio with its frequency bands, every potentiation corresponds to a different transmitter. With respect to human energy levels, my research has shown that each potentiation corresponds to a specific region of the Aura. Samuel Hahnemann, the founder of homeopathy, already knew that low potentiations below D 6 predominantly addressed the course body, while higher potentiations above D 30 influenced the Mental Level.

Besides rage, I found numerous other conflicts such as "Hatred", "Envy", "Arrogance" and so on – 28 in all. On closer inspection, their contents correspond to the deadly sins of the Bible and are archetypal negative human character traits which have without a doubt existed forever. Later on, I toned down such drastic-sounding terms as "Hatred" with milder alternative formulations to make them acceptable to modern man. It took quite a long time for me to track down all the homeopathics that could be associated with the 28 conflicts. The search process consisted of years of a tedious combination of energy testing and repertorizing. In the end, the entire search process was not an endless undertaking, since it was limited by the manageable number of conflicts. Based on tests undertaken thus far on thousands of patients, there do not seem to be more than 28 conflicts.

> In my book *Healing through Energy Medicine* [8], I tried to present a historical development of the concept of evil, i.e. hatred, envy, egotism etc. – the primeval themes that are the subject of the 28 conflict themes of PSE – their presumptive causes and the ideological coping mechanisms and/or the psychotherapy and behavioral

> therapies thereof. This extends from Shamanism to modern psychotherapy and behavioral therapy. In this process, I also delve into modern repression mechanisms for shifting guilt feelings onto others, for instance "an unhappy childhood", a widely-applied ever-popular excuse in modern psychotherapy which is, to my mind, often a morally inappropriate way of wriggling out of responsibility. I believe that a rational integration of all historical models can produce a realistic model, one which I present the broad outlines of in the aforementioned book.

At the first practical testing of the 28 found emotional remedies (Emvita), I noted to my surprise that a by nature very gentle and friendly old woman responded to remedy 9 "Exploding, anger". It would never have occurred to me that this woman had excess aggression stored away in her unconscious. To my tentative question as to whether "Anger, rage" meant anything to her, she confirmed that it did, and explained that she was mainly too good-natured and was much taken advantage of. This left her with a great deal of rage which she, however, kept to herself. I now know that the woman was very likely a Depressive (one might also say a Choleric) character type. The tested remedy was her characterologically determining conflict, which in PSE is known as the "Central Conflict", because it centrally determines a person's character. It later turned out that, with other patients as well, the external impression and the inner life frequently contradicted each other, because people do not reveal their negative socially unwanted feelings, concealing them as best they can by behaving in a polar opposite manner.

As time went on, it gradually became clear that, with the discovery of the emotional remedies in the years 1994 and 1995, the real reason had been found for the revolving-door effect of the Bach Flowers and the homeopathic simple-remedy high potentiations, namely that they were unable to eliminate the conflicts. However, the puzzle was not yet completely solved, since there was not in fact just a single conflict, but rather entire hordes of the most varied conflicts – headed by a "Central Conflict" which must be viewed as the "primary perpetrator". The significance of the emotional remedies emerged bit by bit over time in clinical practice, because the therapeutic effects took effect slowly in most patients. First of all, one conflict after another has to be processed, even though very frequently only a single conflict reveals itself. For many people with complex personalities and chronic physical ailments, conflict resolution sometimes turns out to be quite tedious because in these cases three, four or more conflicts have to be eliminated which are nested within each other like the layers of an onion (cf. Fig. 2.5).

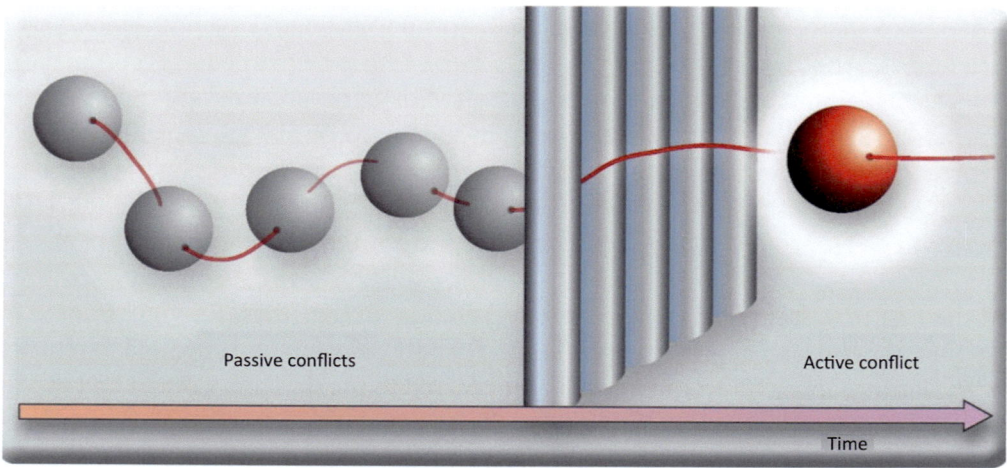

Fig. 2.5 – *Onionskin layers of the conflicts from a chronological viewpoint: one active conflict after another must be broken up in a months-long process; passive conflicts gradually become activated during the course of PSE therapy.*

2.3   Conflict size

With the emotional remedies, I had already discovered the key to detecting and resolving conflicts; still missing was determination of size. My thinking was that if a conflict is energetically independent, then its independence should make it possible to test its size. However, to put forward such a daring hypothesis at all entailed a fairly long learning process, which I would like to describe in what follows. In the end, as a conventionally trained physician, I was convinced enough to consider the likelihood of the independent energetic existence of conflicts. This learning process extended over a number of years, ultimately leading to the development of a testing system which enabled testing for conflict size.

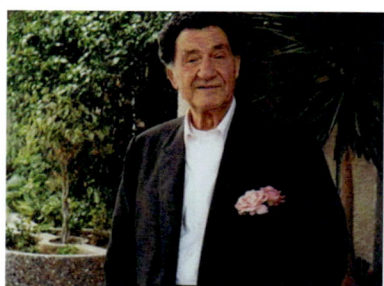

Fig. 2.6 – *The Christian guru Daskalos (Photo: Inge Geissinger, Starnberg).*

Like many of my contemporaries, I at first thought that Shamanism's idea that there exist harmful vampiric demons to be pure superstition, but my opinion on the nature of emotional conflicts changed when I first read the writings of the Cypriot spiritual teacher Dr. Stylianos Atteshlis, better known as Daskalos (**cf. Fig. 2.6**) concerning the "Elemental". I have long greatly admired Daskalos, and consider him to be one of the great spiritual figures of the 20th century. Daskalos teaches a gnostic Christianity which embraces Eastern concepts such as the Aura, the possibility of reincarnation and the practice of meditation. Instead of conflicts, Daskalos speaks of "Elementals", by which he means harmful spiritual entities which arise due to long-held ideas and strong feelings which can lead a long independent life. Under certain conditions, Elementals can leave their conflict hosts and float around freely, able to infest susceptible persons such as children or the mentally disturbed; we say the person is "possessed".

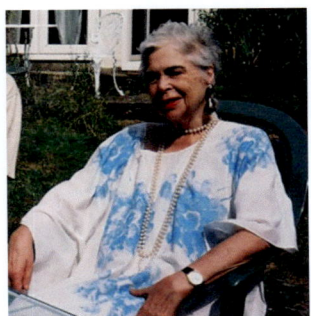

Fig. 2.7 *– Gerda Boyesen (Photo: Peter Bergholz, Otzberg).*

At the same time (beginning of the 1990s), I attended a seminar held by the Norwegian somatic psychotherapist Gerda Boyesen (**cf. Fig. 2.7**). Her work was oriented toward the somatic therapy of Wilhelm Reich, but also made use of mediumistic healing techniques learned from Brazilian healers. In the energy field of a female participant lying before us with her eyes shut, Ms. Boyesen intuitively detected harmful negative energies. She gripped the conflict with her index finger and thumb and slowly pulled the invisible something out of the Aura, while the patient groaned more loudly depending on how quickly the hand was pulling, at the end heaving a sigh of relief.

> I have described the convoluted historical path from shamanism via exorcism to modern psychotherapy and somatic psychotherapy in my book *Healing through Energy Medicine* [8], and I encourage those that are interested reader to read this to find out about the development of the relevant worldviews and views of man.

Ms. Boyesen's technique showed me that Daskalos' Elementals evidently really did exist. It was then logical to assume the same for the 28 conflicts of PSE. In contrast to Ms. Boyesen's hard-to-learn intuitive approach, a great many therapists have succeeded in tracking down and correctly identifying invisible conflicts in the energy field in a reliable manner. Both Ms. Boyesen's technical procedure and Daskalos' gnostic teachings – but also shamanistic methods – make it clear that conflicts represent something independent which can be considered to be actual "living beings" which manipulate us unconsciously and, like vampires, steal our energy.

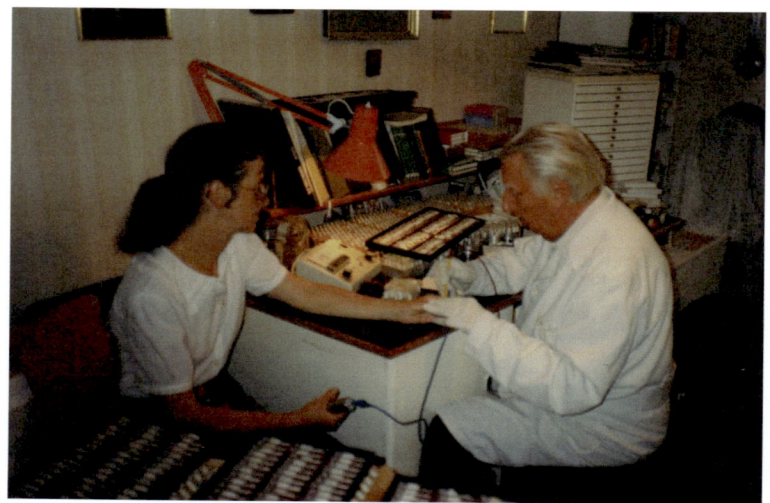

Fig. 2.8 – Erwin Schramm in his Vienna consulting room, testing out medications.

As fate would have it, at this same time I sat in for a few days at the practice of the Viennese physician Dr. Erwin Schramm, a well-known electroacupuncturist (**cf. Fig. 2.8**). From Dr. Schramm, I first learned of his unusual observation that specific medicinal herbs contain energetic information. Edward Bach had already discovered something similar, but that applied to the high-frequency emotional region which responds to certain wild plants, whereas Dr. Schramm had discovered that plants also can have an influence at lower frequencies. This had only been known otherwise in homeopathy, and was at the time a very new insight. I thereupon suspected that vibrations from plant tinctures might be suitable for testing out conflicts. To check this out, I compiled an assortment of a wide variety of plant tinctures. My supposition quickly proved to be correct: after a while, I was able to associate every one of the 28 emotional remedies with a specific plant tincture (**cf. Fig. 2.9**).

Test Substances to Measure Conflict Size	
Chakra 1:	
1. Emotional remedy: Independence	Test substance: Kola nut
2. Emotional remedy: Lack of concentration	Test substance: Ginseng panax
3. Emotional remedy: Helpless	Test substance: Capsella bursa pastoris (Shepherd's purse)
4. Emotional remedy: Extreme self-control	Test substance: Yohimbin (Yohimbe)
Chakra 2:	
5. Emotional remedy: Hectic	Test substance: Papaver somniferum
6. Emotional remedy: Perseverance	Test substance: Kava-Kava
7. Emotional remedy: Show of strength	Test substance: Laurel (Laurus nobilis)
Chakra 3:	
8. Emotional remedy: Isolated	Test substance: Absinthe (Absinthium artemisia)
9. Emotional remedy: Pent-up emotions	Test substance: Deadly nightshade (Belladonna atropa)
10. Emotional remedy: Always wanting more	Test substance: Tobacco (Nicotinea tabacum)
11. Emotional remedy: Hungry for good feelings	Test substance: Pomegranate (Punica granatum)
Chakra 4:	
12. Emotional remedy: Mental overexertion	Test substance: Nutmeg (Nux moschata)
13. Emotional remedy: Withdrawn	Test substance: Passionflower (Passiflora incarnata)
14. Emotional remedy: Introverted	Test substance: Strophantus
15. Emotional remedy: Apprehensive	Test substance: Wild jasmine (Gelsemium sempervirens)
16. Emotional remedy: Panic	Test substance: Common bean (Phaseolus vulgaris)
Chakra 5:	
17. Emotional remedy: Emotional emptiness	Test substance: Chamomile (Chamomilla matricaria)
18. Emotional remedy: Rushed	Test substance: Hops (Lupulus humulus)
Chakra 6:	
19. Emotional remedy: Timid	Test substance: Mate (Ilex paraguayensis)
20. Emotional remedy: Self-sufficient	Test substance: Tiger lily (Lilium tigrinum incarnata)
21. Emotional remedy: Physical overexertion	Test substance: Valerian (Valeriana officinalis)
22. Emotional remedy: Restlessness	Test substance: Balm (Melissa officinalis)
23. Emotional remedy: Tense	Test substance: Musk-root (Sumbulus moschatus)
24. Emotional remedy: Uneasiness	Test substance: St. John's wort (Hypericum perforatum)
Chakra 7:	
25. Emotional remedy: Mistrust	Test substance: Icelandic moss (Cetraria islandica)
26. Emotional remedy: Materialistic	Test substance: Wild grape (Ampelopsis quinaquefolia)
27. Emotional remedy: Unwilling to face reality	Test substance: Henbane (Hyoscyamus niger)
28. Emotional remedy: Wrong thinking	Test substance: Jimson weed (Datura stramonium)

Fig. 2.9 – *Test substances and associated conflicts*

Anyone who takes a closer look at the test substances will be surprised to find many of our culture's consumer drugs there: tobacco, Coca-Cola, hops. These temporarily generate in the consumer a sense of well-being which had not been there previously. Test substances simulate a positive feeling, while the associated conflict represents the negative side of the feeling. Thus, the hops in beer counteract the restlessness of modern civilization, making the beer drinker as calm as a meditating Buddha. The associated conflict is named "Rushed", whereas beer drinkers in their calm mood have all the time in the world. This is why beer ads use slogans that evoke a pleasant mood, a friendly atmosphere, finally, after all the daily hustle and bustle.

Tobacco smokers (associated conflict: "Always wanting more") have the feeling of actually getting more – i.e. the taste of "freedom and adventure" which the tobacco ads promise. Coca-Cola compensates feelings of inferiority (conflict: "Independent") and is therefore particularly popular in a hierarchical dog-eat-dog society where everybody wants to appear to be especially self-confident. There's a reason why Coca-Cola is the highest-selling soft drink in the world, and it helps insecure first world teenagers as well as poor third-worlders feel better and stronger.

One should distinguish between the gluttonous consumption of culture-drugs and self-aware usage of the same, such as when Indians smoke the peace pipe. The peace pipe makes people calmer and thereby more peaceable. On the other hand, the addictive use of culture-drugs unsparingly reveals that an underlying emotional conflict has not been eliminated and now spurs on the addiction, thereby setting in motion an endless spiral.

With the right tincture, a found conflict can be virtually amplified energetically, i.e. test substance 9 for conflict 9, conflict 28 with test substance 28 etc. Amplification means that, instead of the patient, the conflict is temporarily tested, somewhat like the optical enlargement of an object with a magnifying glass. However, the testing has no negative influence on the conflict itself, and does not alter it. Presumably, the plant tinctures in the test agent contain important emotional characteristics of particular plants which resonate with particular conflict contents and thereby energetically amplify them.

Like its conflict host, the conflict has four energy levels, and its energy quantitatively represents that which it has taken from the conflict host (**cf. Fig. 2.10**). However, the two parts cannot be quantitatively added together, since conflicts and humans have differently-sized energy fields, but the comparison still gives a rough idea of how much the conflict has stolen from the conflict host, and roughly how much energy the therapy will restore.

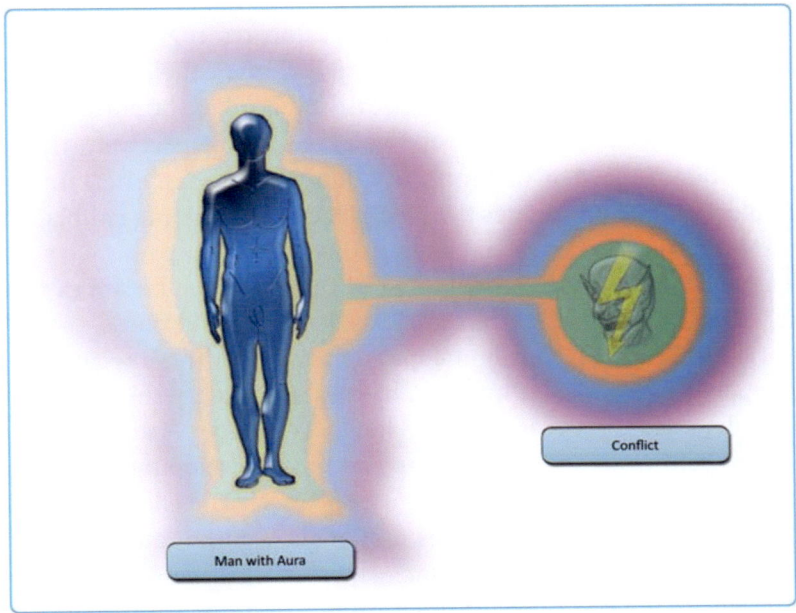

Fig. 2.10 *– Conflict host and conflict share energy fields. The conflict feeds like a vampire on the conflict host. The conflict host cannot access the energy stored in the conflict.*

Most conflicts range in size from 50/50/10/50 up to 80/80/10/80, and unusually large conflicts even go up to 100/100/5/100 (given as percentage values for Vital, Emotional, Mental, Causal). This means that the conflict: has taken, for example, 80% of the Vital and Emotional energy of its conflict host, is only 10% aware and has up to 80% repetitive tendencies. The last characteristic has to do with a repetitive compulsion which goes hand-in-hand with deep-rooted habits and beliefs. The higher the Causal value, the older the conflict and, empirically, the longer it will have to be treated – for instance about 4 to 5 months for 80%.

2.4 Chakras as conflict storage

However, negative emotional conflicts have not only a "geographical" extension inside of the four subtle-energy levels, but also a segmental docking at the energy centers (Chakras). I'd like here to describe how I came to recognize these interconnections. My experience with the Vegatest method had made it clear to me that certain body segments could be long-term energetically blocked in the chronically ill. These segments correspond to the large vegetative plexus or, respectively, the traditional Chakras of Indian Yoga. For instance, in allergy cases, one often finds an upper abdominal block; if one eliminates the block by e.g. stimulating gallbladder activity with certain bitter plants, then the related ailment also improves.

My colleague Dr. Helmut Schimmel was a world-renowned Nestor of nosodes (homeopathic toxins). In the middle of the 1980s, he developed the so-called Meridian complexes (Kern-Pharma) from homeopathic mixtures; these were new compositions which acted energetically on the Chakras to detoxify them. Experience has shown that, afterwards, many nosodes no longer responded. I adopted the principle of operation of Schimmel's nosode therapy as I was developing PSE. Here too, the Chakras are tested and conflict therapy takes place via the energy centers. As with the Meridian complexes, many nosodes no longer respond after the conflicts have been eliminated, such that the active principle is very likely similar. In the meantime, my hypothesis is that a great deal of the nosode vibrations may well correspond to emotional conflicts. A good example is the test nosode Amalgam, which responds to corresponding dental fillings – but also, according to the statements of biologically-oriented dentists, tests positive in cases of emotional stress. I suspect that, in the case of many of those who have presumably been harmed by amalgam fillings, we are dealing with people who have large emotional conflicts who, rather than from amalgam, suffer much more due to their unconscious emotional problems. It is all too understandable that people – and therapists may support them (presumably due to ignorance) – find it more comfortable to externalize their emotional problems and, for instance, shift the blame to a nasty toxin.

> The ideology of subtle toxins shaped many physicians of the postwar generation, such as Hans Heinrich Reckeweg and his Homotoxicology. According to this, people become sick due to internal and external toxins, and the cells are said to become more and more laden (impregnated) with them, leading ultimately to

degenerative and even malignant ailments. One can find similar ideas in the old medicine of the 18th and 19th centuries, as well as in ancient humoral medicine. The entire area of naturopathy and Rev. Kneipp is oriented to the elimination of waste byproducts and toxins. The discoverer of EAV, Reinhard Voll, completed the picture when he at some point identified chemical injection toxins used by vintners as being disease triggers, curing them with homeopathic forms of these toxins. Strictly speaking, these were the initial "baby steps" in a hitherto unexplored region of environmental medicine, and in the 70s it was considered to be very progressive. Like Voll, I soon had thousands of test ampoules containing various toxins and other test substances in my practice. For many years, the search for new toxins was a high priority in daily clinical practice with the Vegatest method. It was the development of PSE that first showed me that, for most patients, toxins represented merely the surface of more deeply situated emotional problems.

My investigations revealed that each of the 28 emotional remedies has a precisely determined segmental relationship (cf. **Fig. 2.11**). Each conflict has a segmental assignment that is identical with the Indian energy centers (Chakras). Experience in clinical practice soon showed that I had indeed found the key to a permanent solution to the problem of segmental blocks – but on closer inspection, it turned out that my insight was by no means new, finding expression in idiomatic phrases such as "anger in one's gut", "fire in the belly"). I had thus rediscovered that which had long been known; I just made it testable in energy medicine and in so doing brought it up into the light of day.

Experience with therapy has shown that conflicts generate an autonomous segmental imbalance which can be related to one of the seven Chakras. The underlying regularity is probably due to psychoenergetic resonances, e.g. as the emotion "Rage" is always stereotypically related to the liver/gallbladder system. We in medicine do not know exactly why this is so, because there are no orthodox anatomical or physiological explanations – or if there are, they have barely been explored. But the reality of these phenomena is confirmed by experience; and everyday speech expresses the psychosomatic correspondences in the form of applicable idioms such as "anger in the gut" or "livid with rage".

By the way, this coupling of Chakra and conflict can also be made use of therapeutically: although conflicts are healed using only emotional remedies, the additional Chakra remedies significantly ease the healing process. For instance, in the case of the conflict "Rage" (Emvita 9), one additionally prescribes the Chakra remedy (Chavita 3),

Part 1 Basics

by which the vegetative disharmony in the upper abdominal Chakra is harmonized, which promotes and eases conflict healing.

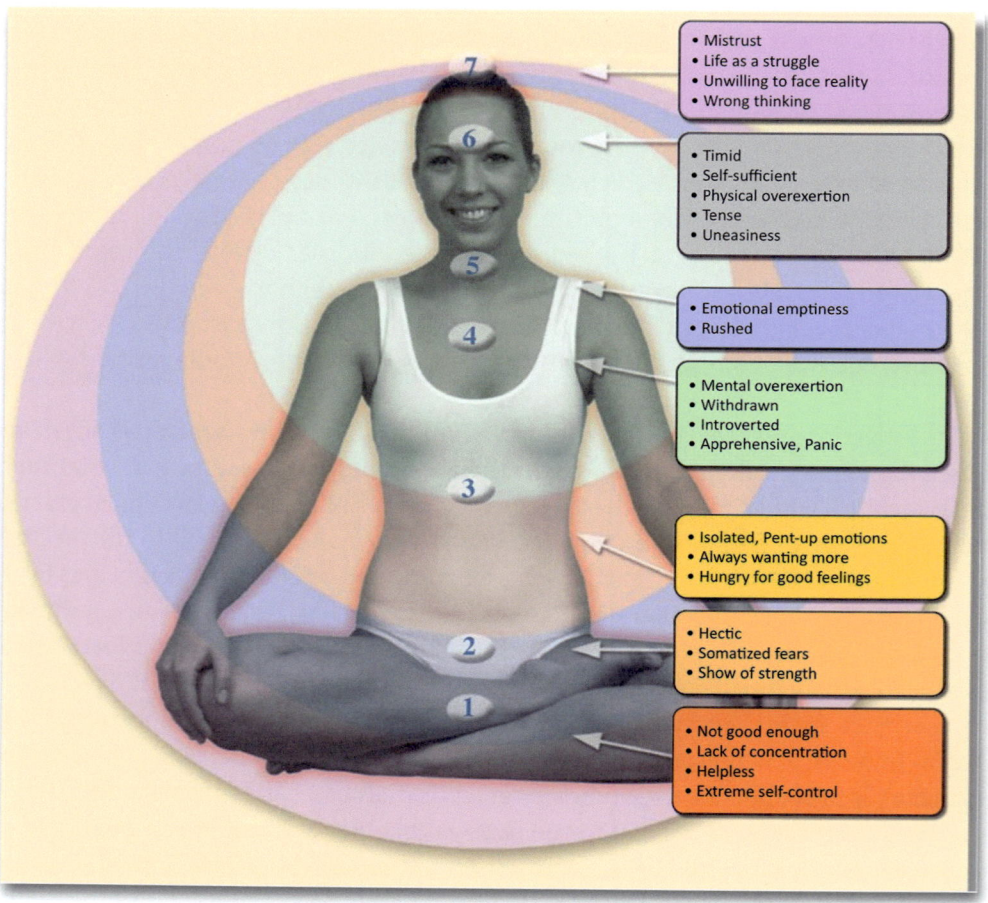

Fig. 2.11 – *The seven Chakras and their associated conflict themes.*

2.5 The Central Conflict

1st Conflict	2nd Conflict	3rd Conflict	4th Conflict	5th Conflict
	8	9 CC	18	23	21

1st Conflict	2nd Conflict	3rd Conflict	4th Conflict	5th Conflict
	8	9 CC	18	23
11 CC	13	24	9	26
3 CC	28	23	14	1
17 CC	16	26	9	6
14 CC	3	10	26	9
	16	11	24	26	23
	1	23	25	5	3 CC
14 CC	23	6	17	27
	7	10 CC	12	3	23
	16	14 CC	17	10	23
1 CC	28	27	11	16
	15	9	23	16 CC	5
	15	10	26 CC	17	3
4 CC	13	26	22	—
3 CC	10	24	15	26

Fig. 2.12 – *Central Conflict (CC) as first, second, third etc. conflict during PSE therapy. Each row corresponds to a patient who was treated for more than 5 conflicts, and for whom the respective emotional remedy was registered as a number, as well as the Central Conflict being highlighted in red. It can be seen that, for about 80% of patients, the Central Conflict is active in either the first or second visit. (From a lecture by Dr. Birgitt Holschuh-Lorang, Expert's Meeting Lake Constance 2009.)*

The "Central Conflict" is a particularly large conflict which is active behind the scenes and constitutes an emotional disturbance factor which leads people to persist in negative emotional situations. The Central Conflict is the largest subliminal energy thief and, in chronic disease cases, is often a crucial cofactor. Thus, in cancer cases, the location of the primary tumor, or region of high metastasis, is frequently identical with that of the Central Conflict. The Central Conflict is to some extent the toughest and thickest onion layer which needs to be peeled away in order to get to the healthy core. Experience with PSE has shown that the Central Conflict must be eliminated in order to achieve deep-seated and lasting healing effects.

I only realized the full significance of the Central Conflict after years of intensive PSE therapy: it was testing thousands of patients which made it clear that the Central Conflict is usually measurable at the very first or second therapy session (**cf. Fig. 2.12**). It is detectable in every 2nd to 3rd patient in the first session; in the second session for every additional third patient, such that after six months of PSE therapy it is visible for 80% of all patients (i.e. after having treated one or two conflicts) and for 90-95% after one to one-and-a-half years (3-4 conflicts). The Central Conflict (CC) is a particularly large conflict that often has energy readings of 80/80/10/80 up to 100/100/10/100. I'll describe how the Central Conflict is tested further on down.

2.6 The four character types

Examining a great many patients revealed that people with the same Central Conflict were characterologically similar. In looking for a pattern, I came across the four character types which had already been known in ancient times, and whose emotional dynamics were first comprehensively described by the psychoanalyst and physician Harald Schultz-Hencke (1892-1953) and his student Fritz Riemann (cf. **Fig. 2.13**):

1. the **schizoid** structure, due to early childhood intention inhibition with respect to closer interpersonal relationship experiences;
2. the **depressive** structure, due to prohibition of oral or oral-aggressive impulses from a very strict upbringing or pampering;
3. the **compulsive/neurotic** structure, due to cutting off the need to take possession or explore the environment;
4. the **hysteric** structure, due to the suppression of sexual impulses at age 4 or five.

> • **Note**
> Schultz-Hencke names, as a neurasthenic structure, an additional subgroup which does not appear in the ancient typology. It is thought to arise from the combined inhibitory experiences of the first five years of life. From the standpoint of PSE, there is no neurasthenic character type, but rather the "easily exhausted" charactertrait is seen in all four types as a nonspecific disease symptom.

Clinical-practice experience with PSE soon revealed that people with conflicts in the third energy center belong to the Depressive character type. The aforementioned example of the woman with the Rage conflict is typical of many. Once I had tested enough patients, I was able to associate each character type unambiguously with a specific energy center (cf. **Fig. 2.14**) – except for the fourth center in the Heart region, which contains elements of all four character types and thus drops out of the scheme.

According to PSE, character is determined by the Central Conflict – an insight which I describe thoroughly in my foundational works *New Life through Energy Healing* [7] as well as *Healing through Energy Medicine* [8]. The Schizoid type has the Central Conflict in the first or seventh Chakra, the Hysterical type in the second or sixth Chakra, the Depressive type in the third Chakra and the Obsessive-compulsive type in the fifth Chakra. The fourth Chakra can contain Central Conflicts of any of the four types. In a later chapter, I go into the character types in great detail, which enable the PSE therapist to offer specific life-counseling in addition to depth-psychological exploration.

Ancient temperaments	Sanguinic	Melancholic	Choleric	Phlegmatic
H. Schulz-Hencke	Hysteric	Schizoid	Depressive	Obsessive-compulsive

Fig. 2.13 *– Antique temperaments and Schulz-Hencke's character types.*

Antique	Melancholic	Sanguinic	Choleric	Phlegmatic
H. Schulz-Hencke and his student Fritz Riemann	Schizoid	Hysteric	Depressive	Obsessive-compulsive
Chakra (except Heart Chakra)	1 & 7 (pelvis & crown)	2 & 6 (lower abdomen & brow)	3 (upper abdomen)	5 (neck)

Fig. 2.14 *– Antique temperaments, Schulz-Hencke's character types and associated energy centers.*

Testing on thousands of patients has since confirmed that, amazingly enough, the old Indian Yoga system of seven Chakras and four ancient personality types yield a perfect overall picture. One may then suspect that we are dealing here with timeless emotional and mental patterns and regularities which express themselves in a strict psychoenergetic manner. Character and Chakra together form a clearly structured and ordered system which enables drawing conclusions in both directions – i.e. from disturbed Chakra with its Central Conflict to infer a particular character type and, conversely, from a particular character type a corresponding Chakra and Central Conflict (more on this later).

2.7 The REBA® Test Device

The REBA® Test Device is indispensable in the application of Psychosomatic Energetics. It serves to determine the charge on the four Aura Levels and the size of the conflict – as well as, at the end of testing, performing a qualitative remedy test which clarifies how much the patient will benefit energetically from a particular therapy. Testing with the device is easy to learn, lasting only a few minutes. At the beginning, I briefly described the procedure, and will get into it more thoroughly later on; right now, it's time to explain why and how the device was developed.

The need for a test device addressing the four energy levels arose during the course of many years working with the Vegatest device, with which the so-called "age levels" were tested. These were mesenchyme potentiations which most closely correspond to the Vital level of the REBA® Test Device. It turned out that the age levels inadequately reflected many states and sensitivities such as emotional burdens. By the way, this restriction applies to practically all energy testing methods, with the exception of mental Radionics and psychokinesiology, in which the therapist asks himself how much energy the patient has. In my experience, these mentally-based tests are extremely unreliable, and only a very few experts have any luck with them, so that an average tester would be totally out of his league. It was therefore desirable to be able to test all four Aura Levels with a reliable device that generated objective signals.

One problem is the way energy is measured. If one measures the extent of the Aura, this varies greatly, even dramatically in the space of a few seconds, so it doesn't tell us very much. This spatial extension, known as "reaction distance", is hardly ever used in clinical practice due to its great variability. My supposition was that the quantitative charge on all four energy levels might yield stable test results, and this turned out to be the case. The Aura charge is like a battery's charge, which also is not constantly fluctuating and whose electromagnetic charge powers a technical apparatus just as subtle life energy does the coarse body.

The History of Psychosomatic Energetics

At my suggestion, in 1997 the biophysicist Dieter Jossner put together the first REBA® Test Device. The name "REBA" is made up of the first two letters each of my first and last name. There are four subtle-energy levels, and since they are resonance-coupled to the physiology of brain waves, one can determine the Aura charge via an ingenious design by measuring brainwave frequencies. It is only the resonant coupling with the physiology of brainwave frequencies that makes this testing so stable.

> **• Note**
> The following correspondences between the energy levels and the four frequency ranges of brain waves (EEG) were arrived at empirically:
> - **The Vital level corresponds to the lowest Delta range (1-3.5 Hz) of trance and a deep sleep;**
> - **The Emotional level to the Delta frequencies (3.5-7 Hz) of dreams and daydreams;**
> - **The Mental level to the Alpha frequencies (7-14 Hz) corresponding to relaxed wakefulness;**
> - **The Causal level to the Beta frequencies (14-30 Hz) corresponding to alert wakefulness.**

With the REBA® Test Device (**cf. Fig. 2.15**), the quantitative percentage charge ("energy charge" or "Aura charge") of the four energy levels Vital, Emotional, Mental, Causal can be tested. At the 0% setting, the device emits a very narrow frequency band, and the entire spectrum at 100%. The more the patient is able to tolerate the stress of the polyfrequency spectrum – i.e. the higher the test results – the more energetically sound the patient. This is thus a **stress test** that functions like a biofeedback test: something imperceptible is registered, and made testable by means of neuromuscular feedback loops. As in other biofeedback systems, one tries for standard values; in the case of PSE, this is accomplished via homeopathic agents.

The **normal values** for the REBA® Test Device are 100% Vital/100% Emotional/100% Mental/40% Causal. Patients may have readings of, say (in abbreviated form): 20/20/100/70. Experience has shown that different testers normally come up with nearly identical results that deviate by 5-10% at the most. The Aura charge is quite robust with respect to short-term influences and yields extremely reliable results.

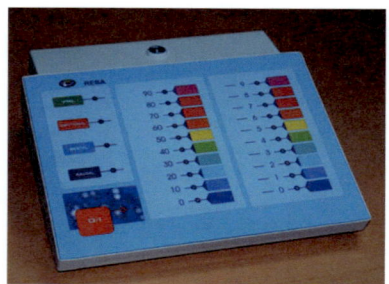

Fig. 2.15 – REBA® Test Device with On/Off switch (red, lower left), 4 energy-level preselect switches and 2 measurement scales – at center 0–90 in increments of 10 and on the right 0–9 in unit increments. For simplicity's sake, values of 99 are taken to be 100%

Using the REBA® Test Device, the patient is exposed to a "polyfrequency spectrum" (as it is known in laser technology) consisting of a blending of a great many different frequencies. This polyfrequency spectrum can be perceived as an acoustical very low-level noise when higher frequencies are switched in. The radiated weak vibrational field extends about 40-60 inches from the device, such that a cable/electrode connection with the patient is not really needed. The device emits waves with a horizontal orientation (like sound waves) and therefore does not need a second electrode to complete the circuit, as an electrical current would. Another advantage to the waves used in the REBA® Test Device is their harmlessness, so that any patient, regardless of basic ailment, can be treated with the device.

New to the REBA device is a tiny component, a new form of Tesla wave coil, in which Mr. Jossner combined two special quartz frequency crystals with a magnet, able to generate not only the customary transverse waves, which vibrate at right angles to the direction of motion (like radio and TV transmissions) but also longitudinal waves, which vibrate along the direction of motion (like sound waves in the atmosphere). Although the longitudinal electromagnetic waves were described and made use of about 100 years ago by Nikolai Tesla, they fell into oblivion because their properties could not be reckoned using the standard Maxwell wave equations. This vibrational form, as yet scarcely researched, is now considered by alternative researchers to be highly significant in the natural transmission of information in living organisms. They represent, as it were, some additional information in electromagnetic radiation and thus a second informational level.

Part 2
Psychosomatic Energetics

3 The Subtle Energy Field

"Life energy" (*Vis vitalis*, ether, Chi, Prana, Orgone etc.) or, synonymously, "subtle energy" is a universally present spiritlike energy flowing through all living organisms; it is invisible to normal persons and is thus far unmeasurable objectively. It seems to be vitally necessary to life itself, since a dead body no longer has any life energy. Since, as we know, scientific logic considers all objectively immeasurable phenomena to be unreal, life energy is from this viewpoint an illusion and not really present. However, this does not agree with the perceptions of countless people since the dawn of humanity: something like life energy has been known in practically all cultures, because people have sensed since ancient times that something like it exists.

Knowledge of the subtle energy field is ancient. Clairvoyant wise men in ancient India (Rishis) about 3000 years ago first perceived the Aura as a colored glowing cloud surrounding people, animals and plants, and they recorded their observations in writing. The "halo" (gloriole) represents a very similar phenomenon associated with spiritually advanced persons, whose life energy is said to glow in the colors violet (indigo), white and gold, whereas the Aura of the average passion-enslaved person is said to exhibit red and brownish colors. The darker and weaker the glow of the Aura, the more unhealthy a person is thought to be, according to the unanimous testimony of many clairvoyants such as Rudolf Steiner and C.W. Leadbeater. One understands how clairvoyance can detect illnesses in advance, and likewise how one can learn a lot about the a person's essence through the Aura. The life-energy-laden Aura is perceived by highly sensitive persons as a bluish shimmering, glowing and vibrating/flowing force.

3.1 Testing the patient's energy field

In Psychosomatic Energetics, subtle energy plays a dominant role. Unlike physically defined energy such as Watt, it is better here to speak in terms of **energetics**. So far, there is no objective measurement method for subtle energy fields (Auras), which means that only biological organisms with their own Aura field can serve as detectors. When one tests a patient's Aura using the REBA® Test Device, it's actually the tester's Aura field which makes contact with the patient's and indirectly reacts to the signals coming from the test device (cf. **Fig. 3.1**).

Like the brain's mirror neurons, which enable us to perceive the feelings of others, it is the reactions of our own Aura which react with the patient's. This view of things has a number of important consequences for the tester:

- Other people can also influence the energy field of therapist and patient, which is why they should keep a distance of at least 4.5 to 6 feet, and best of all not even be in the same room.
- All external substances and fields that exert energetic effects (geo-radiation at the test site, active cell phone in a pocket, medications etc.) can disturb/influence the test field, and should therefore be neutralized or removed.

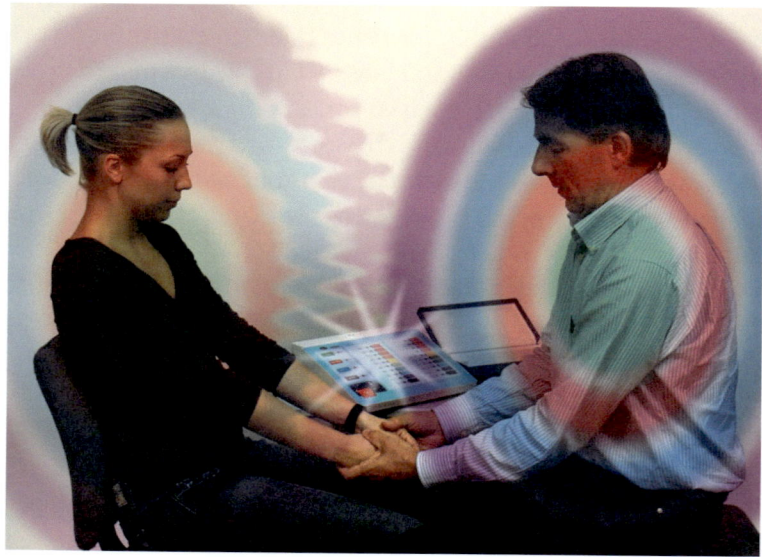

Fig. 3.1 *– During PSE energy testing, the Aura fields of patient and therapist come into close contact with one another. They are depicted here by rings of color. The tester's subtle-energy field reacts with the patient's – which means that he doesn't directly test the patient's Aura, but rather indirectly via his own Aura, reacting to its reaction.*

- All endogenous factors such as the tester's own conflicts can make themselves disturbingly noticed by testing out themselves instead of the patient's conflicts, or the tester's dissonances can falsify test results. Testers should therefore be free of conflicts and be in better energetic shape than their patients.

Understandably, testers should have an energy field that is as neutral and harmonious as possible, so as to enable unadulterated detection and transmission of the patients' reactions. Later on, I will go into the many and varied pitfalls that testers are likely to encounter, as well as the noteworthy elements that make up a good tester.

3.2 The four energy levels

From time immemorial in India, four clearly distinguishable energy levels have been described. They were first perceived more than 2500 years ago by clairvoyant wise men (Rishis) and described in Indian texts.

> • Note
> The four Aura levels vibrate in ever finer gradations, extend out farther from the body and contain ever more complex functions, yet with ever higher psychic degrees of freedom:
> - The Vital level: pure life energy which imparts a feeling of aliveness and strength
> - The Emotional level: harbors feelings and instincts, corresponds to the prevailing mood
> - The Mental level: seat of everyday consciousness and the feeling of oneself; also the seat of memory
> - The Causal level: the deep unconscious, which harbors higher abilities such as intuition and the like

With patients, instead of the "Aura" (which comes across to many as a tad spooky), I talk about the subtle energy field or the layers of life energy which supply the body with living energy and watch over and guide its proper functioning. Picturing plants, which are supplied with light and water by means of light energy, can also be very helpful for patients' understanding. For techno-freaks, there is another image: life energy can be compared to electricity, which powers the activity of a computer (=body). If one has too little of it, then the body suffers. Besides electricity (life energy), software (information) and its storage play a decisive role, one which in part corresponds to the conscious mind, but also the unconscious. Conflicts are then badly coded computer programs which, like viruses, do much harm and to some extent are not at the user's disposal, like a hard disk whose contents cannot be accessed.

Since the charge on the four energy levels can be quantitatively tested with the REBA˚ Test Device, after the therapy session one will want to explain the test readings to the patient and translate the overall result into more easily understandable everyday language. Besides educating the patient, therapists should also understand what the energy levels signify in a medical and psychological respect, in order to deal with them professionally. In the next section, I will present all four levels in sequence.

3.2.1 The Vital Level

Vitality is the level with the lowest-frequency Aura. It is synonymous with the ether body or Ch'i, Prana or Od. This Aura level lies close to the body and only extends outward a few centimeters. It corresponds to overall vitality and a feeling of fitness. At high REBA test readings of 80 to 100%, a person feels fresh, full of energy ("fit") and full of a pleasure-seeking zest for action. At low readings of 40 to 70%, most people will feel ready for a vacation and easily get exhausted. Feeling unwell and tired can (seem to) diminish after years of habituation, and mutate into an apparently normal condition in which one may say: "Actually, I have felt this way my entire life!"

With Vital readings below 30% come feelings of constant exhaustion. Totally energy-depleted persons resemble depressive patients and typically have REBA test values of 10 to 20%. Such people do not necessarily feel depressed, but rather simply empty and lacking drive (like zombies). With genuine depression, on the other hand, the emptiness takes on a decidedly negative aspect which is hard to endure (this is a valuable clinical differentiation characteristic for identifying genuine depression). Even lower Vital readings appear every once in a while, for instance in cases of severe geopathy and enormous conflicts. If I blurt out to a patient with 0% Vital energy: "You have the Vital readings of someone who is at the end of his rope!", I get the answer: "That's exactly how I feel!"

- **Note**
Vitality appears in two forms:
1. **As dynamic vitality corresponding to the everyday manifestation of life energy, and new and**
2. **As a hidden "static vitality" which plays no role in normal life.**

Static vitality is understood to be the same thing as the "inherited energy" of Chinese acupuncture, i.e. an innate gene-coupled form of life energy corresponding to inherited energy reserves. The REBA test measures **dynamic vitality**. Energy-sapping diseases lead to a gradual draining of the "auxiliary battery" in the form of static vitality. To gain an overview here of the course of a disease and its degree of severity – for instance to determine the current survival prognosis of a cancer patient with advanced metastasis, who wants to take a vacation but question is whether his remaining strength will be sufficient – the static vitality can be measured with the following ampoules (contained in the REBA Test Kit):

> **Static vitality**
> Sulfur D1, D30, D60, D200, LM6
> Significance: D1 very low vitality, D30 weak,
> D60 moderate, D200 good, LM6 very high vitality

Children generally have high Vital readings and for this reason exhibit a tireless exuberance when it comes to enjoying life to the fullest. Children with low Vital readings are often nervous, unconcentrated and pedagogically unresponsive, such as in Attention Deficit Hyperactivity Disorder (ADHD). In adults, well-trained in moderation and control of desire, high Vital readings don't lead so much to kicking over the traces as in childhood and the teenage years, but rather to a feeling of well-being, self-confidence and overall interestedness. Healthy and sprightly persons brimming with energy maintain high Vital readings well into old age. The best anti-aging indication is thus a high Vital reading. Although Vital energy is present in all living organisms, it is the predominant form of energy in plants, and so this level is often symbolically represented by the color green (as in the *Psychosomatic Energetics* logo).

3.2.2 The Emotional Level

Emotionality has to do with the "emotional body", which harbors emotions, moods and felt instincts such as sexual desire, territorial defense, personal pride etc. This sphere, higher-frequency than the Vital level, is also present in animals, keeping in mind that, in man, it is increasingly more emotions than instincts, whereas in animals it is feeling-latent instincts which express themselves in the emotional body.

The Emotional and Vital level overlap, which is why someone with a reduced Vital body can feel depressed, or someone with a low Emotional body can feel exhausted. A normal Emotional reading from the REBA® Test Device does not necessarily mean that the person is in a good mood, but rather indicates that the person is fully able to feel emotions, of which sadness is one. Unlike a sick person, however, someone with a normal Emotional reading will soon return to a normal good mood.

Symbolically, the Emotional level is depicted in red, and any "red light district "will show the drunkest fellow where he wants to go – namely into the arms of eroticism. For many, sexuality represents the only avenue for letting out their life energy in a fully unrestrained manner. Sexual pleasure and the erotic are closely coupled with life energy and the emotional body, and constitutes the content of Freud's Libido concept. Yet emotionality means much more than sexuality, since life energy and desire are the expression of a general human ability to lead a happy, self-determined and self-regulated life, which is why children, celibate priests and quadriplegics can also have good emotionality.

For Emotional body readings of 80-100%, a person feels well and is in a good mood. Feeling positive and negative emotions at full strength and showing genuine empathy ("feeling with") means having a healthy, freely vibrating Emotional body unblocked by conflicts. Naturally, a healthy person with a freely vibrating Emotional body will tend over the longer term to be in a good mood rather than having negative emotions. Emotional readings of 35-70% lead to conditions of neurotic unhappiness. By definition, neurosis means making life difficult for oneself, either through inferiority complex, belligerence or anxiety; this type of permanently frustrated state of affairs is always associated with low Emotional readings.

> To my mind, the natural empathy of a free Emotional body unblocked by conflicts represents the most important source of a natural moral sense. Sympathy and helpfulness are therefore natural characteristics of the Emotional body. The question as to whether man is by nature good can thus be answered with Yes – as long as a person remains conflict free. Conflicts are what inhibit natural empathy and give rise to negative, destructive passions and emotions.

Of course, character structure and personal discipline, which is mostly transmitted by upbringing, determines to what extent one "shares" one's frustrations with others, i.e. by being an obnoxious or, in milder form, a boring and frustrated neurotic. From the outside, many people seem loving and good-tempered, but their low Emotional reading has materialized (somatized) itself in the form of headaches, backaches or annoying stiff necks. When such patients are asked "How you feel?", The answer is usually "Pretty bad and miserable, to be honest." thus, people with low Emotional readings never really feel very well, even if they conceal it from others.

Because of the tight coupling of emotions and the immune system, immunological disorders frequently correlate with low Emotional readings. The best known example of this in psychosomatics is neurodermitis, in which an often dominating mother can trigger itching attacks in her child with her strict order "Don't scratch yourself!" After the child has been checked into a clinic and the dominant mother disappears, the itching attacks often disappear as well. In modern psychoneuroimmunology, there are even more numerous examples that show that Psyche and immune system are closely intercoupled. In my research using darkfield microscopy, I noticed time and again that hitherto immobile leukocytes became active again once the Emotional reading recovered. The entire system also improves as the Emotional readings rise, and allergies take a milder course or are dissolved.

Unlike adults, children with low Vital and Emotional values exhibit no symptoms of exhaustion or depression! As we all know, children never get tired and are always good-natured, which has to do with the fact that children normally have high Vital and Emotional values, which evidently represents a protective factor for the growing self. Now if, due to large conflicts, geopathy or other factors, the Vital and Emotional values do happen to go down, children exhibit symptoms of irritability, lack of concentration and asocial behavior. A "fidgety Frank" or hyperkinetic (ADHD) "bratty" child are nearly always suffering from low Vital and/or Emotional values. If the energy situation improves, then all symptoms of fidgetiness, agitation and sullen belligerence disappear.

The Emotional level regulates feelings and behavior not only in humans, but in animals as well. In this, emotional conflicts play a role in humans and pets in that they throttle the energy system and trigger neurotic behavior. With wild animals, on the other hand, freedom from conflict leads to an unbridled enormous reserve of life energy, which can be seen in phenomena such as avian flight and the daylong wanderings of wild herd animals; the more a person resolves his conflicts, the more original life energy is restored. By the way, this applies not just to athletes, who, according to their trainers, experience a powerful performance boost when they resolve their conflicts, but to animals as well. I have heard from horse trainers that Psychosomatic

Energetics is a wonder weapon when used as a performance enhancer. In eliminating conflicts, the animal is not artificially manipulated, as one might rashly assume, but instead reestablishes contact with its original reserves of life energy.

3.2.3 The Mental Level

The Mental level is the realm of everyday consciousness, which, like the Causal level, is only present in humans and not in other animals or plants. Animals have emotional intelligence, which as we know can in many ways be superior to abstract thinking. However, only the human species has the Mental level. It approximately reflects a person's intelligence, such that a less gifted person will exhibit Mental readings of 70% or less. On the other hand, both averagely intelligent people as well as highly intelligent people will all have Mental readings of about 100%. So, based on low Mental readings, one can identify markedly less intelligent people, but normal readings of around 100% cannot determine the intelligence difference of people in this range.

Symbolically, the Mental level is often represented in blue. In content, it corresponds to the feeling of being an individual self and of exercising control of one's person. This also includes memory as part of the self-function. This feeling is missing in people with severe geopathies and/or extremely large conflicts, so that these unfortunate souls then complain of empty-headedness, inability to think and a poor memory. A solitary old man with a Mental reading of 20% complained: "Thinking is so hard for me that it actually hurts!" He lay in bed at night above a strong geopathic zone and had a huge active Central Conflict in the seventh Chakra (cerebrum), which almost completely blocked him on the Mental level. The neurologist which his family doctor had referred him to diagnosed incipient senile dementia, which vanished into thin air after the conflict and the geopathy had been eliminated. Afterwards, by the way, his Mental readings returned to normal.

Another possible reason for low Mental readings is unbearably severe pain. These patients seem peculiarly scatterbrained, with a vague and absent-minded personality, as if a large part of their essence were hidden away somewhere, trying to escape the pain. In some cases, very strong geopathies in the head region lower the Mental reading. The most important cause of low Mental readings, however, is psychosis. This applies not only to classical schizophrenia, but also partial psychoses such as paranoia. Such people are no longer in control of themselves, but rather have become partly or almost entirely pawns of their delusional thinking. One almost always encounters enormous conflicts which have taken on a life of their own and defend their continued existence with all manner of tricks. These patients often tell me: "These drops I'm taking to eliminate the conflict make me very restless and confused!" To some extent, one needs to understand these statements as coming from the conflict's efforts to resist dissolution by upsetting the patient and spreading doubt. If the patient can be persuaded to hang in there and patiently continue to take the Emotional remedies, then the conflict will continue to dissolve and the symptoms will abate until they ultimately disappear completely as the Mental readings rise and the patient sheds more and more of the psychosis.

It is well-known that an intact, emotionally supportive social community fully integrated into everyday life can play an important role in the stabilization of the self in schizophrenia patients after conflict dissolution. By contrast, close relatives of psychotics often exhibit a harmful behavioral pattern sometimes known as the "double-blind", which consists of sending self-contradictory emotional messages which wind up demoralizing the patient. Thus, in the individual case, psychotics not infrequently belong to that small group of sufferers (as do pronounced neurotics) who are not always improved by energetic conflict resolution only, but need additional psychotherapeutic and social assistance.

3.2.4 The Causal Level

The Causal level contains the highest vibrations of all four energy levels, and is symbolically represented by the colors violet or white. The Causal level derives its name from the Latin term *causa* (cause) and, in line with spiritual tradition, has to do with the law of cause and effect (Karma). One also speaks in terms of the deep unconscious which the archetypes are found – roughly universal symbols in mankind's collective unconscious, such as cross, dove of peace, wheel, sun, pyramid and, of course, also the deep basic beliefs of each individual. The Causal level therefore has both individual and supra-individual constituents and corresponds graphically to the "window to the dear Lord" or the presence of the higher self (Guardian Angel) within us.

In the average person, the Causal level typically exhibits relatively low values around 40%. Higher values above 70% correlate with increased intuition, creativity and dynamism. Generally, those with very high Causal readings above 90% are strong personalities and/or extraordinarily sensitive persons who are usually open to parapsychological phenomena and have had personal experiences with clairvoyance, telepathy and/or precognition. People with chronic Causal readings tend to be good healers, simply because a substantially high level of life energy flows through them. I believe that high Causal readings are acquired over the course of many incarnations in which the Psyche suffers through numerous painful experiences and has matured as a consequence. Normally, the Causal reading can only be raised by a few percentage points during the course of a single lifetime.

> Belief in the possibility of reincarnation (rebirth) is surely not shared by all readers. Since PSE is not an ideology, I view the topic predominantly under the rubric of depth-psychological explanatory necessity. One can also interpret reincarnation stories along with their traumas as inner emotional nightmares, and treat them accordingly. Still, reincarnation clears up many inconsistencies of depth psychology, quite apart from the mentally consoling prospect of the eternal life of the individual soul. Whether patient or therapist, those with a negative attitude toward reincarnation can nevertheless work successfully with Psychosomatic Energetics or be healed with it.

Highly developed children with high Causal readings (so-called "indigo children"), which are coming into the world in increasing numbers, cannot possibly have acquired such high Causal readings in this life, but rather apparently have brought them over from earlier incarnations. One thinks of a child prodigy such as Mozart, whose outstanding talent is obvious to all and sundry. Children and teens with high Causal readings often have a hard time finding their way in life, probably because they subconsciously have an inkling of the tremendous personality they had in previous lives – which then makes it hard for them to start all over again in this one. When talking to parents, I graphically liken them to high-HP racecars like Ferrari, which understandably have trouble coping with normal street traffic and are the target of many envious glances. It's not hard to understand why such highly talented children are often misunderstood, e.g. as stubborn and headstrong, shy, arrogant etc.

It is usually advantageous to have high Causal readings. In clinical practice, we see time and again that people with high Causal readings are much better able to cope with and compensate for low energy readings on the Vital and Emotional levels.

Evidently, they are getting something like "emergency power from the dear Lord". High Causal readings seem to generally stimulate the organism's energy flow, which is why people with high Causal readings often have much more energy available than one would expect based on the PSE test results.

The best way to elevate Causal readings is to resolve the inner conflicts. No kind of meditation nor any religious training can have a comparable effect, simply because the flow of life energy is most strongly inhibited by conflicts, and more strongly flowing life energy (Kundalini) most easily unites us with the Divine. Moreover, if one prematurely opens the floodgates of the unconscious by means of breathing exercises, meditation and the like without first having eliminated the conflicts, that can understandably turn out to be very dangerous (Chapter 13.12).

Spiritual teachers warn about madness and severe physical ailments if life energy is allowed to flow freely before first having cleansed oneself and being personally mature enough. In my experience, the wisdom of the organism very accurately shows us through energy testing which conflicts are active at the moment, needing to be resolved. Once such conflicts are healed, it has been my experience that the unconscious opens up exactly as much as needed for a person's developmental level. This leads to tremendous developmental leaps which go hand in hand with a marked elevation of the Causal readings. Thus begins an entirely natural spiritual development which, because it is self-regulating, is risk-free.

3.3 Life energy and well-being

For most people that come to my practice, how well or ill they feel matches up closely with their REBA test results. There are, however, exceptions that one should be aware of.

> • Note
> **Fundamentally, general well-being correlates directly with the quantity and quality of life energy: those who feel generally good and well usually have good energy values.**

People with normal energy readings can also have a bad day now and then, but if they recover on their own, that is a sign of normal energy values. Conversely, those who frequently feel poorly and unwell usually have poor energy values. If these values persist for a long time, the poor condition is often no longer perceived because the difference has been forgotten. This also applies to those who have distinctly limited self-perception, males in particular, who can often no longer objectively perceive the poor state of their condition.

Also, in people with very high vibrations – identifiable by high Causal readings of 80-90% or greater – Aura, well-being and the cells can uncouple from each other to some extent. One proof of my thesis is cases of cancer in advanced spiritual leaders. Cancer often leads to overall feeling unwell long before explicit outbreak of the disease itself. Rudolf Steiner, founder of Anthroposophy and one of the highest-vibration people of the last century, is said to have died of a carcinoma which he knew nothing about for a long time because he was energetically so high-vibration. So if I am seeing meditation teachers and people of that sort who can influence their energy system, I accordingly proceed very carefully (e.g. dealers, mediumistic persons etc.). Moreover, high-vibration persons receive, so to speak, a free extra ration of life energy, such that they often seem to feel better than their actual condition. This applies by analogy to highly disciplined people who often suppress and repress feeling unwell.

3.4   Life energy with respect to circulation and pain states

Desire and happiness are closely coupled with the increased and unhindered flow of life energy, while energy emptiness and congestion lead to pain and feelings of emptiness, rigidity and dejection. The founder of Electroacupuncture, Reinhardt Voll, rightly said: "Pain is tissue's cry for more energy." Blood circulation is directly tied to the flow of life energy, which is why cold extremities and cyanotic regions empirically indicate an energy block. When there is a blockage in the first Chakra, the pelvis and legs are more poorly served energetically, which is why such patients exhibit an above average rate of circulatory disorders in the legs.

The autonomic nervous system is also directly coupled with the subtle energy system, so that a disturbed ANS always indicates a considerable energy block. For example, if a person complains of considerable discomfort in the pelvic region, accompanied by ANS-related concomitant symptoms such as intestinal cramps, sweating and nausea – frequently without any objectively identifiable cause – mainstream scientifically-oriented medicine quite rightly makes a disturbed ANS responsible for it (which by the way, experience has shown, often upsets the patient, who feels insulted as a malingerer). On the other hand, the actual cause, not accessible to objective diagnostics, is almost always found by the energy therapist to be a considerable disturbance of life energy, possibly in the form of a block in the first Chakra and considerably depressed Vital and Emotional readings (as measured with the REBA® Test Device).

4 The Seven Chakras

4.1 Preliminary remarks vis-à-vis "Chakra"

The seven human energy centers (Sanskrit: *çakra*) are tremendously significant in energy medicine. They enable us to more easily understand the actual nature of the disease, thereby making them important decryption keys in the effort to comprehend diseases and emotional disturbances, as well as characterological peculiarities. Because each Chakra has its own distinctive traits and symbolic significance, this makes it easier to discover the actual reason for many disturbances and disorders. Moreover, one also better understands the dynamics and the psychosomatic origin of many disorders when the Chakras are suitably included in one's holistically-based calculations. Therapists who master the language of the Chakras will in time get to know a new and fascinating method which will enrich their diagnostic insights and considerably extend their therapeutic options.

The Sanskrit word *çakra* means wheel or spoke. This designation is based on the fact that clairvoyant wise men (*rishis*) in ancient India saw in the Aura dish-like wheels or spokes arranged from pelvis to head along the central axis. Spiritual tradition has it that the Chakras are relays and energetic transmitters for the universal *Prana* (life energy; an Indian designation used in Yoga) or the "Fluidum" (coinage of the hypnotist Anton Mesmer). In Western mythology, the *caduceus* – which we in the West have adopted as the official symbol of the medical profession, with the addition of two vertically entwined snakes – has been set into association with the Chakras and the life energy which flows through them (Indian: *Kundalini*, symbolically represented as a snake). There are seven Chakras (energy centers) in all, which energetically have a function similar to a house's electrical junction boxes and circuit breaker panel. (**cf. Fig. 4.1**).

PSE research has shown that certain emotions evidently dock energetically with specific energy centers, probably due to similar resonances – as "rage" sticks in one's throat. As the energy center of nutrition and digestion, the third Chakra has the primary function of processing food, but it also "digests" (in a psychoenergetic and emotional sense) mental entities as well, for instance in the form of pent-up aggression and frustration. From a psychosomatic standpoint, therefore, a disturbed third Chakra indicates emotional problems with pent-up rage and swallowed annoyance – as well as, of course, somatic digestive disorders. The Chakras possess superordinate psychosomatic qualities in that they unite energetic, psychological and physical aspects into a whole.

> • **Note**
> the segmental psychosomatics of the seven energy centers finds expression in various idiomatic phrases: "Standing on one's own two feet" is related to the basic trust of the first Chakra in the pelvic region (which, psychoenergetically, also contains the legs).
> - "Stabbing someone in the back" has to do with the second Chakra.
> - "Getting red with rage" relates to the third Chakra
> - "Fear in one's chest" sits in the fourth Chakra.
> - Being upset so much as to have "a lump in one's throat" belongs to the fifth Chakra in the neck region.
> - Expressions like "can't see your nose in front of your face" or "that makes me dizzy" refer to the sixth Chakra.
> - The expression "knock some sense" i.e. into someone's head, has to do with the seventh Chakra.

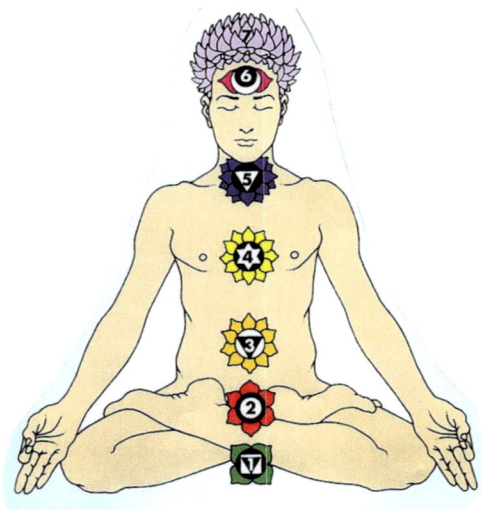

Fig. 4.1 – *The seven Chakras in traditional Indian representation as flower petals (with the thousand petals of the Crown Chakra as the sign of enlightenment).*

4.1.1 Hormones, nerve plexus and stem cells

The Chakras are closely related to the autonomic nerve plexus and to the major hormonal glands (**cf. Fig. 4.2**). Wherever there are superordinate energetic "switching centers" in the organism, one will also find – as per the old hermeneutic saying "as inside, so outside" the same functions on the somatic side.

On a much earlier level than that of the nerves and hormones, one encounters, on the level of developmental history, pluripotent **stem cells**. They guide the growing organism in the mother's womb. Modern medicine is known to have great hopes for these embryonic cell types because they can exert a generally rejuvenating and regenerating effect. Stem cells, as predecessors of the highly specialized somatic cells, have not yet undergone differentiation, so that they constitute something like a universal superordinate "growth capital" for somatic cells.

According to research by the Harvard scientist Charles Shang, a biochemist, biologist and position of Chinese extraction, stem cells constitute an archaic growth system whose regulatory behavior, as well as its distribution in the organism, agrees with both the acupuncture system and that of the Chakras [124]. According to Shang, this is no accident, but rather presumably the expression of a general ordering system. He believes that this is why germ-cell tumors are usually found precisely where the Chakras have traditionally been localized (**cf. Fig. 4.3**). One tendency is detectable: the connection between stem-cell tumors and Chakras points in the same direction as a biographical or evolutionary observation (Chapter 4.1.2), so that, in summary, the energy centers are superordinate regulatory systems.

Chakra	Nerve tissue	Hormonal gland	Superordinate function	Negative emotion	Figure of speech
1st Chakra	Plexus pelvinus	Ovaries/Testes	Reproductive system	Helplessness	"Heart sank"
2nd Chakra	Plexus lumbalis	Glandula suprarenalis	"Negative nutritional system"	Feeling inferior	"Tail tucked between legs"
3rd Chakra	Plexus coeliacus	Pancreas	"Positive nutritional system"	Rage, anger, aggression	"Swallow anger"
4th Chakra	Plexus cardiacus	Thymus	Circulatory system	Fear	'Petrified with fear"
5th Chakra	Ganglion cervicale	Thyroid	Respiratory system	Restlessness, warding off emotions	"Lump in throat"

Chakra	Nerve tissue	Hormonal gland	Superordinate function	Negative emotion	Figure of speech
6th Chakra	Hypothalamus	Pituitary	Involuntary nervous system	Emotional tension, worry	"Splitting headache"
7th Chakra	Cerebrum	Pineal	Voluntary nervous system	Nervous, chaotic	"Going bonkers"

Fig. 4.2 – *Chakras as related to hormonal glands, nerve plexus, superordinate somatic functions, negative emotions and everyday figures of speech.*

4.1.2 Chakras as psychosomatic control points

The father of somatic psychotherapy, Wilhelm Reich, was the first researcher to describe how particular body segments were able to exert long-term control and suppression of emotions.

With the introduction of so-called vegetotherapy in 1930, Reich treated diaphragm blocks in his patients by having them scream and roar, because, in his opinion, their inability to breathe deeply, and habitually speaking in a soft voice, was symptomatic of suppressed aggression. Reich told his patients to strike out with a pillow against an imagined hated oppressor, which they had not been able to defend themselves against in earlier life as helpless children, so that they had stored away the suppressed emotions as muscular tension.

- **Note**

According to Wilhelm Reich, the body segments with control function are:
- Pelvis: Chakras 1 and 2 ("clenching butt cheeks" with disorders such as anorgasmia, dyspareunia, inferiority complex etc.)
- Diaphragm: Chakras 3 and 4 ("holding breath" with asthma, hypersensitive bronchial system, hypotonia and orthostasis, nervousness)
- Neck and mandible region: Chakras 5 and 6 ("gnashing teeth" with bruxism, tension headache, stiff neck, tinnitus, obstinacy, swallowing annoyance etc.)
- Temple and brow region: Chakras 6 and 7 ("I will never get that into my head, dumb as a post" with migraine, thinking and concentration disorders, playing dumb etc.)

The Seven Chakras

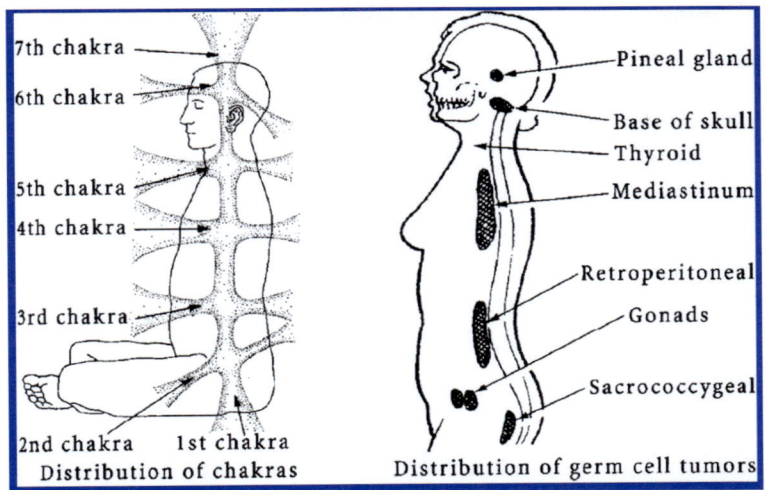

Fig. 4.3 – *The distribution of germ cell tumors corresponds to the sites of the seven Chakras (modified from Shang C.: "Prospective tests on biological models of acupuncture". Evid Based Complement Altern Med 2009; 6(1): 31-39).*

From the standpoint of PSE, one can view Reich's model as a meaningful somatic psychotherapeutic model which can provide valuable insights in individual cases – yet therapeutically PSE parts ways with Reich because emotionally provocative procedures always entail the risk of strengthening already active conflicts or reactivating hidden conflicts. In PSE, we see similar reactions as with so many other far-reaching therapies such as Reich's vegetotherapy, which can be well explained from a somatic psychotherapeutic point of view. Thus, posture and facial expression often permanently change for the better after conflict resolution; people speak with a clear and self-confident voice and become more aware of their body and its needs.

4.1.3 Archetypal significance of Chakras

Back when Chakras were discovered, the holy men of ancient India noticed that each chakra could be assigned specific cardinal psychic traits. These archetypal traits would seem to have a universally valid character that continues to be valid.

> **• Note**
> I would like to briefly summarize the most important "themes" of the individual Chakras (**cf. Fig. 4.4**).
> - The first Chakra stands for the will, power, self-assertiveness, grounding;
> - The second Chakra has to do with self-control, strength and calmness;
> - The third with social interaction, interest in assimilation, satisfaction, the feeling of flow (harmonic streaming);
> - The fourth Chakra symbolizes vibration and identity with oneself and the world, the feeling of being one with oneself;
> - In the fifth Chakra, feelings and thoughts are brought into line; it is also the energetic site of thinking;
> - In the sixth Chakra, the self and its relationship with its own inner world, as well as the alien external world, is regulated, plus it throws open the gate to the inner world (sixth eye);
> - The seventh Chakra operates similarly, but additionally constructs world images – i.e. answers life's sense and order questions.

When discussing the PSE test results, it has proven useful to make use of such archetypal, superordinate concepts such as "entrance, entry, gaining admittance" when explaining the results to patients.

4.1.4   PSE and Chakras

In PSE, seven homeopathic compound remedies (Chakra remedies, trade names Chavita© 1, 2, 3... 7) are tested in sequence to see whether they respond positively in the energy test. As a rule, only one will respond. The disturbed Chakra often coincides with long-standing segmental disorders and diseases, but not always – sometimes it is not until the above/below coupling is established that it makes sense to patient and therapist (Chapter 4.3). The disturbed Chakra can be likened to the main circuit breaker in a home's electrical system; one needs to look for what triggered the Chakra disturbance, and it's usually unconscious conflicts (28 emotional remedies or Emvita©).

There are superordinate emotional remedies for each of the seven Chakras, which are tested in sequence – usually only a single emotional remedy will respond. Because the pre-selection of the Chakra has already drastically narrowed the number of emotional remedies, this considerably shortens the testing procedure: there is no need to test through all 28 conflicts, just the ones for the currently disturbed Chakra. Administering the appropriate emotional remedy as well as the Chakra remedy over a period of months dissolves the conflict in question while at the same time harmonizing the Chakra disturbance. This procedure has proven itself with thousands of patients and is now considered to be a standardized general recommendation for therapists to follow: conflicts heal better when the associated disturbed Chakra is also treated.

> **Special cases**
> It is only when conflicts have mostly been resolved and consequently only provoke mild Chakra disturbances that one can discontinue the Chakra remedies – i.e. if, for a particular conflict, one still tests a conflict Causal reading of 10% and still has half of the flask of the Emvita medication left, but already tests a new conflict in follow-up testing. Then the old conflict can be treated until its Causal reading goes to zero (which has proven to be favorable since it helps prevent recurrence) without also having to take the associated Chakra remedy. One then treats the new conflict, including the appropriate Chakra remedy, but at the same time staying with the old emotional remedy for a little while yet.

Fairly often with new testers, one will note that their patients test out with more than one Chakra, usually two; the testing selectivity of beginners is probably not very pronounced as yet, but will improve as they gain more experience testing. If two Chakras and two conflicts test out, then one uses the remedy test to determine which Chakra and which conflict in the Yin zone achieves the better test result with higher Vital/Emotional readings, then treats only this. Sometimes several Chakras will test out in cases involving strong geopathic fields running along the entire length of the bed. One also sees that sometimes in extremely severe pain cases, but then tests out no conflict associated with the Chakra. In such cases, one should first treat the underlying problem, e.g. eliminate the geopathy or alleviate the pain, so as to calm down the churned-up autonomic nervous system, after which the normal state will return, i.e. one Chakra and one conflict will be testable.

The interpretation of the currently disturbed Chakra has to do with a primary theme which accurately describes the respective active conflict (cf. Fig. 4.4). Sometimes Chakra disorders also coincide with segmental chronic complaints, for instance

Chakra 6 or 7 disorders in migraine cases. If there is an active Central Conflict, then the disturbed Chakra in a sense sets the personality's leitmotif, for instance frustration and pent-up aggression in a depressive character type.

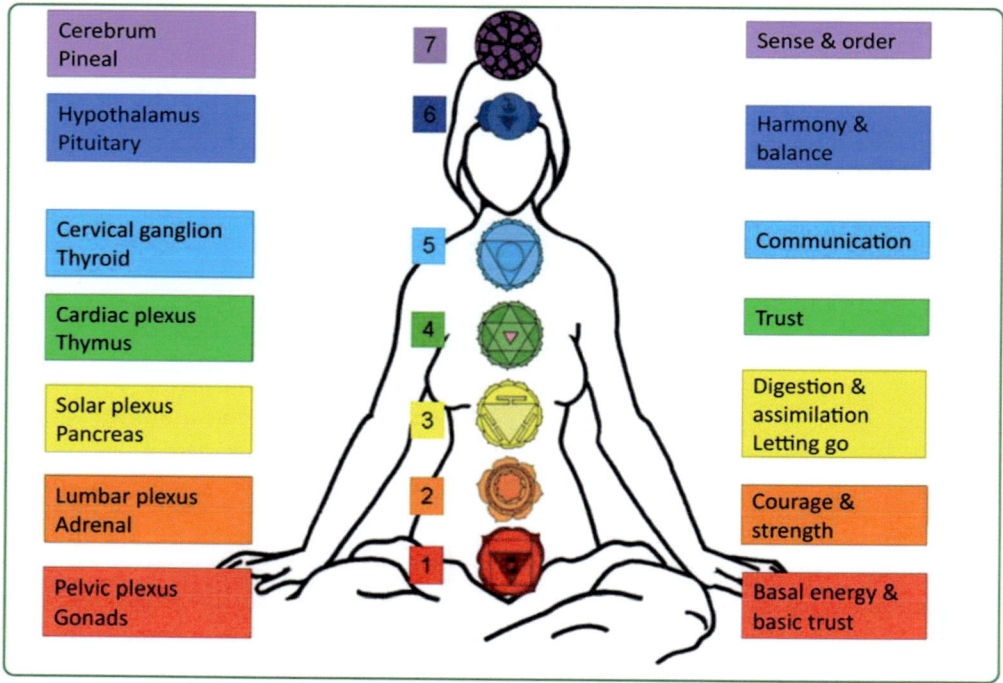

Fig. 4.4 *– Chakras and their significance (from a presentation by Dr. Birgitt Holschuh-Lorang).*

4.1.5 A lifelong journey through the seven Chakras

The layering of the seven Chakras reveals a hierarchical principle which structures each person's individual biography. The Swiss psychiatrist C.G. Jung likens the Chakras to an initiation ritual through which a person, with each higher level, reaches hitherto unknown areas of consciousness. According to Jung, the Chakras reveal a qualitative higher order whose developmental levels each individual, as well as mankind as a whole, passes through. As a child grows up, it also develops energetically in an upward movement from the pelvis toward the head.

The higher mental development of mankind is the basis of some ideas of the American thinker Ken Wilber (*Up from Eden*, who in turn has brought together the ideas of countless philosophers before him – including Teilhard de Chardin, Graves' spiral dynamics). These thoughts are further developed in my books *New Life Through Energy Healing* [7] and *Healing through Energy Medicine* [8]. An evolutionary concept of mankind's development is in harmony with Darwin's evolution of species, and it can likewise be brought into agreement with the idea of individual maturation across multiple lives, which the individual soul possibly passes through (via reincarnation, say).

If one relates the Chakras to age, then it is a matter of mental/energetic powers which are active in every phase of life in different ways: the environment externally stimulates certain steps through which inner psychic contents are brought into resonance and thereby consciousness and maturation. One can speak in terms of a lifelong voyage of discovery which leads man through his energy centers and his unconscious while also gathering experience in the external world. One finds in the Chakras a profound symbolization of the concept "as inside, so outside":

- Small children first discover life energy and begin to live it in a rudimentary manner; meanwhile the first three Chakras are developing. Children stand on their own 2 feet for the first time and develop basic trust (first Chakra), then later differentiate themselves aggressively from their environment (the terrible twos, second Chakra) and, as older children, ultimately "incorporate" the world into themselves mentally and emotionally (third Chakra).
- Teenagers develop love relationships. Romance and feelings of love are said to be associated with the Heart Chakra (fourth Chakra).
- As a mature adult, one lives in society with other people, where one's own personality and that of others play a crucial role. Communication is vocal (fifth Chakra). The central questions of adults, which primarily have to do with the sixth Chakra, are always by nature dialectical, difficult and challenging: What shapes me and what do I shape?
- Finally, in old age, one is confronted with the finiteness of one's individual life – but also with the possibility of a larger spiritual world which reaches beyond the present one. Energetically, old people live in the seventh Chakra. The central questions

are: In the end what does it actually get me? How is all of this actually good? Can I trust the cosmos?

With respect to determining biography, another practical tip: in patient conversations, the Chakra/age correspondences should not be applied too mechanically, since not all correspondences can be precisely related to a person's history. This is a matter of optional assistance in evaluating the test results, and should be thought of more as a cipher and symbol instead of a precise time axis with which the complex psychic processes are summarized in meaningful images.

In the chapters that follow, I will get into each of the Chakras individually, and explain the contents from the standpoint of PSE – i.e. which emotional themes, which conflict themes derived therefrom, which segmentally regulated organ diseases in which functional disorders are associated with a particular Chakra. The associations are based, on the one hand, on well-known ancient Indian esoteric literature and what has since been added to it. Unfortunately, this information source is often of limited help and can indeed at times cause confusion, presumably due to anatomical ignorance, lack of experience and from misguided religious traditions, such as when the sexual function is wrongly ascribed to the second Chakra. To my mind, this is false and is probably due to the hostility to sexual matters in religious circles, which could not stand it if the basis of all life were to be based on pure sexual lust instead of something higher – consequently, it was "hidden away" in another Chakra drawer.

The following descriptions are based on my experiences in clinical practice, and that of other physicians working independently of me with thousands of patients whose Chakras have been tested. This experience has turned out to be extraordinarily valuable and often does not agree with conventional time-honored or esoteric traditions, but rather with Western anatomy and modern depth-psychology theories. As I see it, this clearly shows that clarifying an empirically-guided prejudice-free procedure in a hard-to-access area which has been designated as mystical can nevertheless lead to results which can be designated, to some degree, as scientific and objective.

4.2 Definition of the seven Chakras

4.2.1 First Chakra

The first Chakra is closely related to sexuality and the will to live; its energy is devoted just as much to the struggle to survive as to sexuality. Proliferating genetically through one's descendants is also a kind of survival, even though one is not directly involved; the psychoenergetic origin is nevertheless the same. Body parts with a positive emotional tone, such as the erogenous zones of the genitals (as well as "filthy" areas such as urine and feces) belong to the first Chakra. Thus, the emotional core statements of the first Chakra are:

- "I am who I am (independence).
- I possess (feces/money).
- I melt together (full of pleasure)."

Possession, power, sexual potency and survival are closely related archetypal emotions and strong primordial forces. Those who can feel these forces have basic trust – that fundamental positive feeling of being in harmony with oneself and the forces of nature, and knowing that nature means you well.

The first Chakra has to do with personal pride and healthy self-confidence.

Those who feel helpless and dependent and believe they are not good enough (i.e. suffer from feelings of inferiority) often have a disturbed first Chakra along with the corresponding conflicts. This applies as well for all longer-term disorders and diseases of the lower pelvis, hips and legs. The common ileosacral joint blockages belong to the first Chakra. Also belonging to the first Chakra energetically are most prostate and uterine diseases. Many sexual problems are also caused by energy blocks in the first Chakra. In such cases, one should check with the Organ Test Kit (Rubimed) for the presence of prostate (for males) or uterine (for females) adnexal diseases, which then should be correspondingly treated (Chapter 10.4). Juvenile bedwetting is very often associated with a block in the first Chakra, and it often disappears in the very first night after the associated conflict has been eliminated. (Often it is the conflict "Helpless" or "Not good enough".) Diseases of the urogenital system and the external sexual organs (penis, testicles, vulva), on the other hand, are more likely to be related to the second Chakra.

4.2.2 Second Chakra

The second Chakra is the energetic center of the ability to stand upright (in the sense of getting things done) and the feeling of self; the center, so to speak, of the fully extended lumbar vertebrae. It is also the center of confrontation and dispute and struggles with the environment. The second Chakra is associated with the adrenal gland and its secretion of cortisone and adrenaline – that is, it has to do with the "fight or flight" hormones. The archetypal emotional basic themes of the second Chakra are:

- "I get things done."
- "I am different (better, stronger, special)."

The endocrine gland for the second Chakra is the adrenal. As stress organ *par excellence*, it has a communicative function, since cortisone and adrenaline, on the hormonal level, enable us to confront and deal with the environment. In this, fight or flight in the form of stress, tension, aggression etc. is the key theme here. Moreover, the second Chakra has additional emotional functions, as one learns to moderate one's aggression, to confront and deal with others and establish oneself in a hierarchical social order – in other words, it is all about personal power and one's position within the hierarchy. If the seven Chakras are viewed as stopovers on life's journey, as Rudolf Steiner has suggested (in a seven-year rhythmic cycle), then it is the job of the second Chakra to find its place in society and, if necessary, to fight for it.

The second Chakra is the first energy center if one views the Chakras as upwardly arranged stations of mental maturation in which a process of individuation takes place. While the first Chakra has to do with the naked struggle for survival, the second Chakra is concerned with self-actualization and accomplishment of individual needs. Emotional problems of the second Chakra thus derive from this, as those affected stumble through life: distracted, unconcentrated, lost in thought and "self-lost" so to speak. Those who are not right with themselves cannot really find their social niche, and will therefore feel permanent inner stress. Like the driver of a car in a heavy snowstorm who can no longer see any road signs or traffic signals and no longer knows how fast he is going nor where, this creates extreme discomfort and leads to extreme inner tension and anxiety.

As the site of organ disorders, the second Chakra has three organs in the foreground: kidneys, adrenal gland and intestines. The intestinal flora in particular, with the production of neurotransmitters, feed back in turn to the entire organism, as endorphins such as serotonin and other psychoactive substances influence the entire person. In this, the lumbar spine and the critical region around the fifth lumbar vertebra is a psychodynamic bad-weather area in which the themes of the second Chakra can manifest themselves.

4.2.3   Third Chakra

The third Chakra is the energetic center of the upper abdomen. It stands for every kind of assimilation and digestion, whether material or nonmaterial. The pancreas, whose tasks include splitting up food molecules and supplying body cells with blood sugar by means of insulin, belongs to the third Chakra. The external world is assimilated both somatically and mentally, and the organism derives strength therefrom. As the emotional representative of rage, the gallbladder likewise belongs to the third Chakra, by means of which one fights and stakes out one's territory, like the liver, as the organism's large chemical factory, is representative of personal power. The psychological core statements of the third Chakra are:

- "Part of the world belongs to me and I will assimilate it."
- "I fight for the right that part of the world belongs to me."

The third Chakra (upper abdominal Chakra) has to do with the desire to assimilate matter and energy, and to learn to trust the maternally nourishing nature of the environment. For the first time, the child experiences anger and personal strength, and wants to have its way.

On the energetic level, not only are physical hunger and the subsequent gratifying feeling of satiation imparted by the third Chakra, but also the psychic/emotional hunger for its gratification. Satiation as a physical condition after eating, and satiation as a feeling of comfort or pleasure are psychoenergetically similar. From this one can understand why psychoenergetic frustration can give rise to eating problems.

Insatiability and dissatisfaction can be viewed as the primary sign of all third Chakra disorders. Frustration and emotional dissatisfaction lead to various kinds of addictive behavior, overweight or anorexia. The loss of physical attractiveness associated with adiposity regrettably reinforces the state of emotional frustration, resulting in a vicious cycle of anger at oneself, depression, stubbornness and more overeating, which is hard to break out of – the best way being elimination of the underlying emotional frustration. Every hunt for more possessions can have something to do with a disturbed third Chakra: a lifelong search for intellectual "brain fodder", for spiritual upward development, for material possessions – perhaps a collection of some sort, as long as the search has the irrational and compulsive aspect which characterizes every addiction.

Rage is one of the primary emotions residing in the third Chakra. In Indian mythology it is the darkly depicted goddess Kali who, like the sometimes black-painted Christian Mary, is a coded image for totally energetic absorption and feminine devotion and sacrifice. Unlike the gentle black Madonna, however, Kali is a merciless warrior who, bloody sword in hand, wears a necklace of human skulls. Kali destroys life, thereby enabling transformation, i.e. ultimately creating life. Rage can similarly be cleansing and renewing when one productively frees oneself of something burdensome.

Rage wants to destroy and demolish, just as the digestive juices in the liver (the organ of rage in the traditional Chinese view) destroy complex food molecules by disassembling them into simpler subunits. This is probably why rage has been topographically located in the upper abdomen, because that is where destructive digestive enzymes do something energetically akin to rage, which then by means of resonance generates a kind of energetic magnetism. We thus have here a kind of primitive psychosomatics which finds expression in phrases such as "fire in the belly". However, I think that one should not overemphasize such analogies, for instance by inferring diseases based on presumably hidden emotions. Unfortunately, much pop-medicine or pop-psychological advice does exactly that ("disease as a way"). An overly naïve and superficial disease explanation is often barking up the wrong tree, which only rattles those affected even more through false accusations. Not everyone with cancer wants subconsciously to commit suicide, nor does everyone with heart disease emotionally have a broken heart, while contrariwise in PSE, emotions can indeed have something directly to do with specific organs, e.g. rage with the liver.

Regarding organ ailments, third-Chakra disorders include all those belonging segmentally to the upper abdomen. Particularly frequent from the naturopathic point of view is biliary drainage disruption, which I will go into in greater detail in a later chapter, when I discuss the Organ Test Kit.

4.2.4 Fourth Chakra

The fourth Chakra is the energetic center of the heart (Heart Chakra) and contains the organism's greatest psychic strengths and energies. The fourth Chakra (Heart Chakra) corresponds energetically to a human's center if one imagines the Chakras as layers of an onion (**cf. Fig. 4.5**). Emotionally, the heart stands for the greatest introspection as well as the greatest yearning. Here is where feelings of romantic yearning and melting together with one's lover develop. Biographically, the Heart Chakra is assigned to the teenage and young adult years. The core statements of the fourth Chakra are:

- "I love you."
- "I want to spread out."

The central position of the fourth Chakra in the energy system has its organic equivalent in the vital organs heart and lungs. Proceeding from the organs, it belongs to the thymus, that enormously important immune-system gland which helps immunocytes distinguish between self and other. You might say that the immune system represents the ego in corporeal form, and thus forms a fundamental defensive bulwark in the struggle between the self and its environment. The heart and the lungs play an equally central role: if the heart stops beating or the lungs stop breathing, then the organism dies in short order, which is why all strong fears are directly linked to the fourth Chakra.

Besides a directly tangible surface level, the heart center has a special depth dimension as the center of the Self which touches us in the deepest core of our being. It is a depth-psychological level having to do with the "inner child" and the "higher self". When one is emotionally deeply injured, one withdraws into one's inmost snail shell or is quite beside oneself – both types of emotional conflicts have been observed in cases of disturbed Heart Chakras. "Love of others and love of oneself do not represent alternatives; on the contrary, iy has been noted that all who are capable of loving others can also love themselves." [46] Narcissism as distorted self-love (which doesn't *really* love itself) is therefore likewise a Heart Chakra theme.

Heart Chakra disorders can have an effect on the entire organism and often accompany severe negative symptoms and pronounced exhaustion. Practically any disorder or disease can be influenced by a Heart Chakra disorder. Besides the heart, lungs or thymus, the Heart Chakra has an energetic relationship with the arms, hands and the lower part of the shoulder girdle as well as the mammary glands. When the disturbed Heart Chakra is treated, one often observes particularly strong therapeutic effects – a consequence of the strong overall effect which the Heart Chakra has on the entire organism.

4.2.5   Fifth Chakra

The fifth Chakra, as the energy center of the neck, is considered the superordinate center of human communication. It is here that one finds on an energetic level the rational sense of self, in the sense of the intellect which weighs and considers with self-interest in mind, which enters into cautious negotiation with the environment, always trying to extract the best possible result, optimally dosed and in as perfect a form as possible. The thyroid gland, hormonal regulatory organ for overall internal metabolism, has a similar superordinate function for the entire organism and acts as the metabolism's conductor. The core statements of the fifth Chakra are:

- "Let's talk, and I'll try to explain what I mean."
- "I am in control of myself (as opposed to: I am relaxing/loosening up)."

I am grateful to the Norwegian somatic psychotherapist Gerda Boyesen for the information that the nape and neck region is archetypically related to the father (the mother, by contrast, is located in the third Chakra). The father is psychodynamically the representative of every mental order which stands for control, discipline, law and order, and rational behavior (ultimately for Freud's superego).

The fifth Chakra (Neck Chakra), as an emotional gate, has a sluice function because at this location upwelling emotion and controlling rationality confront each other and must negotiate a solution. If one does not want to cry, one suppresses the uprising feeling in the neck region and promptly gets a lump in the throat or a strangling sensation. Similarly, the neck muscles become tense and one gets a stiff neck. The fifth Chakra, as a control point which equilibrates out rationality and emotion, is thereby an important psychosomatic problem zone because this control point (as the aforementioned example of suppressed crying indicates) is often maintained only with great effort, and the resulting psychoenergetic tension can result in various sorts of disorders such as a lump in the throat, cervical spine complaints, mandibular tension etc.

The struggle between rationality and emotion, the rational and the irrational, duty and "wanting to have fun" is regulated by the fifth Chakra, and right in the middle of this free-for-all sits a clueless "I", like a lost little child that cannot decide what to do. If the outcome tends to favor rationality, then we have overexcited bustling hyperactivity; if on the other hand it tends toward the emotional side, we wind up with a paralyzing emptiness and depressive numbness. Both are bad solutions, which correspond to the two conflict contents of the fifth Chakra, the ultimate result of which is that the self was unable to find a truly sensible and harmonious solution, and is now caught in an emotional trap.

People with a very seriously disturbed Chakra (i.e. the so-called "obsessive-compulsive" character types, about which more later) need to learn to not control themselves so strictly and to savor the joyous lightheartedness and spontaneity of life. These difficulties, along with the annoying inability to give up obsessive control, are well known to those who cannot fall asleep. The more one counts sheep (basically a trick that tries to wrong-foot their obsessiveness by means of exaggerated control – i.e. a paradoxical intervention), the more nervous and wide-awake one becomes, because counting sheep comes across as such a heavy-handed ruse. A person with a disturbed fifth Chakra does not easily give up his agonizing compulsions and extreme strictness. The demand to "Be spontaneous for once in your life!" can be taken as self-contradictory, since one cannot voluntarily undertake to do something involuntarily.

The fifth Chakra has to do with all neck ailments such as angina or hoarseness, as well as the nape, the thyroid and the lower jaw.

4.2.6 Sixth Chakra

The sixth Chakra is the Indian *Third Eye*, a systemic center which brings complex arrangements into harmony. Since time immemorial, the Third Eye has been associated with intuition, the sixth sense and an awakening into awareness of the divine primeval foundation of the world. Anatomically and functionally, the Third Eye corresponds to the autonomic nervous system and hormonal regulation via the hypothalamus and the pituitary/limbic system. This is where those integrated regulatory activities of the entire organism are supervised that obey an independent higher intelligence which is not subject to deliberate influence by the conscious will. The core statements of the sixth Chakra are:

- "Straightening out my needs and those of others;
- Compensating and equilibrating."

Like the second Chakra (with which it has a close psychoenergetic relationship), the sixth Chakra is an energy center in which the process of individuation continues. Here, it has to do with 'self' in the sense of self-actualization and the fulfillment of individual needs, which should be harmonically and evenly coordinated with the environment. Whenever this integration and coordination fails, then the typical sixth Chakra conflicts surface: restlessness, tension, uneasiness, timidity, egotism or compensatory obsequiousness

Somatoform disorders, or vegetative dysfunctions, are typical sixth-Chakra disorders which range from disruption of the sleep-wake cycle and sexuality on up to allergies and functional gastrointestinal disorders. Also, angina pectoris or respiratory complaints, many kinds of headache and lower jaw complaints, tension in the upper cervical spinal region as well as hormonal disorders (menopausal symptoms, PMS, disturbed menstruation etc.) are part and parcel of a disturbed sixth Chakra. Also belonging to the Brow Chakra are the upper jaw, the nose and nasal sinuses, the ears, the equilibrium organ as well as parts of the outer eye (conjunctiva, eyelids), such that corresponding diseases can often be traced back to Brow Chakra disorders.

4.2.7 Seventh Chakra

The seventh Chakra is the energy center for the cerebrum, as analogously the first Chakra represents a kind of grounding to the heavenly sphere – i.e. a spiritual connection between the individual and the cosmos. It is concerned with order and complexity, but above all with something like a well-balanced representation of unembellished reality which freely acknowledges problems as well as one's own negatives and those of others. As we all know, reality is a difficult topic, and ideologies can exert a strong distorting influence in this context.

The seventh Chakra can be viewed as the organism's highest regulatory instance and as the center of the cognitive personality. The pineal gland, a hormonal gland, is closely associated with melatonin and thus to the cosmically regulated day-night cycle which unites the individual with the life-giving strength of the sun and with the rhythms of the universe. The core statements of the seventh Chakra are:

- "Linking my temporal self with the higher unity (environment, cosmos, God)."
- "Looking directly at unadorned reality/orienting myself thereto."

The seventh Chakra (Crown Chakra) has to do with everyday consciousness, the "I" feeling and every day normal reality-based intellectual activity. On the Mental level, one frequently finds misconceptions of reality in the form of imaginary, unreal wishful thinking and unacknowledged pain that the world is much worse than one had ever thought. Basically, such people believe, way down deep, that they are better than everybody else. Greed and mistrust are also typical emotions of the seventh Chakra, in which one prefers the façade of belongings to reality, basically chasing after the façade instead of actual perceptible reality itself, at bottom always thinking ill of everyone.

Disorders of the seventh Chakra always involve false assessments of inner and outer reality, so that illusion gains the upper hand over reality. In line with the statement from Nietzsche [105] that "the dreamer denies the reality staring him in the face, the liar only that which is before others." The person with a seventh-Chakra theme is lying to himself but will not admit it, as per this quote from Albert Einstein [31]: "It is easier to split the atom than break a prejudice." Mistrust, ideological misperception of reality and escapism are thus typical characteristics of a disrupted seventh Chakra, hence one often finds seventh-Chakra conflicts among sectarians and rigid ideologues.

Anatomically, the seventh Chakra corresponds to the cerebrum as well as the upper part of the skull and the eyes. Many brain tumors, as well as many types of epilepsy, seizures and brain-function disorders are often a manifestation of disturbances of the seventh Chakra, as are many psychiatric diseases such as psychoses and all types of psychopathological and other personality disorders.

Part 2 Psychosomatic Energetics

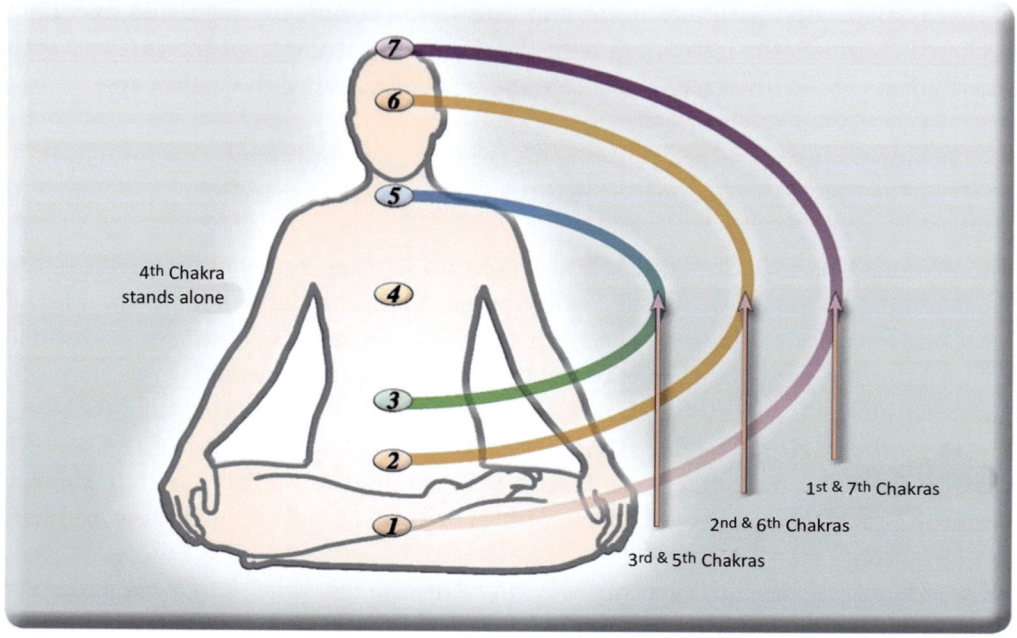

Fig. 4.5 – *Circular relationship of the Chakras to each other (high-low coupling). The fourth Chakra stands for itself and thus forms a human's psychoenergetic center.*

4.3 Chakra interrelatedness: high/low coupling

Practical clinical work with the Vegatest method has shown that cranial foci are often maintained by abdominal foci (H.W. Schimmel). It later turned out that this rule can also be applied to other diseases, as when segmental localized diseases such as a stroke maintain relationships with a chronically inflamed prostate. Now of course a stroke is primarily triggered by high blood pressure, thromboses, sclerotic stenosis, cerebral hemorrhage and the like, but masked inflammatory foci can so aggravate the mesenchymal milieu that such diseases can more easily be triggered and maintained by them. The same logic also applies to Chakra disorders, so that e.g. a first Chakra blockade can thereby maintain a migraine in such a manner that it comes on more frequently.

There is an above/below coupling among the Chakras (**cf. Fig. 4.5**). This arrangement is significant both for explaining disease proclivities (which one wants to make understandable to patients) as well as for likelihood of healing (which one wants to tell patients about). Thus, a patient with a shoulder disturbance can benefit from the elimination of a biliary drainage disorder or a Rage conflict in the upper abdominal region, or one who has suffered a stroke has a lower likelihood of a recurrence if, in addition to being treated with a blood-thinning agent and measures to lower blood pressure etc. also has some pelvic foci eliminated.

Like an onionskin, the center of a human being is located in the Heart Chakra, which stands on its own with no relationship to the other Chakras – which is why it can be called man's energetic center. In view of this onionskin configuration, man is actually not so much a head-governed vertical creature as, energetically, something like a circle or a sphere whose centerpoint is in the cardiac region. By the way, the above/below coupling also applies to two character types: the Melancholic, located in the 1st and 7th Chakras, and the Sanguinic with Central Conflicts in the 2nd and 6th Chakras. Here too, the above/below coupling is active and it explains the psychoenergetics of the two character types (more on this later).

5 The 28 Emotional Conflicts of PSE

In this presentation of the historical development of PSE, I described in an earlier chapter how I discovered the 28 conflicts of Psychosomatic Energetics (PSE) and showed that conflicts are energetically autonomous entities. In the following, I will present a thorough description of the conflict contents and clarify how to picture them, diagnose them, what the experiences have been for particular diseases and how to correctly and completely eliminate them. In order to make the PSE view of things clear at a practical level, I'd first like to outline the remarkable case of a traumatized dog who suffered from bulimia. This case shows how conflicts arise, what consequences they can have and what a beneficial effect their elimination has.

5.1 Example of conflict origin and healing

The following case makes it impressively clear that not just humans, but also animals can benefit from the elimination of their psychoenergetic conflicts:

"On the occasion of a visit to a female therapist, this woman, a therapist-to-be, told me about her dog, who was scratching at the dining room door asking to be let in, but which was not allowed. We were sitting around having coffee and cookies, and we felt really sorry for the poor little thing. He was, in the words of his mistress, a veritable catastrophe, because he would rudely jump right up on the dining table and try to eat everything edible in sight with a total lack of inhibition, if he were allowed to. At some point, the naughty dog was lying down next to me, and I just happened I have the Test Kit with the 28 conflicts and 7 Chakras with me, so I tested them out in sequence by placing the test ampoules near his fur while observing which ampule changed my kinesiological arm-length reaction. Ultimately, I found the conflict "Shock, numbness" in the dog's Neck Chakra.

When asked about the origin of the conflict, his mistress had an interesting tale to tell which made the emotional trauma very understandable. The dog's previous owner was a woman suffering from incurable cancer who, shortly before her death, asked her current owner, a therapist, to adopt the dog after she died. A few days later, the caretaker, called to the house by the other tenants because of the stench coming out of her apartment, found her corpse – and next to it a small half-starved dog. Evidently, the sudden death of his mistress had induced a case of severe shock in him which he has to some extent not been able to "swallow" to this day. Because of the energy vacuum in the Neck Chakra, he had clearly turned into a ravenous monster, trying to satiate his emotional hunger with feeding frenzies – a safety-valve function of eating which, as we know, is not unique to dogs. The rest of the story was even more interesting, for after just a few days of taking the homeopathic drops to dissolve the shock, the dog was once again completely well-behaved, no longer acted hectic and driven, but was completely normal and docile." [7]

I'd like to add that, in the follow-up observation period over many years, the bulimia attacks never again reappeared.

5.2 Conflict formation due to emotional repression and energetic relocation

Emotional conflicts as energy blocks have been known since time immemorial. Aboriginal shamans say that invisible "demons" and "pests" live in the sick person's energy field. In the shamanistic trance state, they are envisioned as poisonous snakes, spiders and the like, and they are said to steal vitality from the sick person, who can only get well after the medicine man has expelled the demons. Many a Hollywood production has dedicated itself to such themes, having to do with vampires and demons – due in part, no doubt, for sensationalistic reasons, but also because people intuitively sense that there is something to these kinds of stories.

These days, we no longer talk about demons, but rather conflicts or dramas. I prefer the term **"conflict"** (from the Latin *confligere*, to fight) which deals with opposing and ultimately unresolvable interests which can arise between people, animals or the environment.

External conflicts lead to internal conflicts, which generate emotionally disturbing experiences that seem so threatening as to be nearly unbearable. They are therefore banished without further ado by the organism as a whole (cf. **Fig. 5.1**). This is exactly the same phenomenon which psychology calls "repression". In order to survive emotionally, the topic is banished from consciousness. In psychotherapy, it is believed that traumas can be healed by bringing them into conscious awareness and achieving reconciliation through something like forgiveness.

The conflict also has a subtle-energy charge which leads, on the energetic plane, to externalization, and which results in a loss of life energy. Like a vampire, the conflict then clings the patient's energy body, living off of its life force. Thus, when someone feels constantly tired and drained of energy, one will usually find conflicts to be the actual subtle-energy cause. Logically enough, only conflict resolution can lead to proper healing and replenishing of the energy reserves – i.e. only in this way can the energy loss be treated causally and permanently eliminated. To some extent, the energetic approach is that of the shaman who dissolves the vampire like conflict and thereby heals it.

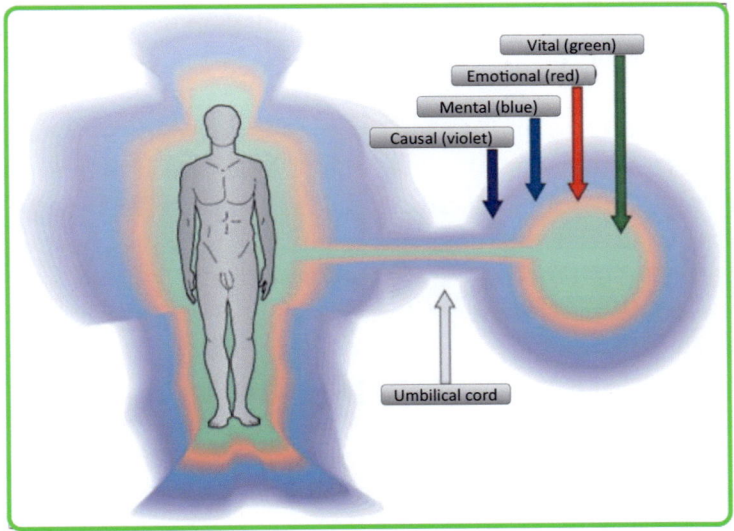

Fig. 5.1 *– Conflict as an appendage of the Aura, connected to the conflict host by an umbilical cord and living vampirically off its energy.*

There is a great deal of tension between the two poles of shamanism and psychotherapy. The psychotherapist sees in the patient someone who acts autonomously – or at least seems to do so on the surface. However, the fact that psychotherapy (through the back door, so to speak) very often views people as underage victims, for instance through the stereotypic hypothesis of an unhappy childhood, is a different story. At any rate, we modern Westerners believe that people have a certain degree of self-determination and are able, within limits, to determine their own fate, at least with foresight as a future project after successful therapy. In our modern, psychotherapeutically oriented point of view, the victim bears a certain share of the blame, say in marital conflicts. The victim is enmeshed in a complex fabric of relationships, which also comes to the foreground in systemic therapies such as Family Constellations.

In shamanism, on the other hand, the victim is totally innocent and at the mercy of envious neighbors, evil spirits and other dark forces. To Western ears, this sounds like making excuses and projection, while, to the shaman, the Western "talking cure" of psychotherapy unpardonably fails to take into account the vampiric aspect of the reality of trauma storage. My summary here is that both therapy systems should learn from each other, and PSE builds a bridge between shamanism and psychotherapy. PSE, to a certain extent, makes use of the best of both therapy worlds, healing conflicts causally by energetically dissolving them.

> In my book *Healing through Energy Medicine* [8], I describe in detail the differences between psychotherapeutic/shamanistic/monotheistic interpretational and therapeutic models, each of which dogmatically claims to be a complete view of man and the world. They thereby force a specific kind of diagnosis and therapy while disregarding alternatives. Since we know that all models have gaps and negatives, it would make sense to combine them, uniting their positives into a new approach – for instance, the way that PSE combines the shamanistic way of resolving conflicts with the advantages of psychotherapy. By the way, the same principle should take place for moral/legal evaluations as well, which I did not go into in the aforementioned book – I am neither a moral theologian nor a jurist – but which seems pretty obvious from a logical viewpoint.

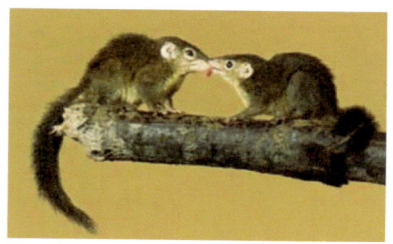

Fig. 5.2 – Tree shrews are popular with stress researchers because they display stress by immediately raising their hackles (Source: University of Heidelberg). (Drawing: Fiore Tartaglia, Göppingen)

The entire process of **conflict formation** can be studied in a well-known animal experiment involving two male tree shrews (**cf. Fig. 5.2**) fighting for control of the same territory. The losing male flees as fast as he can so as to re-attain "peace of mind". However, if the loser is confined with the winner in a cage with a glass partition wall separating them, then his stress becomes permanent and the losing male will be dead in a matter of weeks. The reason for this is that tree shrew males cannot build a conflict which, so to speak, artificially restores peace and thereby saves the life of the loser. The losing shrews are helplessly at the mercy of their emotions, which in fact kill them in short order.

Conflicts are thus, like a measles rash, a kind of protective mechanism or survival program in which the organism gets rid of the harmful agent by externalizing it. The energetic extirpation of the conflict has a protective function comparable to the virus-containing rash – with the difference that viral rashes heal up in a couple of days, whereas the conflict sticks around for a very long time. Evidently, an active conflict at some point sinks down into a semiconscious state in which it only has a subliminal influence, despite which it lives subtly off the energy of the conflict host. Passive conflicts continue to draw subliminally on the host's energy. It's understandable then that conflict-free wild animals have practically limitless energy reserves, and migratory birds can fly for thousands of kilometers, which domesticated animals can no longer do due to their conflicts.

The American trauma researcher Peter Levine has observed in wild-living animals that they play dead in certain dangerous situations and, once the danger has passed, reawaken trembling from a kind of trance. Because of this play-dead reflex, they wouldn't form any traumas (conflicts) and "de-traumatize" themselves, so to speak, with the trembling. However, in the case of the tree shrews, as well as that of the Spanish dog whose case I described, these protective mechanisms are not possible – in the case of the shrew, because it is constantly seeing its rival through the pane of glass; in the case of the Spanish dog, he woke up next to his dead mistress and likewise did not fall into a trance, but rather took in everything fully conscious. It would seem that this is the way it goes for most conflicts which people are forced to undergo in a fully conscious state, who cannot look away nor faint into unconsciousness.

5.3 Conflict storage and activation

Since conflicts can already be tested in newborn children, it may be assumed that various large conflicts arise before birth, possibly originating in earlier lives (more on this later). Evidence of this includes the differing Central Conflicts of identical twins, as well as the statements of mediumistic persons who trace back large conflicts to earlier incarnations as well as to incarnation experiences. Finally, from the viewpoint of PSE, the origin of the conflict is of little consequence since, in this context, one cares relatively little about the conflict contents (compared, say, to psychotherapeutic methods) and they are only discussed in PSE if they have direct consequences in the current life, for instance as character-typical dispositions.

> In the karmically interpreted conflict origin, one can discern a general human question: we humans want to know where the soul comes from, and where it flows after death. To this extent, conflicts are possibly equivalent, in our personal history, to what ancient relics are for archaeologists, something from which we can reconstruct our individual spiritual history. If one posits that conflicts are as formative for our spiritual history as the antique walls are upon whose foundations a city is built, then conflicts from earlier lives are the retaining walls of our ego, which form our character type and our personal worldview. I will take these ideas further in a later chapter.

Conflicts weaken emotional self-perception and steal energy (cf. **Fig. 5.3**). In extreme cases, for instance psychopathy or severe neuroses, one is to a certain extent psychoenergetically repolarized and becomes a regular zombie. Those who no longer correctly perceive themselves, or even carry about predominantly negative emotions, will feel no sympathy for others and will become killers or sadists ("Hell is other people." – Jean Paul Sartre in [120]). For the average person, this course of events is of course much less pronounced, yet nevertheless present, which can be seen in the horrifying social experiments investigating cruelty on command, such as the Milgram experiment [98], in which a majority of the experiment participants, upon being ordered to by a teacher, punished disobedient students (who were actually actors just simulating their death cries) even to the point of administering seemingly lethal electrical currents.

The 28 Emotional Conflicts of PSE

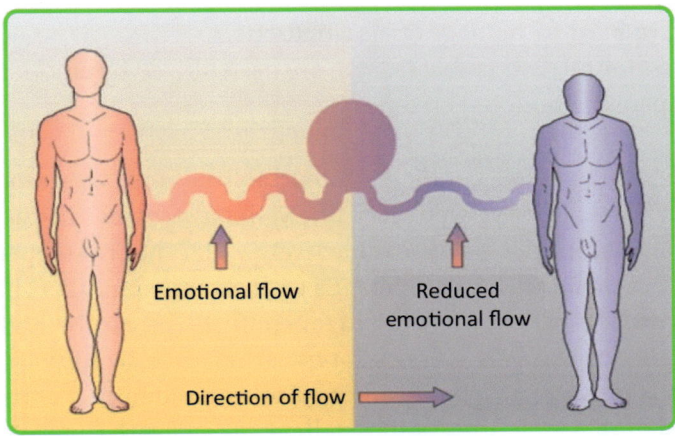

Fig. 5.3 – *Conflict formation and resulting reduced emotional self-image and lack of energy.*

The sequence of events after the energetic formation of a conflict has yet to be investigated; it is still unclear exactly where conflicts are stored and how they become passive. One might presume that conflicts, as mental-emotional misinformation, are stored in the conflict host's Aura field. The conflicts live there in the region of the corresponding Chakra which matches the conflict contents; they are maintained there for their entire life and have no spontaneous tendency to dissolve or shrink. In many persons, the number of stored-up conflicts evidently can be more than twenty, based on the years-long PSE treatments by various different therapists. Once completely resolved, conflicts very seldom return, so the aforementioned twenty or more conflicts always have new contents. The human soul thus evidently has a broad range of stored dramas, and the more complex a person's Psyche, the more conflicts that person will have.

Healthy people needing no PSE treatment have no testable conflicts. Since such people seldom go to doctors, I don't have much in the way of statistics in this context – but I estimate that, from the viewpoint of PSE, at least 70% of all people in the Western industrialized nations have no active conflicts and therefore no need of conflict dissolution.

But when people:
- become ill for some reason or
- feel unwell for a longish time,

107

- get involved in hard-to-manage crisis situations,
- or sometimes, for no discernible reason, are destabilized by emotional drives (puberty, menopause, emotional crisis),

then their previously passive conflicts become active. From the standpoint of PSE, conflicts which become active were very likely already present in passive form, not unlike concealed landmines which only activate when they're stepped on. This can be seen in the fact that even healthy persons with no active conflicts have amazingly many passive conflicts which, when tested for conflict size, exhibit high Causal readings, meaning they are latently present. A typical example, by the way, is the Central Conflict which is present in virtually all people throughout their entire lives, even if it remains passive for a long time. Only smaller conflicts with Causal readings below 60% seem able to arise acutely, but this is just based on isolated observations and is therefore hypothetical.

When a crisis arises, one understandably tends to project the misfortune onto others, making them responsible for one's misery – but the actual reason, in the form of sleeping conflicts, lies in oneself. Of course, that does not imply the contrary, namely that other people should not nevertheless be made morally responsible for their misbehavior, but a greater or lesser part of the problem nevertheless does lie in oneself. It seems to me that it's important to recognize this: on the one hand, it distorts the view of the current problem, in that one sees it through "conflict -colored glasses" (i.e. in Rage conflict cases, everything is rage-tinted, or consists, by way of compensation, of aggression inhibition); on the other hand, one always has a certain degree of blame, and/or one is more or less co-responsible for one's own fate.

> • Note
> **Conflicts going passive cannot be viewed as a peripheral phenomenon of PSE therapy, but rather probably has a fundamental significance in the context of emotional-energetic self-healing and self-regulation. A general rule derivable from this may be formulated as follows:**
> - **Health and well-being simply mean having well-compensated conflicts which have become psychoenergetically passive.**
> - **Sickness and feeling unwell, by contrast, usually go hand in hand with active conflicts.**

> It is not difficult to derive further conclusions therefrom:
> - In trauma management, an emotional conflict going passive presumably plays a very important role, and sees to it that people can forget negatives and find their way back to normalcy.
> - Genuine healing should dissolve conflicts instead of simply making them passive again, since otherwise it could recur later on.

If people get into an emotionally very stressful situation, then passively slumbering conflicts can get activated. In life-changing stress situations such as severe psychiatric illness, painfully experienced loss or life-threatening cancer, the Central Conflict will nearly always become active. "Become active" means that a new trauma, ultimately from the perspective of the old stored-up conflicts, is revived and restored to life through resonance phenomena.

As soon as a conflict has become active and eliminated by PSE, then, as in a multiple birth, a new conflict will turn up in over 90% of cases ("string-of-pearls phenomenon" or "onionskin phenomenon" Fig. 2.5). We don't know why this is so, but it usually seems to be the rule. If PSE treatment is discontinued after the elimination of a conflict, even though testing revealed the next active conflict, then the therapeutic effect is often pretty small. Patients then think, erroneously, that PSE is ineffective. Therefore, in more than 90% of cases, treatment should be performed for at least 10-12 months in order to get good therapeutic results.

For one patient in ten, treating a single conflict is enough; this is usually in the case of persons who are either mentally very simply structured or highly advanced spiritually (with a Causal reading above 70-80%, cf. **Fig. 5.4**). Since PSE conflict therapy always activates new conflicts, it may be assumed that the energetic higher vibration after conflict resolution leads to the activation of old conflicts, kind of like an automobile tire which will exhibit its imbalance when the car is driven at higher speeds. Old negative emotional material is then unable to vibrate at a higher rate and must presumably be disposed of by activation. From another viewpoint, it is something like a psychoenergetic cleansing process similar to a skin eruption due to a viral infestation. Since the PSE view is that it is good to eliminate as many conflicts as possible, the onionskin phenomenon is a great chance to permanently jettison one's old emotional ballast.

Conflict amount until improvement/healing	Duration of therapy	Percentage of patients "healed/markedly improved" per conflict	Percent sum of patients "healed/markedly improved"
1 conflict	4 months	10	10
2 conflicts	8 months	20	30
3 conflicts	12 months	50	80
4 conflicts	16 months	5	85
5 conflicts or more	More than 16 months	2	87

Fig. 5.4 – *Number of patients (as a percentage) who were treated with Psychosomatic Energetics and who reported clear improvement, depending on the number of treated conflicts, as well as duration of therapy. After treatment of any one conflict, only every tenth patient is doing long-term well or clearly better. However, after a year, 80% of patients are improved or cured – and, after another four months, it's an impressive 87%.*

5.4   Conflict uncoupling

Active conflicts can be energetically "uncoupled" by means of certain techniques such as Tapping (Energy Psychology), eye movements (EMDR) and similar trauma-dissolving techniques (psychokinesiology a la Klinghardt), and thereby rendered passive again for a while. From the viewpoint of PSE, one can imagine that the energetic umbilical cord which connects the conflict with the conflict host gets a kink in it: the conflict gets no more energy and goes passive. However, it does not permanently disappear in this process! If one uses PSE to check patients who have undergone such therapy, the conflict size has not decreased (tested with the corresponding emotional remedy), but rather the conflicts are no longer testable for a while (no longer testable with the corresponding emotional remedy, that is). If one waits long enough, such conflicts eventually resurface with their size unchanged.

> EMDR
> EMDR is a good example of how a valuable method can be discovered by sheer chance coupled with conscientious self-observation. While taking a walk, the

American psychologist Dr. Francine Shapiro noticed that agonizing thoughts concerning a personal separation suddenly disappeared and did not return. She recalled having involuntarily moved her eyes quickly back and forth when the disturbing thoughts arose in her mind. From this, Shapiro developed a treatment concept that ties together eye movements with specific psychological treatment strategies. Usually, a number of sessions are necessary for a good outcome. EMDR is based on the theoretical concept that traumas are possibly visually wired into both halves of the brain, and become uncoupled due to the eye movements of EMDR. After the first publication, the procedure was intensively researched, and there are allegedly more controlled studies into EMDR than any other trauma treatment method. EMDR is finding use especially for ailments such as posttraumatic stress disorder in cases of simple traumatization (e.g. due to accident or rape) but also complex traumatization in childhood or adulthood (e.g. war veterans or victims of child abuse).

Psychokinesiology
The quality of conflict interpretation goes up the closer one gets to the subconscious, as well as with the effort of the therapist to turn off his own perceptual filters and simply looks at what arises out of the unconscious. In psychokinesiology, all the named conditions are fulfilled, i.e. it is quickly doable, it recognizes conflicts well (here they are called "unresolved emotional conflicts (USK)", inexpensive and easy to implement. But psychokinesiology has two decisive drawbacks vis-à-vis PSE.
First, it has a relatively large test uncertainty which has to do with the phenomenon of mental testing, since as soon as testers mentally frame certain questions, the error rate rises dramatically for many of them. Much better results are obtained if one works with test ampoules and a test device, as Psychosomatic Energetics does. This way, it is much easier to ease into a relaxed Alpha state and one gets markedly fewer errors. For this reason, many experienced psychokinesiologists combine Psychosomatic Energetics with their own system.
The second downside of psychokinesiology has to do with its lack of therapeutic efficacy, since as a practical matter the conflicts are merely uncoupled. Dissolution with colored glasses, succussion of particular acupuncture points, eye movements (EMDR) or other virtual procedures is, experience has shown, impossible over the long term. With patients who have previously undergone such therapies, I always

> find that they still have large conflicts. It is thus a good idea to always eliminate conflicts fundamentally and energetically using the Psychosomatic Energetics method.

When conflicts are uncoupled and made passive, this gives rise in the patient to rapid symptomatic improvement, but the conflict has not been really eliminated, i.e. what one has here with a mock healing. The procedure is reminiscent of shielding for geopathy, with shielding mats, copper rings, grounding and the like to simulate cleansing, but the actual problem is not eliminated. In the view of PSE, therefore, every form of conflict decoupling is only an adjuvant to PSE therapy. This is practically used as such by some therapists, who use the rapid effect of tapping and similar procedures so that the patient will quickly feel better, while in parallel the conflict is properly eliminated by means of PSE. From the viewpoint of PSE, there is nothing to be said against such a procedure; in fact it can be welcomed, because it increases compliance and lessens suffering.

5.5 Conflict consequences

From the PSE point of view, conflicts have two effects:

- energetic-vampiric and
- mental-emotional consequences.

I'd first like to talk about the **energetic consequences** which the conflict has from the viewpoint of the person who has it. From now on, I shall refer to this person as the "**conflict host**" and his energy readings as "**personal readings**", the emotional conflict as "**conflict**" and its energetic readings as "**conflict readings**". There are also animals who have conflicts, but they are of course not persons. I ask the reader to kindly overlook these linguistic lapses, since the terminology has established itself in the meanwhile, because the great majority of PSE patients are, after all, human beings. By the way, when it comes to animals, one should keep in mind that "animal readings" do not include either Mental nor Causal readings: only Vital and Emotional readings are testable.

Because the conflict lives off the energy of its conflict host, it weakens the host like a vampire would (**cf. Fig. 5.5**). With large active conflicts, the weakening can be considerable, say with readings of 10/10/100/60 for the conflict host and 70/80/10/80 for the conflict. Thus, the conflict energy readings do not yield comparable magnitudes which one could simply add to the conflict host readings. This is erroneously done by many therapists in order to make the expected therapeutic effects clearer and thereby impress the patient, but it is not right because the readings are not comparable. This can be seen in a case in which, after elimination of the first conflict with initial readings of 70/80/10/80, a person then has personal readings of 60/70/100/60 (the initial readings being 10/10/100/60). If both sets of readings could simply be added together, the expected personal readings would be 80/90/110/140 – which is mathematically impossible because percentage values absolutely cannot exceed 100%. But it is also illogical because, as I have said, conflict readings and personal readings are, in principle, two different things.

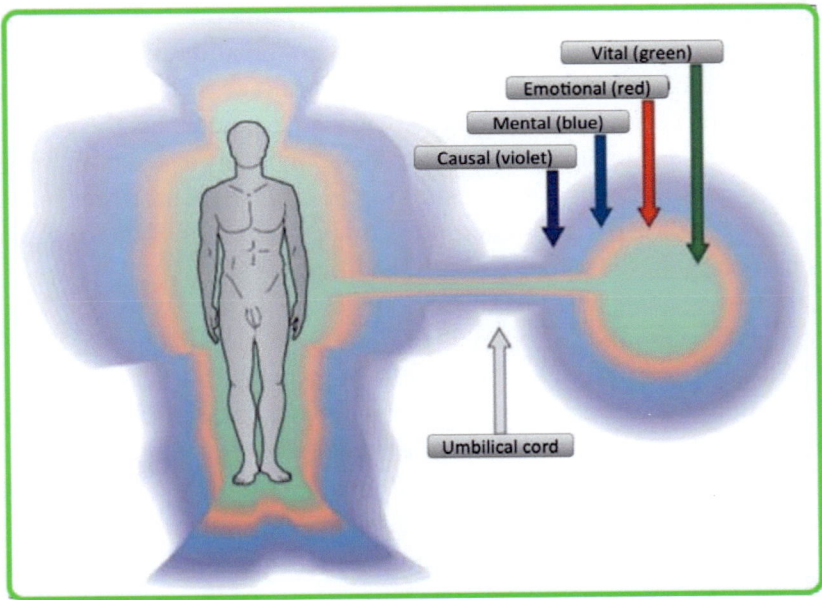

Fig. 5.5 – *Like the conflict host, the conflict has four energy levels and is energetically connected to – and nourished by – the host via an umbilical cord (vampire effect).*

At this point, I'd like to set the record straight about something: several times, I have compared the conflict to a vampire, but the metaphor doesn't work to the extent that conflict host and conflict are, strictly speaking, the same thing: the conflict merely represents a segregated energetic region which is not directly accessible to the conflict host – but it is by no means something separate. Secondly, the conflict is, with respect to content, not independent, but rather a repressed emotional portion of the conflict host. Still, the vampire comparison works to a certain degree, and it makes the psychodynamics of the process easier to understand: one has no access to an important portion of one's life energy and, annoyingly, supplies the inaccessible part with even more of one's own energy, which the conflict post then lacks.

PSE **distinguishes between active and passive conflicts**. The latter cannot be tested directly; at the most, the size of a conflict can be determined with the corresponding test substances (**cf. Fig. 2.9**). Passive conflicts should not be treated, as experience has shown that this evokes strong negative reactions such as feeling unwell, uneasiness, dizziness etc. PSE therapists let themselves to be guided by the wisdom of the organism: only active conflicts should be treated and, more precisely, only those which trigger an improvement, in the remedy test, of low Vital and Emotional readings (or, if the Vital and Emotional readings are 100%, do not make them worse). To check this out, one places the remedies in the body's so-called Yin zone, i.e. the pelvic region.

Placing a particular Emvita and Chavita which previously tested positive in the Yin region of the patient's pelvis simulates taking the remedy. There are three possible reactions to testing the patient's energy readings under the influence of the placed remedies compared to the initial PSE test readings:

- If the patient's Vital and Emotional readings get noticeably better, it means that the placed medications will be the right healing agent; this is most frequently the case (in about 98% of cases). Typically, the personal readings improve markedly from vital/emotional 20/20 to 60/70 or even 100/100.
- If the Vital and Emotional readings only improve a little (about 10-20% each), then often something is missing, possibly an acute agent (more on this later). If the acute agent is added, then the readings go up, or else something else has been overlooked, such as geopathy. Such a test reaction seldom appears (about 2% of cases), but of course it can nevertheless come to pass, and then one should maybe have the patient come in at shorter time intervals to check up on tolerance; the readings often improve the second time around.
- The Vital and Emotional readings stay the same or get worse. This happens very infrequently, roughly one patient in two hundred or even less. In most cases, one

turns for a while to other types of therapy, such as with only one acute agent, or eliminates a geopathy acting as a blockage.
For testers whose Vital and Emotional readings remain the same more often than normal or get worse, it's possible that their own untreated conflicts might be a factor. Another cause can be therapists' concerns about side effects, which they project, in a sense were, into correspondingly unfavorable test result, which then suggests a seemingly cautious dosage.

Besides energetic weakening, conflicts can noticeably influence a person's thoughts and feelings. One particular conflict will generate a repetition compulsion in the conflict host, which ends up with the conflict theme in question being re-staged over and over and thereby strengthening the conflict:

- For example, I have found anxiety conflicts more frequently than normal in patients who engage in risky sports. Those who like to experience fear have deep-rooted fears.
- Overweight persons feel they are unsightly and thus live with a permanent feeling of dissatisfaction, which in turn strengthens their conflicts in the third Chakra such as "Always wanting more, being frustrated". Those who are frustrated secretly see to it that they remain frustrated.
- A woman has a Rage conflict theme and ends up time and time again with husbands who beat her. Those who carry around rage provoke mistreatment and abuse. The logic of the unconscious self-destructive program must by no means be turned around in the sense of "You have bad luck because you carry negative energy around with you." After all, there is an unknowable percentage of senseless accidents and coincidences for which we never know when and to what extent they will affect things. Accidents constitute the well-known assurance that we live in a free and unpredetermined world, and they of course also find their expression in things such as strokes of fate and runs of bad luck.
- A businessman with the conflict theme "Always wanting more" provokes, through his reckless business practices, situations in which his line of credit is maxed out, and ultimately he has to beg the bank manager to raise his credit limit. Those who risk too much, risk someday losing everything.
- A man with the theme "Helpless" always winds up with overbearing wives who make him look like a ridiculous henpecked wimp. Those who feel helpless inside subconsciously want to be belittled by others, so that their low self-image can be confirmed.

The above example show that, through potentially harmful or self-destructive actions, people can contribute to keeping alive their unconscious negative programs: "I try really hard, I do, but then I give up once again" says the overweight person with the theme "Hungry" (emotional remedy 11). He doesn't spend much time with justifications and, as a depressive character type, immediately admits his total culpability. Psychologists characterize the depressive's willingness to admit guilt as a masochistic tendency having to do with an unconscious self-punishing predisposition – a masked form of aggressiveness directed at the person himself.

The situation is quite different when it comes to the hysteric, who likes to wangle his way through things and is extremely averse to admitting faults or shortcomings. "From the bottom of my heart, I wish no quarrel with anyone" protests the curmudgeon with the Central Conflict "Show of strength", who is always getting into situations in which he feels exploited and badly treated, never noticing his complicity in the matter. In his view of things, it is always the others who are in the wrong, since he has only the best of intentions, and it must be an odd quirk of fate that he always meets up with exploiters and bad people. He never realizes that he unconsciously picks fights with others because he always wants to gain the moral high ground. The reason for this is a strong unconscious feeling of inferiority which gnaws at his self-image – which, however, he can never admit no matter what the cost.

The hardest ones to catch on to are negative programs which – as can be seen in both the above examples – become character-typical traits. This will be discussed when we get to the topic of the Central Conflict and character types. In those cases where people are totally blind to their own shortcomings, we proverbially speak of "looking for spectacles perched on your nose". In such cases, any outside observer can clearly see that the overly good-natured, reckless, mistrustful, exploitative or frustrated person is digging his own grave, totally unaware of his self-destructive activity.

5.6 Uncovering the 28 unconscious emotional conflicts

When patients come in to be examined with PSE, I first have a chat with them. However, the conversation doesn't offer me or the patients a specific suspicion which conflict is active at the moment. This is no surprise to the therapist, since one has to know people intimately for a long time in order to be acquainted with their unconscious conflict themes – which plays a role, say, when spouses are usually already familiar with character types and their associated problems. Since I have spent only a few minutes with the patients (maybe longer if they have come a number of times for treatment), experience has shown that this still isn't enough to foretell the patients' conflicts; there's no getting around testing with PSE. The compound homeopathics used contain high potentiations which correspond to the current emotional main problem and thus respond in the energy test.

The **cluelessness of some patients** is remarkable, who almost always miss the point if they have read a book about PSE and found in it a conflict that they feel is suitable and consistent for them. Where does this ignorance come from? Because conflicts are part of the unconscious, it couldn't possibly be any other way, since otherwise the conflict would be deprived of an important part of its defensive bastions. After testing, patients almost always confirm that the conflict theme is correct. One may conclude from this that conflicts must be tested with PSE in order to be reliably detected, since they are otherwise too unconscious to be able to be put into words – i.e., they are stored away nonverbally.

Having read about the 28 emotional themes of PSE, skeptics attribute to the so-called **Barnum-** or **Forer-Effect** the fact that patients deem the conflict theme to be correct. As a successful circus manager, Barnum made sure that his program had something for everyone. This is also the reason why ambiguously formulated horoscopes offer something that seems to apply to any person, in such a way that nearly every person feels individually addressed. Psychology calls this deception the Barnum Effect. However, this effect does not work with PSE: patients complain to me about colleagues whose conflict testing was not accurate. If the Barnum Effect were effective in PSE, then there would be no such complaints.

I do not tell patients – because I want to maintain solidarity with my professional colleagues (and because my professional oath as a physician says that I must) – is the fact that these colleagues are always the same few names who are known to be poor testers. Possibly these untalented colleagues will someday find a reason to no longer use PSE in their practice, thereby solving the problem. In addition, word-of-mouth works against them. I would like to add here that the same complaints from patients are also expressed regarding incorrect character type assignment, where the same subpar colleagues once again miss the mark: character types, unlike horoscopes or comparable "wishy-washy statements", are clearly distinguishable from one another; one is either this or that, and never anything in between.

> We try to counteract these negative experiences that we have had in the past through a strict training program with practical and theoretical exams when training people to become "Certified Energy Therapists" (the official designation for PSE practitioners). Unqualified therapists harm not only themselves and on occasion their patients, but also, through their poor quality, ultimately diminish the esteem of the entire method.

The patient can almost always do something with the conflict contents and recognizes in them the current central emotional theme. This often deeply moving Aha! effect favorably affects the therapeutic relationship in several ways: the patient feels understood to the depths of his soul and is grateful for that, just as the entire relationship with the therapist is experienced as being deeper and more meaningful. For the therapist (but of course for the patient as well) it is usually very worthwhile and important to investigate the effects of the unconscious conflicts on the current life history and to derive appropriate conclusions there from.

The conflict theme which has been found holds a mirror up to patients. Telling them the PSE test results calls for a great deal of professional experience and a sure instinctive tact, so it is no surprise that PSE is particularly well thought of by the more experienced professional colleagues. As a therapist, one needs a good measure of life experience as well as psychological talent to be a master practitioner of PSE. PSE holds up to patients an unadorned emotional mirror, one which makes negative personal characteristics visible, which is not always pleasant to hear. For example, overweight patients with a depressive exhaustion symptomatology learn that they have an unconscious conflict with the theme "Frustration". Not all patients are emotionally mature and honest enough to acknowledge their complicity in their fate, and then make productive use of this knowledge. PSE is thus not suited for all patients, and can be quite an emotional challenge for many of them.

The essential difference with other methods of conflict interpretation is that PSE says that the conflicts are already present when a traumatic situation arises, being activated, woken out of a kind of hibernation, by the current trauma. Even traumatic childhood experiences activate pre-existing conflicts, so that we may assume that we come into this world pre-supplied with individually differing conflicts. When conflicts are interpreted in this context, this then shifts causality, since all of a sudden it's no longer the evil parents or unloving spouse who are responsible for the current difficulties, but instead they are mere triggers of already-present conflicts. One is thereby again responsible for one's own conflicts.

It goes without saying that we therapists do not harp on the self-made nature of a patient's fate, and it would be very bad indeed to wag a moralizing index finger. For one thing, it's not our job to lecture on morality, but it would also be inappropriate because the patient, from the PSE viewpoint, has to some degree become the victim of unconscious programs. It is thus sheer bad luck when the patient performs a conflict program's commands – at least to some extent relatively involuntarily. Of course, one may discuss in the individual case how big the self-contribution is to the patient's fate. As an advocate of the individual soul which can consciously choose its goals, I plead for a certain measure of self-guilt, but how much that might be is ultimately a matter for the individual and his conscience in private, and not to be discussed with his therapist, who is completely unsuitable for this.

The question of influencing self-harmful behavior is nonetheless of great interest to the therapist of course, quite aside from whatever moral or legal aspects there may be. Experience with many hundreds of patients has shown that addiction problems, for instance, become controllable the moment a conflict is reduced or eliminated with the aid of PSE. I therefore don't tell the patient what (not) to do (and if I do, then indirectly: "You shouldn't eat so much" or "You should quit smoking"), but instead treat the conflicts. We therapists need to modestly realize that the patient very likely knows best what to do and not to do, and if he nevertheless does not, it's due to the aforementioned unconscious conflicts – which we therapists are of course busy eliminating. With that, we have done our part, and the rest will almost always be done automatically by the newly autonomous patient.

Knowledge of the conflict contents is very important to the patient, as I have already said, since, after all, it makes the negative behavioral and emotional scripts, by which the patient unconsciously lives and suffers, very clear. The therapist's art consists of elucidating these conflict contents. The following descriptions of conflict contents are based, on the one hand, on the homeopathic medication pictures of the individual components of the 28 emotional remedy complexes, and further on practical experience with many thousands of patients. Understandably, the whole process is a continuing developmental work in progress, always needing new viewpoints, formulations and supplementations, so as to be consistent and correct for as many patients as possible.

5.6.1 First Chakra conflicts

> The following conflict descriptions are excerpted from my book *New Life through Energy Healing* [7] as well as the new addition of the PSE review manual [13].

The first energy center in the lower pelvic region connects us via the legs and feet with the ground, just as it stands emotionally for grounding and independence. A disturbed first Chakra has to do with a lack of grounding, disturbed self-confidence, identity problems and a lack of basic trust.

Conflict No. 1: Independence
One does not feel good enough, has identity problems. Primary emotional orientation, in the sense of sufficient self-confidence, is lacking. Basic trust has been mislaid or was never there in the first place. Frequent tendency to melancholy. The world is experienced as bad. Often among children with early childhood shocks such as divorce, death of a parent, neglect, unwanted child. In cases of unhappy childhood as, for instance, after the birth of a girl, the parents had been hoping for a son and heir.

Lack of inner strength to cope with the burdens and stresses laid upon one. Incapable of perceiving one's own strength. One feels smaller than one really is and tends to close other people out and not enter into any real relationships.

Conflict No. 2: Lack of concentration
The person concerned wants to be anywhere but here. One is not really here, one does not know what one's calling is. This conflict also applies in the case of an inner opposition to being in this world at all. One's own life is only lived halfheartedly and not with complete conviction. One does not trust oneself to show what one is capable of. In stressful situations and those where one's abilities and strength are to be tested, one tends to withdraw. Tendency to postpone things or do them unwillingly.

Such persons often seem unapproachable and featureless when others meet them socially. One is not aware of one's strength. Only a fraction of the possibilities within oneself are realized. Way down deep, one is stubborn in the sense of passive resistance.

Conflict No. 3: Loss of control, helpless
One feels helpless and completely paralyzed. The stronger the demands, the more incapable one feels of any solution whatever. Life is experienced as a never-ending struggle. In the past, particularly during childhood, one was seldom allowed to be oneself and always lived in total dependence on others. One was never seen as that which one truly is. In one's social environment, one only feels accepted when one does justice to the role expectations. One tends to live as a puppet and a proxy for others. One has learned from experience that living out one's own talents, strengths and needs is punished, one therefore does not believe oneself capable of anything whatsoever anymore.

One tends to sluggishness and immobility, has the tendency to scheme, to be indecisive, to be a tactician, to keep things vague, to postpone everything until the last minute or, in the extreme case, even to give up entirely.

Conflict No. 4: Extreme self-control
One does not permit oneself to grow and live one's own life. One was restricted in the normal juvenile joys of expansive self-expression and was possibly too strictly raised. There are frequently problems with sexual identity. One wants to rescue a destroyed family environment through good behavior. One was subject to overly strict discipline at too early an age, and even as a child acted like an adult to others. One tends to repress feelings and impulsive behavior, one blocks one's emotions or those of others.

Only compulsion, reason and proper behavior have top priority. One demands one's own strict view of life from others as well. One is afraid of giving into one's own spontaneity, freedom and *joie de vivre*, because one associates that with great danger for oneself and others.

5.6.2 Second Chakra conflicts

The second Chakra has to do with attaining the individual's interests in a social context.

Should one fight or flee, expend more energy or less to reach one's goals? Those who don't know this become restless and disoriented, struggle frantically, or compensate weakness with a show of strength.

Conflict No. 5: Hectic, nervous

Nervous and driven, upset and restless. Physically very tense, with a tendency to react to inner stress with physical symptoms (somatization). One's accomplishments are well above average; one is ambitious and often overactive. Tendency to obsess on perfection. One gets the depressing impression of never quite getting there and hardly ever being able to cope with something. One strives for recognition from others, because one has an overly high inner standard. One feels responsible for the lives of others. One thinks that one only deserves to exist if one drives oneself to outstanding performances, believing one will lose control if one does not stay in harness and remain alert. Incapable of rest and relaxation. One would like to be present everywhere, so as not to miss anything and to extract the maximum from life.

Conflict No. 6: Perseverance

Tendency to cloak anxiety in physical complaints (somatization). From the outside, one seems calm and collected, but is frightened inside. One fears for one's inner security and one's life, but is unwilling to admit it. One has to seem strong and courageous to oneself and others. Feeling of constant overstress, whereby at bottom, one feels very weak, constantly exceeding one's limits.

One is incapable of saying no to new demands and therefore often ends up getting saddled with more than one can cope with. One is too weak to withdraw from overexertion and allow oneself the necessary rest. One believes only being loved and accepted if one does one's duty. One believes that only strong and capable persons have any right to live. Showing weakness and being downhearted means having no right to an existence

Conflict No. 7: Show of strength, stubborn

One's actual existence does not agree with one's self-image. One feels secretly insecure and inferior, but hides behind a façade of ostentatiously strong self-confidence. One does not let it be seen on the outside how it looks on the inside. The actual symptoms and problems remain in the dark, as one confuses and deceives others. One gets oneself tangled up in contradictions, constantly alternating between feeling strong and weak, thereby coming across as unpredictable and inscrutable to others. Another behavioral variation can consist of cutting others down to size in order to seem big oneself. The large external stresses and the actual inner strengths are in blatant contradiction to each other.

5.6.3 Third Chakra conflicts

The third Chakra has to do with becoming satiated and satisfied by assimilating the environment, by being externally nourished materially and emotionally and thereby made satisfied. One takes what one needs and wants by sheer force of will. When the third Chakra is disturbed, it leads to aggression inhibition and frustration. One withdraws from the world and always wants more than one gets.

Conflict No. 8: Isolated
Emotionally, one lives as if on an island among strangers. One would like to make contact, but somehow cannot approach the others. One feels alone and cast out, even though there are many people all around. One does not have any opportunities for communicating with the others in any satisfactory way. The resulting feeling of isolation leads to inner paralysis and lethargy. One therefore does not even try to oppose the intolerable situation. One becomes emotionally very still and lifeless.

Conflict No. 9: Pent-up emotions
One tries to win the sympathy and affection of others by means of an especially friendly and obliging nature. One constantly orients oneself on the needs of others, and tries to satisfy their desires. In the process, one denies one's own goals, which leads to subliminal resentment and eventually to a mountain of unfulfilled wishes. What others think of one is extremely important. Always playing the victim magically attracts exploiters. One subconsciously gets other people to behave egotistically toward oneself. One tends to exceed one's limits and overtax oneself. One imagines that someday in the future, one will be richly rewarded, but in reality this never happens, giving rise to even more disappointment. One suffers from a nagging feeling of dissatisfaction and a great deal of rage. One is quick to get annoyed and angry, since one's tolerance level for frustration is low. Thus, such people often get stuck in anger instead of hazarding a new approach.

Conflict No. 10: Always wanting more
Thanks to a nagging feeling of dissatisfaction and a deficiency of positive feelings, one is always wanting more from life. Way down deep, one feels poverty-stricken and needy. One has come to the realization that everything in life involves hard work if one has anything and wants to make something of oneself, since nothing is ever

given to one. However, that which one has or has achieved is never enough, so one has to do even more. Good luck and great fortune are presumably just around the next bend in the road, so one becomes a driven person. One's own self image tries to hide the inner hunger from oneself and others, by outwardly projecting the opposite. The hunger for more life can consist of piling up material or immaterial objects and energies. There is often also the desire for more depth and intensity in life, but this is never truly satisfied.

Conflict No. 11: Craving good feelings
One is deeply dissatisfied and empty inside. The misery of frustration easily gives rise to a counter-reaction which consists in the refusal to perceive one's own frustration and to act in a lighthearted manner. From the feeling of constant emotional hunger there develop unreal fantasies and a nagging feeling of drivenness. One tends unconsciously to bring about situations so as to repeat frustrating experiences and to be rejected, for instance. Many fall into a servile role in order to experience secondhand satisfaction by giving others satisfaction, but that is not really fulfilling, and one simply gets even more miserable. Occasional susceptibility to addiction and dependence of various kinds.

5.6.4 Fourth Chakra conflicts

The heart represents the energetic center of the *Self*, an emotional core of individual perception and personal development which has to do with loving trust, mental strength and playful/spontaneous self-actualization. If the Heart Center is disturbed, it triggers a feeling of total retreat, of being trapped, and a paralyzing and, in the long run, exhausting disorientation, behind which are concealed great fears of being injured or annihilated.

Conflict No. 12: Mental overexertion
One thinks that one can, by an effort of will, monitor and control all one's feelings. The need for control is valued above spontaneous expression of feelings. However, due to the fact that more than 80% of human communication is wordless – i.e. takes place in the unconscious – one winds up constantly overtaxing oneself and so cannot keep the multiplicity of impulses under control. One quickly gets tired and then

feels unable to concentrate at all. One begins to suspect having taken on what is "actually an impossible task" and has a tendency to take inner flight. This tendency has a paralyzing effect and engenders an inability to fully concentrate mentally on the matter at hand. Thoughts of sorrows or failure predominate and there is a lack of trust in oneself and others.

Conflict No. 13: Withdrawn, deeply wounded
One feels deeply offended and that one will never be able to get past a severe injury and insult. Rejection by a counterpart who has not responded to these feelings has hit one very hard. One feels not only injured, but humiliated as well, made an object of derision. One withdraws from human contact because one expects no good to come of it. One begins to erect walls around one's sensitive soul and withdraws like a snail into its shell, deep into one's inmost self.

Conflict No. 14: Introverted, compulsive
One has isolated oneself from the outside world and feels imprisoned and helpless behind walls. One's thoughts go around in circles and one feels ever more miserable. The separation from others is not felt to be protective; instead, one feels a violent compulsion and permanent pressure. One's emotional freedom of movement is extremely restricted, so that one becomes suspicious and timorous. The oppressive feeling can become physically or mentally perceptible. Often, the reason for the emotional retreat can be a strong emotional shock which, at the time, one considers to be insurmountable and far too formidable. One then immures oneself in a psychic fortress – which, however, eventually comes to be experienced not as protection but rather as compulsion.

Conflict No. 15: Apprehensive
One feels left alone in a world which is felt to be threatening. Deep inside, one feels fearful and would most of all like to go into hiding. The threat can consist of huge worries which weigh too much on one's heart and whose consequences now paralyze one's initiative. Because of one's own weakness, one thinks that the heart might simply stop beating at any instant. One is cramped and constantly tense. There is a very deep fundamental fear, which can be focused on real-world objects, yet which is also experienced diffusely and quite generally. In this process, many people develop a fear of fear itself, which can be viewed as a kind of self-amplifying emotional "echo".

Conflict No. 16: Panic
One is overwhelmed by an overpowering fear of death, like a gigantic tidal wave. One is unable to put up any resistance to this powerful fear, and instead feels completely paralyzed. It feels as if one's time has come and that it is all definitely over, so that one can no longer have any clear thoughts at all. One feels unable to avoid the inevitable catastrophe. In one's mind, the fear takes on monstrous dimensions.

5.6.5 Fifth Chakra conflicts

The neck region – the control center where the confrontation between intellect and emotions, rational and irrational, duty and desire – has, as an energy center, two conflicts which are extreme opposites with regard to content. If the confrontation tends toward the rational side, this creates a conflict with a hyperbolic and rushed bustling activity; if it tilts toward the irrational, there arises a conflict with a huge inner emptiness and rigidity.

Conflict No. 17: Emotionally blocked
The neck region, as the "gate to the feelings", can stifle uprising emotions in such a manner as to engender a condition of complete emotional rigidity. One is then totally dominated, coldly intellectual, as if nothing at all affected one anymore – almost like a robot. However, it is actually the case that the repressed feelings are simply deep-frozen, and have not really disappeared. Often, the upwelling feelings are bound up with emotional shocks and great inner terror, so that the psychic play-dead reflex instinctively ensures survival. With such a blockage of feelings, one has very limited access to one's emotions, whereas rationality seems to keep on working unhindered. This can lead to the person in question reporting dispassionately about horrible events, leading listeners to think that it doesn't make any difference to the person. The truth is that the person is in a state of emotional shock which separates emotions and intellect from each other, giving rise to this false impression. Many patients with this conflict feel an enormous inner emptiness with a very depressive feeling-tone which can last for a very long time.

Conflict No. 18: Rushed
In the neck region, the "gate to the feelings", strong impulses and drives can rush forward like a flash flood, so that the frightened feeling comes up so suddenly that

one feels literally overrun by it. Since too many intense impulses and contradictory desires are all active at once, one comes across to others as rushed, too tightly wound and rather disorganized. Many compensate inner fears through tension, perfection and control in the form of compulsive behavior. One suffers from the fact that one cannot make oneself clearly understandable. One tries and tries to get the listeners to finally grasp what one is trying to get across, speaking more and more hastily. There also often arises an inner unrest which is not perceptible on the outside. People with the theme "Rushed" thus often outwardly come across as very calm and relaxed, since they so skillfully camouflage their inner unrest.

5.6.6   Sixth Chakra conflicts

In the sixth energy center, a person's individual needs are coordinated with the environment. As in the second Chakra, this involves a complex regulatory system, but basically it is once again a matter of "fight or flight". The typical conflicts of the sixth Chakra, such as Restlessness, Tension, Uneasiness, Timidity, Egotism – or, by way of compensation, subservience – appear when the harmonic equilibrium breaks down.

Conflict No. 19: Timid, faint-hearted
The actual root causes of a lack of resolve are, first, the fear of making mistakes and, second, the hope that a better option might yet come along. Maneuvering around and being undecided are based on an inability to weigh clearheadedly the relative pros and cons of various possibilities and then resolutely opt for one of the options. One instead timidly tries to satisfy everybody and to avoid any confrontation. One tries to act diplomatically, without noticing that one is suppressing one's own impulses and wishes. One goes around in circles without making any real progress.

Conflict No. 20: Self-sufficient
One feels the immediate environment to be an exclusive expansion of one's own person, and thus mainly circles around one's own interests and desires. One believes that one can do everything oneself, and in fact better than anyone else could. This self-sufficiency can degenerate into narcissism, yet remain concealed behind a façade

of modesty. Way down deep, one is unsure of oneself and feels unloved, trying to compensate for that with an oversized self-love. Some people with this conflict suffer severe mood swings and are irritable because they are under so much emotional tension.

Conflict No. 21: Physical overexertion
One feels harried and drained, because one overtaxes oneself so much. One is constantly exceeding one's limits and thereby harming oneself. One has the feeling of always having to be doing something and not being able to give oneself a break. One suppresses one's own needs in the effort to be the best. Way down deep, one feels unloved and worthless, so that one exerts oneself in having to have something to offer to others. One tends to be physically driven and tense, and in the extreme case this can lead to auto-aggressive substitute activity. Sometimes long-lasting pain states are found, as well as other warning signs in the form of somatizations or behavioral disorders pointing to permanent emotional overexertion.

Conflict No. 22: Restless, mentally hyperactive
One feels inside as if one is under constant pressure, whereby one's thoughts never settle down. Ideas buzz around incessantly in one's head, stirring things up into a state of inner unrest and drivenness, because one has too many worries and fears. One would most like to settle everything at once. One is worried about missing something crucial. One has a constant feeling of uncertainty and great worry, is irritable and feels driven.

Conflict No. 23: Tense
One feels constantly tensed up and unable to relax. This can manifest itself in the form of involuntary tics, writer's cramp or muscular tension e.g. in the cervical spine, as well as in a cramped way of speaking, gnashing of teeth and intestinal cramps. Sometimes, the tension manifests as exaggerated discipline and overdone diligence. From the outside, such persons often seem particularly friendly and well-adjusted. The emotional background to the tension is based on an overly strict Superego. Often in childhood, an age-inappropriate correctness and self-discipline was expected of one. As with the other similar conflicts of the Brow Chakra, the tension is actually based on a fear of making mistakes. Basically, one is too unforgiving and strict with oneself even before any mistakes have been made.

Conflict No. 24: Uneasiness, discomfort

One feels unwell in one's own body, as if wearing uncomfortable clothes that are the wrong size and therefore pinch and press everywhere. The body is felt to be a source of indisposition and, in the extreme case, even of pain and suffering. All possible manner of disturbing unpleasant sensations can be present, as if the head or hands were too large, the neck muscles way too heavy or the spinal column deformed. One's mood swings from hopelessness all the way over to obvious depression. One feels unbalanced, since everything is unpleasant and most of the body is in pain. The predominance of physical symptoms often leads to the underlying depressive basic mood being overlooked. It is, however, the negative psychological mood condition which generates the physical symptoms. The unease and discomfort is based on a deep-seated feeling of emotional frustration. One is dissatisfied or even hopeless. Deep inside, one feels unloved or unlovable.

5.6.7 Seventh Chakra conflicts

The seventh Chakra provides a realistic depiction of the world, portraying the individual's place in the world reasonably and to scale. Through this energy center, outlooks and feelings are sensibly and contextually correctly dispensed with respect to those of others, so that the individual and others are both realistically portrayed. Disturbances of the seventh Chakra leads to misjudging reality in the form of imagined and surreal wishful images, and the unacknowledged pain that the world is much worse than one had thought. Acquisitiveness and mistrust are typical emotions of the seventh Chakra: the façade of ownership is prioritized over reality and one fundamentally suspects the worst of anyone and everyone.

Conflict No. 25: Mistrust

Based upon disappointed experiences, one believes that others basically have it in for them. One imagines oneself surrounded by a hostile environment with the explicit goal of doing one harm. In this process, one overlooks one's own share of the blame, projecting everything negative outward. People with this conflict sometimes play the clueless innocent and take insufficient precautions, whereby they are easily disappointed by others, thereby reinforcing their mistrust. The American billionaire J Paul Getty put his finger on the insoluble problem of mistrust when he said: "If you trust a person, a contract is unnecessary; if you don't trust him, then a contract is useless."[42] If one is too mistrustful, then (as in the case of the useless contract) one is, deep in one's heart, truly hopeless and disappointed. One often observes in those with deep-seated mistrust a fundamental lack of basic trust: everything is called into question (including the presence of this conflict!), everything is dissected with a critical eye and reduced to its component parts. One refuses to open oneself up emotionally, as though one were thereby to lay oneself completely open and totally defenseless to someone or something.

Conflict No. 26: Materialistic
People with this conflict often have a great fear of change; it is very hard for them to let go of things and behavioral patterns, and to hand something over. Possessiveness can also relate to possessing particular convictions, such as believing that one is among the very few who really know "what's what". One can accumulate knowledge or spiritual values or good deeds as possessions, yet deep inside a gnawing feeling of frustration will continue to exist. One is constantly searching about and, way down deep, not really satisfied. There is often an extreme tendency to prioritize external factors such as possessions and the maintenance of a façade over inner values. In the extreme case, it can lead both to an obsession with impoverishment as well as avarice, miserliness and a dog-eat-dog mentality.

Conflict No. 27: Unwilling to face reality
One cannot stand reality and banishes it from one's perception. One is like a good actor who transports the audience to a strange marvelous world, and helps them forget their own misfortunes – except that in this case spectator and actor are one and the same. We're speaking here of fantasy: tuning out reality can encompass subsets of reality, as one, for example, may over- or underestimate the importance of certain others. However, one can also feel that one's entire reality along with all of its negative aspects is so unpleasant that one undertakes a flight into a dream world.

Many tune out parts of their inner or outer reality and flee into dreamland or *ersatz* worlds. Underlying this are emotional misery and intolerable frustrations which, in the overall emotional situation, generate a dark and unpleasant basic mood from which one seeks to escape out of sheer will to survive.

However, it does not change the basic problem, just one's standpoint, when one acts as if one were partially existent in other realities. If one tries to flee from the pain which is inseparably linked with being alive, then one strangulates one's own vitality. One needs to realize that the pain only constitutes a limited reality, and that life itself is much larger than the pain.

Conflict No. 28: Wrong thinking
Right thinking leads to an awareness that is in accord with both external and internal reality. Now if, by contrast, one entertains false ideas which are rejected by the inner voice (the conscience of the true Self), then one of necessity betrays oneself. The same happens if one denies external reality. The basic problem with wrong thinking is the refusal to acknowledge reality as such in order to derive truthful and sensible laws of consciousness. One then tends to dogmatic thinking, as if obsessed and possessed by particular convictions. One is not prepared to deviate from one's opinion even if that means having to put up with restrictions and inconveniences.

6 The Four Character Types

> Watch thy thoughts, for they become words. Watch thy words, for they become deeds. Watch thy deeds, for they become habits. Watch thy habits, for they become thy character. Watch thy character, for it becomes thy destiny.
> This passage from the Talmud describes, unmistakably and clearly, the nature of character and what it leads to, namely to self-responsible destiny. However, from the standpoint of Psychosomatic Energetics, the following should be added to the beginning of the passage: "watch thy unconscious dark sides which have triggered an emotional trauma, for they become thoughts."

After many people had been tested using Psychosomatic Energetics, it emerged that identical personality types have specific conflicts in common.

> • Note
> In the search for an appropriate ordering system, the ancient character types Melancholic, Sanguinic, Choleric, and Phlegmatic have proven to be ideal. They correspond energetically to a Central Conflict in the Chakras:
> - 1 or 7 (Melancholic, Schizoid)
> - 2 or 6 (Sanguinic, hysteric)
> - 3 (Choleric, depressive) new are
> - 4 (Phlegmatic, obsessive-compulsive)

> • Note
> The psychotherapist Christa Mewes uses the following terminology: recluse type (schizoid), sacrificing type (depressive), orderly type (obsessive), actor type (hysteric).
> The East-Berlin child psychiatrist Gerda Jun designates the four character types as contemplative (Schizoid), emotive (depressive), archaic (obsessive) and dynamic (hysteric).

So if someone has an active Central Conflict in the first Chakra, he is assigned the Melancholic character type. This is almost always confirmed during the initial interview, when, for instance, a Melancholic behaves rationally, likes to be alone, has trouble warming up to others, strategically arrives at solutions faster than others, to name a few cardinal symptoms (cf. Fig. 6.1).

With the aid of Psychosomatic Energetics (PSE), one can reliably determine character type. Normally, ascertaining personality calls for intensive and lengthy depth-psychology investigatory work, but with PSE it can be done in a short time. I'll explain in detail in a later chapter the specifics of how this is done. Energy testing makes possible not only the clear identification of unconscious conflicts – for which psychoanalytic methods usually take a very long time – but also allows the therapist to reliably determine character type in each case.

One key question is what all this character diagnostics is supposed to be good for anyway, since patients don't normally seek out alternative-medicine practitioners in order to have their personalities revealed and the associated consequences explained. One needs to explain to patients what the advantages are with respect to choice of career and partner, as well as deeper self-knowledge and many other important questions which can thereby be answered comprehensively.

The need for **self-knowledge** is a modern phenomenon whose importance is constantly on the rise. As modern man's demand on himself, the topic was first worked out and formulated so well by the Roman philosopher-emperor Marcus Aurelius, that 2000 years later, it still seems up-to-date: one should work on oneself, purify and restrain oneself in order to become a genuine and happy person. According to him, wisdom (mental maturity) and happiness are synonymous concepts which go hand-in-hand. The French poet Antoine de Saint-Exupery wrote: "The Earth bestows more self-knowledge on us than books do, because she offers resistance – and it is only in the struggle that man finds himself." [118]

The struggle with the world, of which the poet speaks, has a positive aspect: the resistance lets us feel what we are rubbing up against and thereby allows us to develop a personal identity. We get frustrated, betrayed, disappointed, enraged and sad, and in this manner we learn things about our self. The struggle with the world generates emotional conflicts which act as striking surfaces for the Self, like a matchstick on a rough surface, which bursts into flame only when rubbed on it. Thus character is the end product of a long maturation process which, however, because of its normality as a second nature, for the most part we are completely unaware of, like the famous eyeglasses one cannot find that were on one's nose the whole time. It represents an ancient human need to really get to know oneself at some point, and characterology offers the best entry point.

Besides self-knowledge, characterology has other benefits as well. Since particular character types have specific talents, preferences and dislikes, knowledge of character type enables deriving appropriate **life counseling**. A Phlegmatic character is better served by archival activity or an office job than a sociable type such as a Sanguinic, who would be better off as salesclerk or teacher. In large companies, these typologies are used to place people in positions which are a good fit for them, but it is obviously a big gain in knowledge for persons to be informed about their strengths and weaknesses. One also has better knowledge, for instance, about which partner with which character type best matches one's own when it comes to a long-term relationship, since some types get along better with each other than other type combinations do.

By knowing one's character type, one can develop a better understanding of others, who at times "march to a very different drummer" than one's own. Since almost all emotional conflicts are social in nature, this opens up a new level of understanding for patients. Patients will better understand why a Choleric partner more often says yes and backs down in a quarrel, but also know that the partner's swallowed aggression continues to have a subliminal effect in the form of depressive moods, grumbling etc. Or the patient will understand what nourishes the rivalry with a Sanguinic colleague, which ultimately has nothing to do with oneself, say because the colleague feels one to be incompetent, weak etc., but rather because Sanguinics feel themselves to be so, down deep, but refuse to accept their weaknesses. If, then, they wind up at some point winning a competition, then they have shown us all up, but their rivalry was fed by a hard-to-endure feeling of their own weakness.

- **Summary**

I would like once more to summarize the significance of the character types:
- Each character type has specific weaknesses and advantages. Knowing one's character type helps one better know one's weaknesses which, as part of one's personality, normally cannot be properly discerned.
- The elimination of the Central Conflict does not automatically help one become a better person who feels and acts more authentically and more lively, but rather calls for an effort on one's part. Before one can develop, however, one needs first to grasp what the weaknesses actually consists of before one can get to work on overcoming them.
- Different character type combinations get along more or, respectively, less well with one another (more on this later).

- For children, each character type has a different optimal upbringing method (Chapter 6.8).
- Certain character types are essentially masculine, but sexual identity can still be feminine (or vice versa).

6.1 Basic laws of PSE characterology

- **Note**

There are four basic laws of psychoenergetic characterology which PSE users need to be aware of:
1. **Between the seven energy centers (Chakras) and each of the four character types there are fixed regularities such as that, e.g. for Cholerics, the Central Conflict is located in the upper abdominal Chakra.**
2. **People can be classified as to type based upon their psychoenergetic polarity as emotional, feelings-based (feminine) or rational, intellect-based (masculine). Two character types are emotionally (Sanguinic, Choleric) and two are rationally (Melancholic, Phlegmatic) polarized.**
3. **It is very important to differentiate between prototypical character "raw" forms and the more common hybrid types.**
4. **There exists between two respective character types a certain similarity (Schizoid/Choleric as well as Sanguinic/Phlegmatic). Each of these constitutes a pair in which one part occupies the foreground and the other the background.**

In the following chapters, I will get step-by-step into the four basic laws which make PSE into a clear and logically graspable system. Two of the basic laws are **psychoenergetic in nature**, namely that the Chakras can each be related to a specific character type, and that each character type has either masculine or feminine polarity. The **classification of the Chakras** meets the basic condition for PSE energetic testing of character types, while also enabling deep access into the essence of the characters.

Polarity says whether one's basic feeling is dominated more by intellect or by feelings. In addition, the polarity points out what is underdeveloped and thus needs developing. Those who work with polar therapy, moreover, get information on what the optimal therapy is. For example, Yang types are in greater need of relaxation (Yin) whereas Yin types more need toning up and strengthening (Yang). When it comes to polarity, keep in mind that biological gender does not necessarily have to agree with characterological polarity. A woman with masculine polarity will have a harder time of it in life because others will sense it and instinctively reject it – this applies, turned around, for men with feminine polarity. Explaining this is often a great psychological relief to patients, because they realize that there's nothing they can do about it.

The best way for beginners to get familiar with character types is by way of the **raw forms** which can be recognized right off the bat. Clearly discernible raw forms are often strikingly original and expressive people, such as the pronounced Sanguinic with a theatrical manner and a visually impressive outfit who likes to quickly win everyone over. In our modern division-of-labor society, raw character forms are found less and less, because the modern contemporary is expected to act autonomously and be guided by intellect, be compassionate and warmhearted, exciting and energetic all at once, as well as orderly and thrifty. While the imperative of the "fully integrated personality" (which, according to the Berlin psychiatrist Gerda Jun, unites all typologies in itself) becomes ever more strongly the socially desirable norm, i.e. generates strong pressure to conform, the negative traits of the character types become more and more undesirable.

These days, most people are **mixed types** of various different characters, i.e. they have a little of everything, and yet the primary character type sticks out clearly enough. The ones that are hard to classify are very simply structured people and very harmonically integrated characters. One thing that helps in learning characterology is determining the character type of a person whom you spontaneously don't like very much whose behavior you find particularly reprehensible. As a rule, they will be the antipodal raw form to your own character type with strongly negative elements. Thus, a Schizoid will consider the raw-form Hysteric to be unacceptable, or the Obsessive will find the extreme Depressive to be quite impossible; logically enough, the converse applies as well.

When classifying characters, gender, age, nationality and the like can make things more difficult, for instance because inhabitants of southern climes tend toward a Hysteric personality, Scotsmen or Swiss come across as Obsessive, Scandinavian males, by contrast, seem diffident and Schizoid. Women basically tend to seem motherly (Depressive) or charmingly beguiling (Hysteric) (dominatrix-whore-complex), whereas men tend to seem strict (Obsessive) and principled (Schizoid). Still, with a little bit of pre-experience, one can recognize the respective character types, and only have to take the difficulties into account in order to come to the appropriate conclusions.

> • Note
> In the four character types, there are two ideally compatible balanced pairs which secretly resemble each other and exhibit a hidden affinity:
> - Behind every Depressive character there is a Schizoid person (and vice versa)
> - Behind every Hysteric character there is a masked Obsessive person (and vice versa).

When there is healthy mental maturation, a Schizoid person more and more takes on a Depressive character. In my book *Healing through Energy Medicine* [8], I explained this with the example of the Melancholic-Schizoid character of Albert Schweitzer who, as a benefactor of mankind, developed ever more Depressive-solicitous characteristics. In a couples relationship, the compensating character type is the ideal partner, the so-called "better half". This means that Albert Schweitzer would best have married a woman with Depressive polarity, who would have taught him even better what it means to be caring and empathic than he already was, while the Schizoid husband would have taught his Depressive polarity wife the strict clarity of the Melancholic, who does not put up with just anything and who can now and then just say no.

6.2   When to talk about character type and when not to

Generally, a high patient Causal reading has proven to be a helpful indication when exploring the issue of the patient's character type. With high Causal readings, experience has shown that people more readily talk about their character type, since their acceptance of such delicate topics is greater. It makes basic sense to discuss fundamental personality issues only with characterologically well-grounded and emotionally developed persons, since a certain degree of mental strength and maturity is called for in order to realize the inevitability and difficulty of the character question and to be able to deal with it in a psychologically sensible manner. This is often the case with high-vibration persons, so that, empirically, an initial favorable impression plus the aforementioned high Causal reading suffice as guiding principle.

The character type discussion is not infrequently experienced as a "holy moment" by therapist and patient alike. When a person opens up, knowing character type can offer a particularly deep glimpse into the Psyche. The insights gained thereby are often as shocking as they are liberating – on the one hand, because, of course, deep inside we know very well our weaknesses, but on the other hand would prefer not to acknowledge them. Comparable to the nonverbal status of unconscious conflicts which I mentioned in the preceding chapter, we're aware of our character type, yet don't want to admit it – like a shell game con man, our own subconscious tries to leave us in the dark because this is a matter of repressed emotional reality which we want to hide from our self. But it is only after we've accepted our weaknesses that we can work on and overcome them.

Discussing character type is a first step. The dissolution of the Central Conflict can help and offer support, but the actual work must be done by the patient; as therapist, all I can do is simply point them in the right direction of personal further development.

Particularly during emotional crises, knowledge of character type helps one make one's peace with particular character traits and accept them as part of reality. Mature and self-aware persons wanting to grow emotionally can gain valuable inspiration from knowing their character type.

For many patients, the character type discussion does not help very much, for instance those who vehemently reject anything having to do with "psychic" issues, or who are very simply structured, so that complicated topics such as personality theory directed at them with simply bewilder them. However, despite these reservations, it is worthwhile in such cases for the therapist to be informed, since patients can be treated in a more accurately targeted manner if the character type is known. For instance, a Phlegmatic needs a different kind of patient management than a Choleric.

6.3 PSE diagnosis of the four character types

There are two testing techniques in Psychosomatic Energetics for determining the Central Conflict and thereby identifying the character type:

1. A big conflict (say 80/90/10/80) is tested, and the question is whether it's the Central Conflict (CC), so the Brunler-Bovis ampoule is placed in the Yin zone of

the pelvis. If a previously positive test ampoule for a large conflict still responds, then it might be a Central Conflict. The patient is then asked about so-called core characteristics (**cf. Fig. 6.1**) which fit the tested conflict; if the patient says yes, then it is the Central Conflict.

2. The Character Type Test Kit can provide a reliable classification even if no Central Conflict is actively testable. The test uses five ampoules (Diencephalon as well as 4 character type mixtures; for procedure, see additional information in the box). After testing, the patient is also asked here about so-called core characteristics (**cf. Fig. 6.1**) which must fit the tested conflict; if the answer is yes then it really is the right character type. This testing is almost always confirmed, otherwise the test has been done wrongly.

> **Character Type Test Kit (5 ampoules)** — First, the Diencephalon ampoule is placed in the Yin region. The Character Type Test Kit also contains four Emvita ampoules, each one associated with a corresponding character type (c: Choleric, p: Phlegmatic, s: Sanguinic, m: Melancholic). The four test ampoules c, p, s, and m are tested in order in the REBA Test Device (e.g. P for Phlegmatic contains Emvita 17 and 18, C for Choleric Emvita 8, 9, 10, 11 etc.). Whichever ampule responds positively indicates the corresponding character type.

3. In a further testing step, and as a continuation of the procedure described under 2 above, one can also determine the corresponding Central Conflict. To do this, the Brunler-Bovis ampoule is placed along with the Diencephalon ampoule in the Yin region and the emotional remedies belonging to the associated character type just determined are tested in sequence (e.g. Emvita 17 or 18 for an obsessive type); the Central Conflict then responds – even, by the way, if it has already been treated and eliminated by PSE. The reason this is so could be explained with an instinctive-seeming impregnation which the Central Conflict evokes, which evidently lingers like an old scar even after total conflict dissolution.

The tests steps presented above reliably determine character type practically every time. It should be kept in mind that the test result must agree with reality if it is to be considered reliable – i.e. agree with the core symptoms which reflect the patient's actual situation. Some testers have asked me whether or not there can be multiple

Central Conflicts, but whoever asks such a question does not correctly understand PSE: every person has only one character type and consequently only one Central Conflict. To be sure, it can happen that a number of large complex will continue testable when placing the Brunler-Bovis ampoules in the Yin region, and thereby simulate a Central Conflict (this is known as "pseudo-CC" or "Side conflicts"). However, since there can only be one Central Conflict, the question of the core characteristics very quickly reveals whether, for a given patient, it really is the Central Conflict or not. As I've said before, character traits are strikingly different and are therefore to be kept clearly separate from each other, so that, with the proper questioning technique, this is easily possible and always ends up with an unambiguous result.

Sanguinic	Melancholic	Choleric	Phlegmatic
• Lively-sensual and irresistible • Empathizes well with others • Enjoys deeply • Easily enthused • Avoids commitment	• Somewhat reserved • Rationally oriented • Strategic • Has trouble warming up to others	• Outwardly aggression-inhibited • Thoughtful-altruistic, socially well-adjusted • Empathic • Emotionally warm	• Loves structure and order • High standard of perfection • Likes well-structured developments • Rationally oriented

Fig. 6.1 – *Typical core characteristics of the four character types.*

> • **Note**
> The hypothesis of multiple personalities is a myth, and one which I have never encountered in over 30 years of clinical practice. The well-known American psychiatry Pope Allen Frances (in charge of the DMS 4 *Manual of Psychiatric Diseases*) has made a similarly scathing statement [3].

With the Character Type Test Kit, there is no longer any need to wait for the Central Conflict to emerge, which can take a long time for patients with well-being and good health; this now can be determined right on the spot. Therefore, the Character Type Test Kit may be used even after longer-lasting PSE therapy, out of curiosity if the character type has not shown up or if one has failed to determine the character type during the course of PSE therapy. Since the question of character type is very centrally significant if one wants to know oneself better, this seems justifiable to me. Another key question relates to the issue of the characterologically right partner or the characterologically right occupation for upcoming training – which also seems like an opportune time to be investigating character type.

One can of course ask if it makes sense, and doesn't maybe represent crossing a line, for a therapist to want to answer such types of fundamental vital questions – to which my reply is that knowledge is seldom harmful, and in fact potentially more useful; besides it is of course up to each individual to make use of new knowledge or not. One may doubt that an unfavorable result in a character type test might keep a couple from staying together any longer, but it would be a good prospective investment in one's future to keep a lookout for a characterologically ideal partner. The same thing applies in essence when it comes to education and career, where character-compatible work promises much more fulfillment.

6.4 Description of the four character types

6.4.1 Melancholic

In ancient times, Schizoid characters were called Melancholics. With respect to patients, one should use the term Melancholic rather than Schizoid. Inside, they feel themselves to be independent, self-confident and proud persons, not unlike Napoleon, who outright radiated self-confidence when he crowned himself Emperor (cf. **Fig. 6.2**). Whether Napoleon was a Schizoid, however, remains unclear (I rather suspect he was a Hysteric), but he nevertheless symbolizes particularly well the actual self-image of this character typeThe first Chakra stands for basic trust, the seventh energy center for a trusting mental order. Both can be disturbed in a Schizoid, either due to lack of basic trust, weird and unreal images, mistrustful ideas and generally by not being very well grounded. Melancholics like to go it alone, in the process dwelling on their own thoughts. For them, thoughts and ideals are very central, which is why Melancholics like to search for Grand Unified Theories. Typical occupations are physicist, astronomer, philosopher or theologian. They are interested in the essential, while gossip gets on their nerves, i.e. cocktail party chitchat and small talk are not their thing. Melancholics are fundamentally serious people interested in the Big Issues.

Many Melancholics are intellectually oriented, sometimes even intellectuals, whereby the intellect is utilized as a weapon and to create distance, for instance through incisive argumentation, a know-it-all attitude, cynicism etc. To those around them, they often seem arrogant and aloof. Less intelligent Schizoids can appear in other unpleasant roles such as household tyrant; sometimes they are sociopaths or psychopaths. Schizoids often have few or no friends, and are bad at warming up to others, since empathizing with other people is very hard for them. As good strategists, they are often found in leading positions, but have trouble with people management. Schizoids are more susceptible to schizophrenia than others, but this psychiatric disease is also encountered in other character types. The same applies with modification to Depressive, Obsessive and Hysteric (i.e. manic-depressive) characters.

The best partner for the Melancholic is the Depressive type because the Depressive supplies the emotional warmth and thoughtfulness which the Melancholic lacks and needs. Conversely, the Depressive learns from the Melancholic how to draw boundaries and use the intellect. A relationship with a Hysteric is intolerable, since they have completely different life models and fundamental convictions. For the Sanguinic, pleasure and happiness are very important, whereas for the Melancholic it is serious endeavors that don't necessarily have to bring pleasure or joy, but which are felt to be fulfilling and giving meaning. A relationship with an Obsessive-compulsive is neurotic because for this type even the individual steps toward a goal are important (typical saying: "The journey is the reward."), While for the Schizoid, only results count (typical saying: "Winning isn't the most important thing, it's the only thing."). However, both Obsessive and Schizoid are intellectually polarized and thus even so have certain things in common.

For the Schizoid, being swamped with emotions and sensory impressions is often threatening, such that many people of this type lead a relatively uniform lifestyle which from the outside tends to look

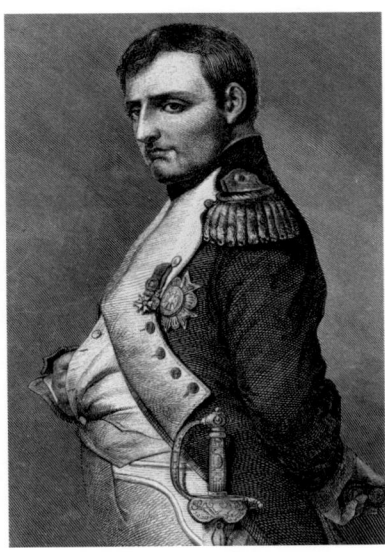

Fig. 6.2 – Napoleon, the very model of a self-assured person (Jean Auguste Dominique Ingres: Napoleon on the Imperial Throne. Paris, Musée de l'Armée).(© bpk/RMN – Grand Palais/ Emilie Cambier)

rather boring. One should keep in mind, however, that Melancholics have a lot of inner stimulus and love to be lost in thought, and so it by no means feels boring to them. For instance, a writer – who had been a spy and because of that spent a long time incarcerated – once told me that his prison time had been the best part of his life: there, he had been able to dwell undisturbed on his thoughts

Typical occupations or hobbies of Schizoids include lighthouse keeper, solitary global traveler, author, philosopher, conspiracy theorist (Howard Hughes, L. Ron Hubbard, Etc.), but also strategic CEO, pilot and inventor. Some well-known representatives of this character type include Albert Einstein, who loved dwelling on his thoughts and ideas and who admitted that he was miscast for the role of husband (His laconic comment was that he was a "one-horse carriage".). In the current crop of politicians, the German Chancellor Angela Merkel is probably a Schizoid, as was the German Chancellor Konrad Adenauer, the banker Josef Ackermann and the software developer Bill Gates. Because of his great charisma, Steve Jobs was probably more an Obsessive or a Hysteric, which would also cover his ruthlessness and his aesthetic fanaticism, whereas to a Schizoid the appearance of a product would take second place; that and how it functions would be the primary thing.

A classic Melancholic was the American actor John Wayne, who in his rough-shod manner represented the stoic loner who, as a leading figure, unswervingly went his own way, holding tightly to specific basic convictions. Another typical Schizoid is the American actor Charles Bronson who, playing the strong silent type, does not like to give interviews (small talk again). If you believe his own words, Bronson has no friends: "I don't have and I don't need any friends."

A third classical type is the taciturn and gruff Clint Eastwood, whose biography is typical of a Schizoid: as a child he was considered shy and introverted, he attended ten different schools and in 1948 dropped out of college. He has worked as a lumberjack, boilerman, gas station attendant and stockman. Eastwood has seven children from two marriages and three extramarital relationships. "I don't see myself as a conservative, but I'm not ultra-left either. I like the Libertarian attitude of simply letting everyone be. Even as a kid, I got annoyed at people who wanted to tell everybody how they should live." Of all the James Bond portrayers, the British actor Daniel Craig best incorporates the masculine hard and solitary Schizoid. Hermits with their hairshirts, whose external appearance is fairly unimportant to them, and who earnestly and diligently study holy Scripture – i.e. dedicate themselves to that which is truly important – are typical Melancholics.

Women with a Schizoid character type are often accused of being "mannish", typically for instance someone like Margaret Thatcher, the former British Prime Minister. This British politician is famous for unswervingly going her own chosen way despite all the strikes and mass protests during her reign as prime minister. As a Schizoid, she ruthlessly pushed through her political agenda. It has been my experience that the masculine role in lesbian couples tends to be this character type. Schizoid females, such as Condoleezza Rice, often live alone. In the case of Angela Merkel, her first profession (physicist) as well as her strategic political talent and her long-term perseverance and intellectual orientation coupled with relatively little charisma, indicate a Melancholic character. For all three Schizoid female politicians, the idea of passing a jolly and sociable evening seems less likely than having a serious and contextually significant political discussion with them. For it really to be fun, on the other hand, Hysterics would be more suitable (Chapter 6.4.2).

6.4.2 Sanguinic

With patients, the recommended term to use is *Sanguinic* (from the Latin *sanguis*, blood) because they are passionate people whose blood boils easily. A large portion of the charming attractiveness of this character type is evoked by the subliminal eroticism that they radiate. Following the motto "Sex sells" (**cf. Fig. 6.3**), their erotic quality represents the actual secret of this character type, since nothing fascinates people more than sexual attractiveness. In psychoanalysis, the dryer term is "Oedipal problem complex" for those who tend to be constantly trying to seduce others erotically. Of course, the eroticism is not usually explicitly noticed, particularly not for those of the same sex, but rather it's that many Sanguinics seem to others to be particularly nice, sympathetic, understanding, amusing and charismatic, attractive, cultivated or in some other way fascinating.

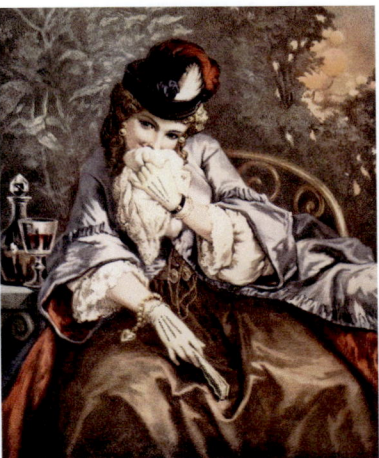

Fig. 6.3 – *This painting of the coquette (i.e. a maiden of easy virtue) clearly depicts the sanguinic's erotic, flirtatious nature. (The Coquette. Lithograph from a painting by Gustave Doré) (©bpk)*

Both the second and the sixth Chakra have to do with regulation. This is expressed psychoenergetically by how much energy one wisely invests in each instance in order to get something, and how one rations one's strengths. Behind this are hidden mental qualities such as self-discipline, order, thriftiness, modesty, reasonableness, and impulse restraint, with which this character type can, constantly or occasionally, have a hard time of it.

With more highly developed people of this character type, the aggressive and rivalry factors are frequently in the foreground, because Sanguinics secretly feel that they're not good enough in every respect, i.e. not beautiful, talented, attractive, amusing etc. They often have very weak self-esteem which, however, they never admit to because they are at great pains to conceal any personal weakness from others. Hysterics have the unfortunate tendency to overextend themselves all the time, literally burning the candle at both ends. People of this type try to extract the maximum from every occasion and opportunity. Therefore, Sanguinics are often among the last to leave a good party, so as not to miss anything.

One of the charming traits of hysterics is their ability to win people over. This can be accomplished through good looks, likeliness, wittiness, erotic signals and many other qualities. However, the empathetic tendency of hysterics by no means originates in any true thoughtfulness (as with the Depressive character type), but rather it always has to do entirely with themselves. Just as with the previously discussed Schizoids, they can behave egotistically, but in this case it is basically that others are the guilty party, because they are masters at talking their way out of situations and argumentation, and they never admit error if at all possible.

Sanguinics tend to confuse the real world with their imagined world, and to view both as equally valid realities which can, if needs be, be appropriately modified in the blink of an eye. Many conmen and swindlers (also as concerns titles), as well as hypochondriacs can belong to this character type. Typical of them is the inability to deal appropriately with resources of whatever kind (physical and mental strengths, money, credit cards etc.), because they always want to extract the maximum from anything and everything, letting themselves be carried away by spontaneous enjoyment and painting a rosy vision of the future instead of acknowledging reality.

Sanguinics are very sensual (key phrase: "wine, women and song") and live life to the fullest. They love to play and are excellent communicators. Many people of this type really enjoy life and can quickly become enthused about something – but on the other hand, their strong emotional polarity can flip their mood to the exact opposite, and they become very depressed, disheartened and with no hope for the future ("singing hallelujah, in the depths of despair"). Hysterics are often very demanding and always try for more than one would normally want to give them. A very essential Hysteric character trait is their outsize love of freedom, since committing to something signifies, to them, at some point making a mistake and thereby revealing a weakness – but also not to be able later on to decide differently. They worry about becoming permanent captives of their decisions, and that is felt to be disadvantageous.

A classic female representative of the Hysteric character type was the American actress Marilyn Monroe. One can see very well in her the fragile self-esteem problem of this type, for Marilyn thought she was not very attractive and even homely. To this day Marilyn is considered to be the epitome of the seductress. Other famous Sanguinic actresses include Bette Midler, who well expresses the life-loving, bubbly and comedic aspects of this type. The actress Angelina Jolie, on the other hand, stands for the dominatrix aspect of the higher-vibrating Hysteric (power woman), who always want to be counted among the winners and whose arrogance resembles that of the Schizoid type. In the pop singer Madonna, one can see the tendency to call attention and be provocative come what may, as well as morphing between the innocent woman-child (which Marilyn Monroe embodied), and the oh so cool vamp (like Angelina Jolie). Basically, most actors, singers and other professional self-promoters belong to the Sanguinic character type, but one should not derive any stereotyped rule from this.

Male Sanguinics include as a classic example the rock singer Elvis Presley, whose erotic pelvic activity had millions of women swooning in ecstasy, and whose charisma continues to work to this day. Michael Jackson exerted a similar fascination, although he was not the Don Juan type like Elvis, but rather the eternal youth (like Peter Pan). As a mature person, the American singer Frank Sinatra represented the prototype of the typical Hysteric, able to captivate everyone with his singing and charisma, but who also frequently had problems with drug addiction (as also did Elvis Presley and Michael Jackson) and was considered in his private life to be inconsiderate and egotistical (these also the often unlovely characteristics of Hysterics which, however, do not have to develop every time).

Adolf Hitler can also be designated as a demonic example of the Sanguinic (more information on this in my book *Healing through Energy Medicine* [8]), who, because of his severe personality disorder can only dimly be recognized as an example of this character type. Typical of Sanguinics is their ability to win people over, especially in public appearances, as Hitler did, completely fascinating people with his speeches. Another characteristic trait is that they often mix up their fantasy world and the real world. Hitler, for example, bought a lottery ticket when he was a young man, and was so certain of having the winning ticket that he spent a lot of money in the days before the drawing – but, to his great disappointment, he did not win the prize. It is characteristic of Sanguinics to tend to mix reality and imagination and also often be susceptible to magical thinking.

6.4.3 Choleric

With patients, one should refer to the caring or Choleric character type, where the latter designation indicates that it originally (historically) had to do with a gall-weakling – which, however, has nothing whatever to do with a violent temper (from the Greek *chol*, gall (bladder)). The fact that Cholerics are nevertheless sometimes choleric is mainly a taboo topic among Cholerics themselves. The image of a dying person with a farewell letter expresses the tragic basic sensibility which shapes the life of most depressive character types (cf. Fig. 6.4). As with the Melancholic, the basic feeling of Cholerics tends to be tragic in nature. Depressive types have their Central Conflict in the third energy center, the upper abdomen, the center of interaction with the environment which this energy center primarily represents psychoenergetically.

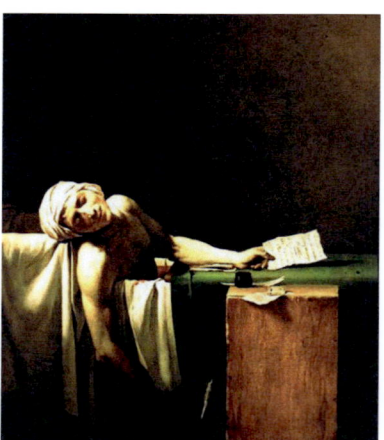

Fig. 6.4 – Jacques-Louis David: The Death of Marat, 1793 (Brussels, Musées Royaux des Beaux-Arts de Belgique).
(© bpk)

Besides the social component, the third Chakra deals psychoenergetically with giving and defending. Depressive types often want to give away too much and cannot defend themselves sufficiently, i.e. often feel like a child wanting to do right by everybody, feeling themselves to be totally harmless and innocent, having to suffer at the hands of evil forces, whereby (understandably) a lot of aggression can build up.

Depressive types have somewhat fatherly or motherly aspects, often thereby something harmless in their nature and at times even somewhat childlike. It is important for depressive character types that things go well for other people, even if in the process they are themselves disadvantaged. They are particularly good at empathizing with others. Unlike Sanguinics who do things for their own advantage, depressives are truly empathetic, to the benefit of others. Depressives are usually very friendly, exhibit a great deal of sympathy and worry anxiously about what others think of them. The worst thing for depressives is to be deserted by people who are dear to them and to fall, lonely, into a huge depression, whereby, as emotional persons, are basically the victims of their own strong emotions. Depressive characters defend themselves through constant moaning and complaining, as well as a feeling of helplessness for which they blame those around them for not helping them enough nor standing by them. One often observes in them longish depressive episodes, as well as somatic equivalents, e.g. in the form of overweight, chronic pain, exhaustion etc.

Typical Choleric occupations are social in nature, such as social worker, nurse, doctor or clergyman. Many people of this type are involved in charitable facilities, and are about as idealistic as Schizoids. They like to give their support to helpless creatures such as animals or children, and might, for example, run a facility for stray cats. Because of their anxious emotional nature, which strives to establish stable relationships, one often finds them as civil servants or government officials, as well as occupations in which the people are known for their exceptional faithfulness, unobtrusive work habits and conscientiousness – or, typically, are in fact **not** known for those very traits!

A typical example of the Depressive character type was the comedian Oliver Hardy (of the comedic duo Laurel and Hardy), who radiated good-naturedness, emotional warmth, a fatherly or comradely warmth and a certain air of innocence. One can well imagine asking a favor of him and not being turned down, that Mr. Hardy would be a good-natured and trustworthy neighbor whom one could rely on. Depressive character types – like the also very sensory-oriented and emotionally polarized Hysterics – have a weakness for sensual pleasures and like to eat, so that, like Oliver Hardy, quite a few of them tend to overweight. Another example was the jazz trumpeter Louis Armstrong who, as "everybody's darling" also very well incorporated the warmhearted and friendly as well as the wouldn't-hurt-a-fly harmlessness of this character type. Another good example was the German actor Heinz Ehrhardt, who basically played the endearing, constantly overstressed *paterfamilias* of a (usually very large) family.

Depressive/Choleric females tend to radiate a warmhearted, motherly and pleasant Aura as a means to be likable to others. Unlike the Hysteric character type, this is not done calculatedly in order to gain some advantage, but rather in order to truly help other people, even if it's to their own detriment. Depressive character types in social situations basically stay in the background, wear modest clothing and hairdos, very little jewelry etc. With Choleric women, one can well imagine asking them for a favor and not being turned down, but in fact getting their full attention.

6.4.4 Phlegmatic

The Phlegmatic or obsessive-compulsive, rigid or orderly character type is represented in the picture by a medieval merchant whose strict and precise attitude is clearly visible (**cf. Fig. 6.5**). The Greek term *phlegma* means skin/mucous membrane, so a rough translation would be something like "mucous membrane weakling". Modern usage makes "Phlegmatic" synonymous with sluggish and lazy – which of course nobody wants to be, so that when patients one should refer them to the original meaning of mucous-membrane-weakness. One can also talk about the orderly character type who likes clearly recognizable structures.

For the Obsessive type, the Central Conflict in the fifth Chakra has to do with control of the voice (expression) as well as emotions in general, so that the neck can be viewed as psychoenergetically a kind of safety valve and control center between body (emotions) and head (intellect). The Obsessive character is a control freak that cannot let go. It is very hard to voluntarily give up control in order to attain spontaneity, as can be seen in the example of trying to will oneself to go to sleep. For Obsessives it is comparatively very hard to overcome their obsessive need to control; think of the well-nigh impossible (because self-contradictory) command: "Now be spontaneous for once!"

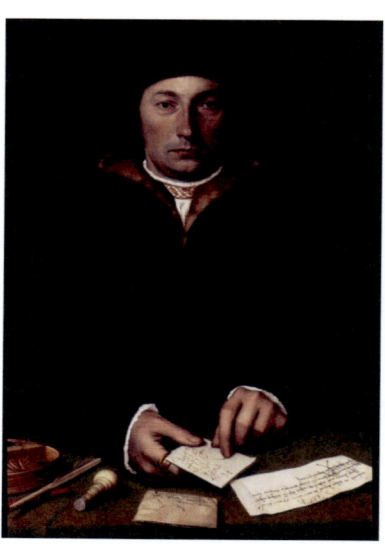

Fig. 6.5 *– Medieval merchant as the image of the obsessive-compulsive character type (Hans Holbein the Younger: The Merchant Dirck Tybis of Duisburg. Vienna, Kunsthistorisches Museum). (© bpk/Hermann Buresch)*

In terms of archetypes, the Obsessive is associated with the role of the strict and rational father who lays down the law. In terms of segments, the neck stands for the paternal principle of law and order, while the upper abdomen has a symbolic relationship to the nourishing mother, the energy center of the Choleric. Hiding behind the obsessive need for control of Phlegmatics is the fear of being overwhelmed by unknown forces, becoming disorderly and confused. Phlegmatics thus feel the world to be a dangerous and chaotic place which one must hold in check with all the means at one's disposal.

For the Phlegmatic character type, the individual steps toward a goal are very important, so they tend to lose sight of the goal itself. Their perfectionist standards are so high that they themselves can hardly meet them. One of the essential traits of this type is the desire for everything to proceed in a structured and orderly manner, and for the logic behind a process to be clearly discernible. Decision trees are thus a typical invention of Obsessive character types, who find it helpful – as they do all kinds of structures, organizational patterns, hierarchical operational instructions and the like. Something only seems right and sensible once they have identified the logic, systematic order and structure, which is why Obsessive characters tend to divide things up into hierarchies, to arrange them in order, to file them away and to organize them into a system. Typical occupations are therefore archivist or bureaucrat. For the Compulsive character type, archives and collections are essential because they are meant to bring order and harmony into an unruly and threatening environment.

Obsessive characters are often very respectful of authority – as they, conversely, can then act out their subliminal aggression sadistically by mercilessly punishing violations of the law. As intellectually polarized characters, many of this type come across in a social context as somewhat aloof, matter-of-fact and down-to-earth. The friendly, personally somewhat innocuous type of the Compulsive character is represented by the American actor Jack Lemmon, famous as the finicky house-husband constantly scurrying about with a dustrag after his chaotic roommate Walter Matthau. The German comedian Loriot and his Swiss colleague Emil Steinberger have both satirized pedantic types which humorously represent the fussy eccentricity of Compulsives, their know-it-all attitude, passion for order, small-mindedness etc. which are always a rich source of absurd comical situations. Oddly enough, the most conspicuous character trait of Compulsives is that they are inconspicuous (like the Choleric), whereas absurd comical characters more tend to be Schizoids or Hysterics.

6.5 Tips for practical character diagnostics

Because character diagnosis enables extensive access into the depths of the Psyche and thus also far-reaching conclusions regarding the respective personality, one should proceed with caution. It should become a habit to categorize each character type carefully and without hasty prejudgment. The core symptoms should fit and the patient should fully agree with the selected character type; this also applies to members of the patient's immediate family. Should some of them happen to have come along to the appointment, it has often proven beneficial and helpful to ask them to attend the discussion of the Central Conflict – of course, only if the patient agrees to this.

Questionnaires (reproduced in the back of the PSE manual) can sometimes be helpful as well, since there the respective character type usually stands out clearly. I have not tried out other classification systems such as the enneagram, but it seems likely that there will be some overlap with a number of models described in my book *Healing through Energy Medicine* [8], where they can be read about. Basically, character diagnosis is somewhat like a court trial based on circumstantial evidence, i.e. the more that characteristic features and shady sides hold true (**cf. Fig. 6.1**), the more likely the correctness of the tentative diagnosis.

It is sometimes difficult to classify people, especially if the mother is an antipodal character to that of her child. In this context, one should know that parents and children almost always have the same character type. There may be exceptions, but I have not yet seen such, though the number of family cases I've tested out is still quite small. Usually, marriages involving antipodal partners are very tension-laden and very problematic; as a rule, they end in divorce.

Character Type	Schizoid	Depressive	Obsessive (OC)	Hysteric
Antique typology	Melancholic	Choleric	Phlegmatic	Sanguinic
Polarity	Yang	Yin	Yang	Yin
Affected Chakra	Base Chakra, Crown Chakra	Upper-abdominal Chakra	Neck Chakra	Kidney Charka, Brow Chakra
Basic emotional tendency	Rational	Emotional	Rational	Emotional
Basic emotional characteristic	Independent	Empathetic	Obedient	Lively
Biggest fear (per Riemann)	Existential	Isolation	Transitoriness	Commitment

Fear compensation	Too isolated and defensive	Too willing to conform	Too rigid and insistent	Wanting too much to be free
Frequent emotional shadow	Megalomania or (compensatory) too shy, know-it-all, totalitarian	Too enraged or depressed, extortionate, frustrated, resentful	Stingy, lazy, inflexibly conservative, pedantic, anxiously rigid	Rivaling, self-centered, too lust- and pleasure-oriented, dreamy, fanatical
Classical prototype	Lone wolf	Do-gooder	Pedant	Don Juan
Typical occupation	Pilot	Social worker	Bureaucrat	Actor

Table 6.1 *The four character types, their characteristics and dark sides.*

Now, if a child comes from such a marriage and has an antipodal character, especially vis-à-vis the mother (such as: child Hysteric, mother Schizoid), the child is instinctively forced to hide its true character and, say, pose as a Schizoid or, as an auxiliary reconstruction, a Depressive so as to be loved by its mother – which the child will do intuitively from a very young age. In my experience, this kind of psychic deformation leads to a lifelong neurotic development due to an extensive denial of its true personal core. Whether – and how – such people can be helped at all remains an open question. With respect to character type diagnosis, it is understandable that, when it comes to such neurotic persons who hide their true character type, it is extremely difficult to arrive at a correct classification – or else they will reject it because their true character type could very well be unknown to them.

Sometimes certain classifications are rejected because the character in question doesn't seem prestigious enough (example: the "suspenders-wearer" image of the Obsessive character). One should be clear on this and also tell the patient that no one character is better than any other, that each of them has its upsides and downsides, and that besides, ultimately all men are equal, in that the core no longer has any neurotic structures in the form of character structures, so that value judgments at some point become superfluous anyway.

One fairly seldom finds a **Central Conflict in the Heart Chakra**, and then mostly in spiritually advanced persons. Often such a Heart-CC appears in particularly poignant tragic cases. Treating the Central Conflict then often turns out to involve particularly intense psychic transformation and especially beneficial therapeutic effects. One sees cases involving the CC in the Heart Chakra mostly in spiritually advanced persons who otherwise no longer have any CC, or very heartrending illnesses and difficult phases of life. As in the more usual character type classification cases, the patient confirms the respective core symptoms (**cf. Fig. 6.1**) and the Central Conflict response despite the Brunler-Bovis ampoule.

> The assignment of the Central Conflicts in the Heart Chakra are: 12 Depressive, 13 Schizoid, 14 Obsessive-compulsive, 15 Depressive, 16 Hysteric. Since so few patients ever have a Heart Chakra conflict, this assignment list should be viewed as provisional.

6.6 Emotional growth in characterology

Every character type has its own set of limitations which shape (and to some extent limit) a person's entire life, how they think and feel and their possibilities for acting and reacting. Deep inside, every person has a matrix of the true self (inner child) which integrates all of the character type's personality traits, and which wants to express itself. Consequently, every person, at some point in life, more and more has an unconscious tendency, as soon as they have noticed a shortcoming and begun to suffer from it, to characterologically rise above themselves and to express their true self. In this manner, they hope to feel more authentic, more lively, happier etc. (more on this in my book *Healing through Energy Medicine* [8]).

Every character type has negative traits which have to be overcome before a person can grow spiritually. Only then does a harmonious psychic growth process begin with the goal of developing the positive characteristics of the ideal partner (Schizoid-Depressive and Hysteric-Obsessive). This growth step is preformed in all humans and thereby can be well implemented, since, after all, they are actually already very much like the ideal partner. With PSE, one can in this context give patients useful advice as to which appropriate characteristics should be developed. PSE treatment can itself aid in opening up spiritually and initiating maturation, but the brunt of the labor must of course be carried out by the patients themselves. Thanks to PSE, people get to know their so-called "shadow" and can accept and integrate this spiritual element as they decipher the hidden messages of the Psyche. They can exercise these new abilities in everyday life, rise above their personality limits and at some point become human(e)ly more rounded and integrated.

> **• Note**
> Harmonious spiritual maturation consists of learning to develop the positive characteristics of the ideal partner. It is good for Schizoids to try to develop the positive personality traits of the Depressive character (their ideal partner), and the converse applies to Depressive types. Hysteric characters should build up the personality traits of the Obsessive-compulsive character, just as, turned around, Obsessive characters should learn to develop Hysteric personality traits:
> - Schizoid: emotions, sympathy, perceiving body and heart
> - Depressive: think and act rationally, say no, keep and maintain boundaries
> - Hysteric: think and act rationally, accept boundaries and orders
> - Obsessive: accept feelings, become more spontaneous (go easier on oneself), accept chaos and spontaneity as inevitable

As previously explained, spiritual maturation is a spontaneously initiated process in higher-vibration persons so as to feel more authentic, more lively, happier etc. and so as to be able to live better and more authentically. Every character type represents a negative pseudo-solution through which spiritual impulses and emotional/social characteristics are tuned out. Since each character type involves being set into either an emotionally or rationally oriented lifestyle, it is only the development of the character traits of the ideal partner type which can lead to becoming humanly whole (cf. **Fig. 6.6**).

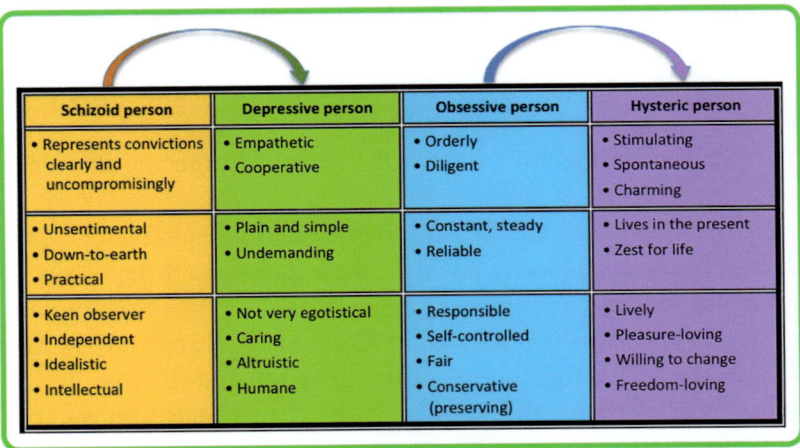

Fig. 6.6 – *Emotional maturation as the development of the characteristics of the ideal partner.*

The drive toward emotional maturation does not come from any conscious decision to become a "better person", but rather is based on the subliminal discomfort of feeling in some manner incomplete. For instance, someone might have the feeling of "not living right", "wanting to make more of myself" or "wanting to live out a secret desire" (from patient statements). The discomfort causes the individual to then search for solutions, and it can serve as an impetus for ongoing personal development. Character maturation usually makes people happier as well as more productive, creative and sociable. It is thus an advantageous win-win situation for one and all.

6.7 Partnership

Knowing the respective character type is a good idea when dealing with social relationships. This applies to child rearing, which should apply different methods based on the corresponding character type of the child (more on this in Section 6.8), but also and above all when it comes to closer interpersonal relationships, especially married couples. Since the various character types have preset sympathies and antipathies among each other (which cannot be permanently changed), knowledge of the corresponding character in the choice of ideal partner for a good relationship seems to be quite essential and, strictly speaking, indispensable.

In contemporary society, the choice of an appropriate life partner is one of the greatest and most important challenges in life. Unlike earlier times, when social conventions and economic necessity had inclined toward marriages of convenience, marriage nowadays has become a core institution meant to guarantee personal happiness and satisfaction.

In any partnership (**cf. Fig. 6.7**), the following apply to specific character types:

- Many types get along well together (marrying the same character type)
- Others actually get along ideally (ideal partner e.g. Schizoid-depressive Depressive or Hysteric-Obsessive)
- Others maintain a neurotic relationship (Obsessive-Schizoid or Depressive-Hysteric) – i.e. everyday life together is sometimes good and then again bad
- Finally, the fourth group can be designated as completely opposite or opposing (Schizoid-Hysteric and Compulsive-Depressive) – i.e. over the long-term they always get along badly.

Experience with hundreds of married couples who have been examined with PSE over the years, and in which character types have been determined, show clearly that happily married couples strictly follow the guidelines laid down in Fig. 6.7. I have yet to see a single exception to this. The divorce rate in first-world nations, which has been oscillating around the 50% mark, can also be held up as striking proof of this. PSE testing has shown that only half the couples are well matched. If couples meet randomly and thus are evenly distributed among the four types, and if one furthermore assumes that the four character types appear at the same percentage, then there is logically a 50% chance of divorce. After 5 to 7 years at the most, one has had enough of compromises and files for divorce.

Own character type	Schizoid	Depressive	Obsessive	Hysteric
Opposites (attracting) = ideal partnership (+/−)	Depressive	Schizoid	Hysteric	Obsessive
Identical natures = friendly but often non-erotic (+/+)	Schizoid	Depressive	Obsessive	Hysteric
Similar character traits = (neurotic) (−/+)	Obsessive	Hysteric	Schizoid	Depressive
Opposites (repelling) = often unhappy marriage (−/−)	Hysteric	Obsessive	Depressive	Schizoid

Fig. 6.7 – *Relationships of the four character types in partnerships.*

Although the plain downhome couples logic "birds of a feather flock together" is technically correct, it doesn't go far enough, because the identical-character type partner is just the second-best choice, since it lacks psychoenergetic compensation – i.e. both are polarized either Yang or Yin, which becomes boring over the long run. Nevertheless, the rule of thumb is on target, for even the best matching pairs such as Schizoid/Depressive or Obsessive/Hysteric form similar couples, because, as I've said, every Schizoid is secretly a Depressive character etc. Therefore, from the viewpoint of PSE, the proper formulation is: "one should marry a partner which is like one's own (positive) characterological shadow."

Consequently, the ideal partner (Schizoid/Depressive or Obsessive/Hysteric) does indeed represent the well-known "better half". The ideal partner offers the emotional qualities lacking in oneself, because they're a part of one's unconscious shadow. Moreover, ideal partners balance each other out because one inclines toward Yin and the other Yang. This energetic tension is important for long-lasting sexual attraction and has a generally harmonizing effect, meaning that one feels better with the partner than without.

Dysfunctional relationships sooner or later lead to increasing disappointment because the fundamental differences are simply too big. Usually, they end in divorce after 10 to 15 years at the most (check out the divorce statistics in modern societies). Thus, it would be an important future project, beneficial for all concerned (humanly, socially, erotically and financially), if character type could be unambiguously determined before the wedding. That should be possible to do using the PSE Character Type Test Kit – provided that those seeking partners would agree at all to something as unromantic (although certainly long-term beneficial) as a character type test.

6.8 Child rearing

The Schizoid child and the Schizoid teenager feel like miniature Napoleons inside. It's not easy to teach these self-confident little Caesars anything because they think they don't need it. An indirect approach is therefore necessary, providing inducements via role models that promote learning through imitation. Because Schizoids are strongly influenced by ideals – of which, to be sure, children and young teens often do not yet have much understanding – one can begin here at least for the 12- to 14-year-olds and above.

Hysterics always tend to kick over the traces and to be competitive, in the process of which they can hurt themselves in the extreme case, so they definitely need clear boundaries to be established. A strict (but not unloving!) pedagogical style would thus be ideal for them.

The **Compulsive** character is under great internal pressure and so quickly feels overwhelmed and, disheartened, gives up. Here, modest goals must be set, accompanied by constant encouragement and praise.

This also applies, in somewhat modified form, for the **Depressive** character as well, who always wants to do right by everyone, and who can in the process quickly wind up an inner dead-end situation with seemingly no way out, one from which he can be extricated with encouragement and disclosure of small steps whose successes then increase courage.

> **• Summary**
> The following teaching styles, each adapted to the appropriate character type, can be recommended, but they each need to be fitted to the individual case as well, in order to avoid doing more harm than good:
> - The Schizoid child needs a nondirective style (Montessori, Rudolf Steiner School etc.).
> - The Hysteric child needs clear boundaries.
> - The perfectionist (Obsessive) child sets the personal bar too high (and then sometimes becomes fainthearted and "lazy").
> - The Depressive child tends to procrastinate and easily feels overwhelmed (provide encouragement and clear arrangements).

6.9 Getting to know the character types

Besides dealing with unconscious conflicts, confronting one's own character type represents an important life task which can better explain many processes in daily life and in interpersonal relationships which would otherwise take place instinctively and unawares. Knowing one's character type can also promote reconciliation with specific character traits of oneself and others, and derive appropriate life tasks therefrom. Self-knowledge is the very beginning of a process: only by knowing one's character type can one also better understand others.

To be able to deal successfully with character types as a therapist calls for about 2 to 3 years of intensive practical study, during which one tests hundreds of patients and discusses with them those of their character traits and problems in their life history which can only be properly explained and understood through the typology. In addition, it is helpful to determine the respective character types of oneself and people with whom one is closely associated, and then to quietly observe the types in the real world. In time, one comes to understand that there are very many variations, compensations and overlaps of character traits, and yet the respective important character contours are nevertheless always preserved.

Books are another good study aid. A standard work is the slim volume by the Munich psychoanalyst Fritz Riemann on the basic forms of fear. In my opinion, it has little relevance for daily practice, but it contains an excellent philosophical approach to understanding the far-reaching implications of characterology as a kind of metaphysics and worldview. As a pure textbook, *Personality Typology* (Persönlichkeitstypologie) [77] from the business administrator Hans Jung has proven useful, as it well describes the ABCs of the theory. Because character types also come up in businesses and factories, it is understandable that psychological advisors of human interchange also fall back on characterology – often making use of a different terminology but ultimately making the same statement. For patients, characterology is made clearly understandable in my two books *New Life through Energy Healing* [7] and *Healing through Energy Medicine* [8]. A very excellent book is one by the psychotherapist Christa Mewes: *Character Types – Who is Compatible with Whom?* [97] which is highly recommended for patients.

Other typologies generate a great deal of confusion because they seem to use completely different concepts, but which ultimately, upon close inspection, turn out after all describe characteristics comparable to the ancient characterology. Currently in academia, the dominant **Big Five Model** is considered to be the most useful in the context of modern psychology. It measures character traits using five values: neuroticism, extraversion, openness to experience, agreeableness and rigidity. Some traits can be unambiguously related to one of the four character types: 1. Melancholics (and Sanguinics) are open to experience, 2. Sanguinics are extroverted, 3. Cholerics are agreeable and 4. Phlegmatics are rigid. The only trait found in all types is meuroticism with the features anxiety, insecurity, nervousness – which makes it worthless as a differentiation factor. My limited experience with the Big Five Model shows that it is a step backward compared to the ancient temperaments, since it waters everything down and since self-statements elicited by questioning can often be misleading: introverts and shy people often have a strong core character (e.g. Melancholics), while externally brave seeming extroverts are often introverted and anxious inside (e.g. Sanguinics), such that questioning can often lead one astray.

- **Note**
Of course, the symbolism of characterology is found not only in humans, but ultimately in all possible aspects of reality. The Munich psychotherapist Fritz Riemann was one of the first to demonstrate that with cosmic phenomena:
1. The earth orbiting the sun (circulation)
2. The rotation of the earth on its axis (spin)
3. The force of gravity (centripetal)
4. Centrifugal force (centrifugal)

> Translating these basic impulses into appropriate Riemann psychological terminology, it has to do with:
> 1. Social conformity (Depressive type) and at the same time
> 2. The desire for individuality (Schizoid type),
> 3. The desire for permanence and stability (Obsessive type) and
> 4. The desire for novelty and variety (Hysteric type).

Riemann [115] writes: "Therefore, according to this cosmic analogy we would be subject to four fundamental standards which, in varying forms, pervade our entire life and, in ever new ways, need to be answered by us." And so, according to Riemann, these are basic elemental forces which guide both the Psyche and the cosmos.

Now of course one can take these analogies even further and discover characterological phenomena everywhere in life, whether political parties, schools of art or hobbies. In Table 6.2, I have tried for a typical categorization which should help develop a sense for the essence of each respective character type. The risk of any arrangement of this sort consists of drifting into prejudices and stereotyped arbitrariness. One should therefore use such categorizations only as rough clues, and not interpret them to literally: not every globetrotter is a Melancholic nor every Green Party member a Sanguinic.

6.10 Does character type trigger specific disease susceptibilities?

In ancient medicine, each character type was associated with an excess of some humor, such as too much blood for the Sanguinic (called a "plethora"). It is indeed true that I have determined in clinical practice that Sanguinics often suffer from hypertension, stroke and, with their ruddy complexion, "head plethoras"– but this does not represent an exclusive trait of this character type. It might well be that the ancient Greek physicians had not been particularly good statisticians, added to which the population figures were statistically too small. The disease susceptibilities of the character types, such as ostensible skin/mucous membrane ailments among Phlegmatics or gallstone tendencies in Cholerics, are more in the realm of medical folklore when applied to today's diseases, and more correspond to mesenchymal metabolic inclinations. So, in the PSE Organ Test Kit, biliary drainage disorders play a key role, and in this context Melancholics and Cholerics (from Greek *chol*: gall) are clearly overrepresented.

	Melancholic	Choleric	Sanguinic	Phlegmatic
Political parties	Liberal democrat (neoliberal), anarchist	Social democrat	Communist, Green, Pirate	Values conservative
Sciences	Philosophy, physics	Social sciences, medicine	Dramatics, theater arts	Mathematics, systematics, archiving
Musical genres	Country, jazz	Choir music, blues	Opera, rock	Military music, Classical canon
Musicians	Bob Dylan, Eric Clapton, George Harrison	Mahalia Jackson (blues singer)	Cecilia Bartoli, Madonna, Queen, John Lennon	Herbert von Karajan
Art genres	Expressionism, naïve art	Romanticism	Baroque	Classicism
Painters	Giacometti, van Gogh	Goya	Picasso, Salvador Dali	Leonardo da Vinci
Authors	Goethe	Johanna Spyri (Heidi)	Schiller	Thomas Mann
Hobbies, interests	Travel, astronomy	Group tours, choirs	Opera, theater, dancing, singing	Audiophile, gadgets, robots

Table 6.2 *Character types in everyday life.*

6.11 Basic aspects of Central Conflict treatment

The Central Conflict usually has a Causal reading of 80-90% and therefore calls for 4-5 months of therapy with the appropriate Emvita and Chavita. It is recommended that the conflict be reduced to 0% Causal reading, because the Central Conflict steals considerable amounts of energy. One should instruct the patient to inform close family and friends that, during the first few weeks of therapy, there might be increased irritability, mood swings etc. related to the dissolution of the Central Conflict. Because during this time one is often emotionally quite labile, one should not undertake any life-altering decisions such as quitting one's job etc. During the treatment period, there might be vivid dreams and sometimes strong somatic discharge reactions as well.

In many cases, treating the Central Conflict leads to a big therapeutic breakthrough. People become emotionally more open and gentler, while at the same time their resilience increases. They can behave with greater self-assurance and develop more *joie de vivre*.

7 Character type and Karma

Many historical memory traces get lost in the depths of the individual subconscious which we know nothing about, such as buried early childhood experiences. Some of these buried memories are said to stem from earlier reincarnations of the individual Psyche. As we know, many psychic pathologies cannot be traced back to childhood or early childhood experiences, nor to genetics, so many depth-psychology therapists opine that they stem from earlier lives. There are numerous good indications that favor this hypothesis, which I would now like to briefly introduce.

The question as to the historical origin of deep psychic traumas is by no means mere academic hairsplitting, for if there truly are traumas from former lives, then that has manifold consequences. The question as to the actual primary cause of traumas would have to be recast – which would not call into question any conventional theories thereby, but merely expand them considerably. Theological questions of morality and restitution would have to be reexamined. The familiar concept of the Psyche would have to be completely rewritten, and the image that we normally tend to have of ourselves as individuals would be radically altered. However, I don't intend to get into all of this here, I just wanted to mention the issues.

Certain karmic traumas seem to have clearly defined conflict patterns which can be reconstructed somewhat in the manner of an archaeologist. Just as many of today's buildings have been erected on the ruins of older ones and copy their form, the individual Psyche (e.g. in the form of the character and certain formative basic beliefs) seems to be based on specific old traumas. Those who do not believe in the possibility of reincarnation are free to view such traumatic experiences as something like depth-psychological nightmares, akin to a Grimm's fairy tale. Yet no matter where they originate, the aforementioned psychic traces remain effective, and in fact often in unhealthy ways such as fears or negative character traits, so that it's worthwhile tracking them down and eliminating them.

7.1 Reincarnation and depth psychology

In the Christian West, reincarnation is one of the taboo topics. Although people in all cultures around the world believe in reincarnation, this is not the case for modern Western man, for two reasons: Christianity and Science. Both of these worldviews consider impossible the idea of the continued existence of the individual Psyche after death, with continued existence in the form of multiple incarnations. The Christian and scientific paradigms influence the thinking of the great majority of the modern Western population. However, attitudes and ideas are slowly beginning to change, with more and more people considering reincarnation to be possible.

My experience has been that the number of patients who are now open to topics such as reincarnation is growing. A number of them report their own experiences of having lived before, either from waking dreams or déjà vu experiences. Such patients often have high Causal readings in PSE testing, which experience has shown considerably facilitates access to karmic recollections. More and more people, unafraid and ideologically uncommitted, are getting interested in such themes and are searching for an answer.

When dealing with the topics reincarnation and depth psychology, four critical questions arise:

- Why do modern therapists busy themselves at all with a topic that has such a strong religious aspect,
- which evidently can hardly be objectified,
- which at first glance hardly seems to have any effect on the current life,
- and which, moreover, strikes one as therapeutically outlandish?

In the following, I'd like to explain why these four questions can nevertheless be positively answered. I want to show that there are good reasons for therapists to deal with the topics of reincarnation and karmic traumas. There are many cogent indications favoring earlier earthly lives of the individual Psyche whose logical stringency and abundance are impressive. If one considers traumas from earlier incarnations to be possible, then, in the view of regression therapists, the topic is especially important because the old injuries would continue to have an effect. Because they do so into the present, they should be detected and eliminated. There are thus good reasons to busy oneself with this controversial topic.

Some important trailblazers of modern reincarnation have made it possible for modern man to deal with such themes without prejudice and non-ideologically. Access to earlier lives is hidden deep in the unconscious, so that one cannot normally remember or, if so, then only very vaguely. It therefore calls for special psychological techniques such as trance or hypnosis to descend into the deep and strongly repressed levels of the Psyche (the technical term for this is "regression"):

- **Depth psychology access** – Having established contact with deep psychic levels, psychiatrists such as the Swiss Carl Gustav Jung first considered reincarnation to be possible (Eranos Conference Ascona 1939). The British jungian Roger Woolger, after World War II, was a significant pioneer in modern reincarnation therapy.
- **Hypnotic access** – The American medium Edgar Cayce first reported on earlier lives in hypnotic trance around 1901. After he woke up, he was very shocked by it, because his mediumistic messages could not be squared with his traditional worldview as a devout Christian. The tool of hypnosis later turned out to be helpful in countless cases to bring recollections of former lives into the light of day.
- **Drugs** – Hallucinogens have led to drug experiences such as described by the British author Aldous Huxley (in his well-known book *The Doors of Perception* [69]), in which people in a trance frequently experienced scenes from earlier lives.
- **Meditation** – During deep inward contemplation, scenes from former lives rise up in many people. The first to describe this was, as we know, Gautama Buddha, the founder of Buddhism.
- **Transpersonal psychology** – Transpersonal psychology developed out of the experience with hallucinogenic substances. Here the attempt is made, using trance techniques, holotropic breathing (deliberate hyperventilation), ecstatic dancing, drugs etc., to penetrate into deep psychic levels.

One special form of therapy is reincarnation therapy (known as "regressions"). Besides everyday motives such as curiosity and the spiritual need to learn about one's survival, such techniques show that, with deep regression, a strongly transformative healing process can be triggered.

7.1.1 Evidence for and against reincarnation

I would next like to address the question as to what credible indications there are for the phenomenon of reincarnation. One should, as a critical contemporary, differentiate credible from untrustworthy stories. Many recollections that arise under hypnosis turn out to be **untrustworthy**, although most people are of the opinion that everything which arises under such circumstances is true. Under hypnosis, the Psyche can, involuntarily and without being aware of it, create imaginary creatures that are hard to distinguish from real ones [128]. Follow-up tests show that these are cases of cryptomnesia, i.e. recall of forgotten books, movies etc. that a person had seen as a child or teenager. Also, spontaneous recollections from adults have turned out, upon closer examination, not to be real. Critics therefore basically consider all recollections to be false, which I think is going too far, since there are credible indications of the existence of earlier lives.

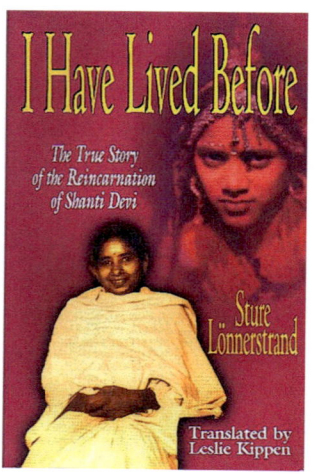

Fig. 7.1 – Front cover of the biography of Shanti Devi.

Credible evidence of earlier lives is often found in children between the ages of 3 and 6, when they can still genuinely recall earlier lives. If their statements are checked, in many cases one finds correct information regarding names of earlier family members, persons who had done them harm in an earlier life, details of family secrets and other personal things that no one except e.g. the former husband could have known. The case of the Indian woman Shanti Devi (**cf. Fig. 7.1**) in 1930 was one of the first cases to be a global sensation. The concept of reincarnation, widely accepted in India, was impressively confirmed in her case, which gave the founder of modern India, Mahatma Gandhi, a good opportunity to document scientifically some old time-honored religious traditions.

The late Scottish psychiatrist Ian Stevenson [128] after World War II investigated thousands of children's cases worldwide who recalled their former lives. In cases of violent death in an earlier life, Stephenson found deformities or birthmarks/pigment anomalies at locations which coincided with the acts of violence. A majority of the cases he examined involved violent death, which presumably favored the later recollection of the earlier life. Many of the cases exhibited, in their next incarnation, pigment disorders, noticeable skin anomalies or deformities which precisely agreed with the karmically inflicted injuries.

7.1.2 Consequences of former lives and mixed therapeutic experiences

Based on the investigations of Ian Stevenson, former lives have a formative effect on the current one [128]. According to Stevenson, habits and personality traits, as well as appearance, seem to be passed on, as are fears and other emotional traumas. There is a particular affection for loved ones from former lives; on the other hand, regarding the murderer, when a child has been murdered in an earlier life and meets him again, there is a strong dislike even if the child is seeing this person for the first time in its current life.

Additional credible evidence includes recollections of former lives by adults, which turn out upon investigation to be correct. According to Roger Woolger, the majority of all strong fears are karmically conditioned: for instance, someone who drowned in a former life now has a panicky fear of swimming or boat rides [137]. The Jewish Rabbi Gershom has investigated numerous cases of Americans who report having been Jewish in a former life and murdered in a concentration camp (described in his book *Beyond the Ashes* [49]). One woman with asthma traces her illness back to the karmic trauma of the gas chamber.

According to Roger Woolger, re-experiencing karmic traumas might have a psychic strongly cathartic and transformative effect. After such experiences, people have completely readjusted their lives. The psychiatrist Stanislav Grof reports that, after LSD psychotherapy of cured alcoholics or depressives, they regret their suicide attempts and have gained a positive attitude towards life [54]. In the 1970s, great hope was placed on reincarnation therapy. It was believed that many chronic emotional problems could be permanently healed with this method, because it got down to basics and triggered strong catharses. Now, however, clinical practice has been yielding conflicting and somewhat negative experiences. The initial therapeutic euphoria has faded for many therapists; within the therapeutic community, reincarnation therapies have not experienced the breakthrough which many had hoped for. There are two reasons for this: many of the scenes experienced in a hypnotic trance cannot be verifiably confirmed, i.e. they are based on unreal fantasies which discredit such procedures. Moreover, cathartic procedures can be emotionally destabilizing over the long run (up to and including psychoses), and negative emotions can be reinforced.

7.1.3 Psychoenergetic dissolution of karmic conflicts

With this as background, the question is whether there are any alternatives and what these might achieve. Diagnostically, Psychosomatic Energetics, unlike hypnotic and similar procedures, exhibits numerous advantages. Its results are not falsified by flights of fantasy, i.e. with qualified testers, it delivers reliable and reproducible results. Thus, the contents of Central Conflicts, which in my view are karmically conditioned, frequently agree with mediumistic pronouncements and transpersonal experiences. PSE is gentle and leaves old negative emotions untouched, so that the negative effects of provocative techniques can be avoided.

PSE postulates that a particular strong emotional trauma (Central Conflict) fundamentally shapes the Psyche. Based on this trauma, it is believed that permanent effectual character traits develop over the course of many incarnations (psychological term: "character types"). With PSE testing, the Central Conflict, and thus the character type, can be determined, which would seem to make possible a clear diagnostic statement concerning the old karmic traumas. Using a Character Type Test Kit, both the character type and the associated Central Conflict can be reliably identified.

The dissolution of the Central Conflict often proves to be a particularly strong healing impetus during PSE therapy and, compared to other conflicts, triggers especially strong healing reactions. The advantage of PSE therapy is that the emotionally strongly repressed conflict and its extreme negative emotions do not need to be made conscious, as is the case with the usual reincarnation therapies, but rather are gently and nonverbally eliminated with the aid of homeopathic high potentiation mixtures (Emvita).

Those who are emotionally stable can deal consciously with old emotional traumas from earlier lives once the determinative karmic themes of the trauma have been uncovered by PSE testing. Of course, very few will be able to recollect the old trauma, but there is the option of transpersonally interpreting the 28 PSE conflicts in an empathetic manner (more on this in my book *Healing through Energy Medicine* [8]). My hypothesis is that this way the actual basis for certain negative characteristics of a person's character can be uncovered and understood, and then consciously changed.

Roger Woolger learned that many of his American patients led a life full of privation in a former incarnation. They now try, in their current existence, to compensate the old trauma of material poverty through a lavish lifestyle. Behind this is their unconscious fear of having to miserably vegetate and starve. In such persons, PSE often finds conflicts such as "Always wanting more, frustration", which likely have a karmic cause, as well as a Depressive character type which in a certain sense has preserved the old slave mentality. If the conflict is eliminated, the feeling of constant frustration disappears. Patients can see that the unreal aspect of these old traumas no longer have anything to do with their current lives, and reorient themselves. They can rid themselves of outdated negative personality qualities through conscious work on themselves and develop more self-confidence, with the therapist supporting them in this.

7.2 Reincarnation and PSE – a new transpersonal approach

Reincarnation continues to be a highly controversial topic, and there will probably never be objective proof of it. Because of the volatile nature of this area of research, it is unfortunately very little investigated scientifically. Nevertheless, there are numerous indications from research, for example by psychiatrist Ian Stevenson, that unconscious emotional traumas can originate in earlier lives. It has been my experience that more and more people sense that they have lived more than one time. For this reason, reincarnation should definitely be discussed, if one is dealing with the deep levels of the unconscious. It goes without saying that this does not involve a declaration of faith in it, but rather the non-ideological idea that would like to make the individual ultimately responsible for his own fate, thereby being able to reinforce human freedom and personal responsibility.

Dealing with deep emotional levels which might possibly originate in earlier lives involves certain risks. Imagined earlier lives can, upon inspection, turn out to be flights of fantasy, which can cast doubt on regression therapies in general, and can lead one astray into false conclusions, i.e. that one must atone for past misdeeds, which can promote unconscious self-castigating tendencies. Moreover, strongly cathartic psychotherapeutic techniques can also disastrously reinforce negative emotions. Reincarnation therapies are thus a Pandora's box, which should only be used with the requisite circumspection and a great deal of experience. PSE offers a therapeutically gentle yet effective alternative, which also offers good diagnostic options for analyzing the contents of emotional injuries from former lives, and deriving from oneself corresponding positive conclusions.

7.3   Karmic conflicts in PSE

My activity with the topic of "reincarnation" began simply enough because most of my patients were unable to recall any cause for large conflicts, even though they confirmed the correctness of the conflict contents. This raised the question of where their conflicts originated. At some point, cases began accumulating of patients who recognized the conflict contents during regressions into former lives. A number of mediumistic patients of mine likewise confirmed that large conflicts are often karmic in nature. This raised a suspicion, albeit quite a vague one. Closer analysis then showed that large conflicts are found even in newborn babies, whose mothers had no explanation for the conflict contents. So where were they supposed to have come from? A genetic cause was also ruled out, because identical twins had different Central Conflicts, although they often had the same character type.

The riddle was solved when patients in reincarnation-therapy sessions (regressions) or spontaneously – i.e. via nightmares and visions – were able to recall the contents of these large conflicts. What they reported agreed with the tested conflict contents and evidently came from their earlier lives. Normally, one no longer recalls this kind of karmic content, because they lie too far back in the past. These contents are called transpersonal because they go beyond the current individual self. A few of my patients have detailed memories of the origins of large conflicts which likely correspond to the Central Conflict.

For instance, a patient described a nightmare and wanted to know whether its contents could have something to do with his Central Conflict, which we shortly before had found with the aid of Psychosomatic Energetics. The man's deep unconscious was presumably wide open due to his schizophrenic psychosis, so that buried karmic recollections were able to rise up. He had been suffering from this disease for a long time, and looked me up in order to try out alternative medicine besides chemical medications and psychotherapy – which, after more than one year of PSE therapy, proved to be successful.

He told me that in the nightmare he found himself on an ancient field of battle. Based on his description of the uniform and the conditions, it was possibly a Mesopotamian or ancient Egyptian battle. In the crucial scene, the man was forced to experience, during his death agonies, vultures pecking away at his flesh in the gaps between his metal armor and leather straps, while the sun burned mercilessly in the sky. All around him lay many others dying who also suffered horribly. To be alive and be helplessly at the mercy of the entire situation corresponded with his conflict theme. It also had to do with the feeling of completely losing his mind, which also corresponded with his psychiatric ailment, and also matched his character type.

My conclusion was that, in this earlier life and in the face of the threat to his very existence, the trauma led to the development of a Central Conflict in the seventh energy Center. In view of the horrible experience, he was in danger at that time of going completely insane, and after his reincarnation into a new body, he developed a Melancholic character type. For the Schizoid character, there is a deep characteristic rift between body and soul; this seems understandable as a protective mechanism, considering such a trauma. It's not hard to understand that somebody like this can lose basic trust – typical for the Melancholic character. The patient was no longer able to trust the good forces of life because he had been to gruesomely killed, and he became, at the core of his being, mistrustful and cautious.

The psychotherapist Roger Woolger, who studied under C.G. Jung and made a name for himself as a reincarnation therapist, names some typical psychic injuries which come to light during regressions and which appear particularly often in conjunction with certain disorders and diseases:

> *"Uncertainty and fear of abandonment are often bound up with recollections of pre-existential abandonment in childhood, separation during a crisis or war, loss of parents. The people in question also frequently experience being sold into slavery or being set out to starve during famines etc. Depression and lack of drive: these feelings are often bound up with pre-existential recollections of the loss of a loved one or parents, unsettled sorrow, thoughts of suicide, desperation as a result of war, massacre or deportation. Material difficulties and eating disorders: people who suffer from these difficulties often recall during regression an existence in which they starved or lived in times of economic chaos or inescapable poverty. External features: anorexia, bulimia, obesity, accidents, violence, physical brutality are usually bound up with recollections of battles during earlier lives as soldiers, with re-experiencing unresolved power struggles or broken-off adventures. These symptoms often appear in young adults, i.e. at an age when – historically – many young men have died in wartime."* [137]

The psychic injuries cited by Woolger to my mind correspond most of the time to the Central Conflict. In one regression, a woman, who in PSE testing exhibited the Central Conflict "Always wanting more" (emotional remedy 11), was able to recall having starved to death in an earlier life. It was exactly this conflict theme that was likely the emotional message which her starving organism had stored up as a key message: "I must have more (than nothing) in order to survive." In real life, people such as this often suffer from eating disorders and frequently become overweight, because they unconsciously believe they would otherwise starve again.

These ancient psychic injuries from former lives probably have such an enormous effect on the current life that they should be viewed as one of the essential causes of much suffering, disease and probably also social behavioral disorders. My experience with Psychosomatic Energetics points in the same direction. If one wants to find the actual causes of psychic and emotional problems, one should therefore look for them in earlier lives, where, in a manner of speaking, an endless train of specific psychic injuries was set in motion. In view of the above, one can understand that people are characterologically forever (de)formed by this Central Conflict – for many, "forever" signifies subsequent incarnations.

8   The Acute Agents

In Psychosomatic Energetics, there are four homeopathic compound remedies that are called "acute agents" because they are used for acute ailments. In this section, I would like to explain how these special agents can be turned to good account in daily practice – even without the application of Psychosomatic Energetics (PSE). As the designation "acute" makes clear, we are talking about medications for use in acute cases, which can either be indicated on a purely symptomatic basis or administered adjuvant to PSE therapy – for instance, to better get through the initial phase of an anxiety disease case.

> These acute agents are available by prescription as globuli or drops in 50 mL vials, and are marketed by Rubimed AG (Switzerland) as well as Rubimed B.V. (EU region).

8.1   Anxiety

The most important acute agent is, without a doubt, Anxiovita (available in Switzerland as Kava Kava comp.). As a targeted homeopathic compound remedy for anxiety states, it has proven itself in cases of panic conditions, test anxiety, social phobias and other forms of anxiety or fear. The usual dose is 12 drops twice daily, or for acute ailments five drops or globuli every 30 minutes. For hundreds of patients, the experience has been that it usually works reliably and rapidly, so that it can be used as a preventative emergency agent in anxiety cases. This also applies to situational anxiety such as just before an exam, where it also has a preventative effect.

Years of experience have shown that Anxiovita is a specific for anxiety and can be used in this context diagnostically as well. When it is regularly tested energetically in a general-medicine practice, i.e. via the kinesiological muscle test, one might notice with surprise that it responds for more patients than one would've expected based on the anamnesis. Yet upon closer inquiry, it has to do with anxiety patients who, due to subliminal apprehensions concerning, say, close relatives or job security, are experiencing inner stress which is making them uneasy and tense, which then often leads at some point to the typical anxiety symptoms. Such patients report on exhaustion, tension, pain, uneasiness etc., in which the symptoms described are based primarily on anxiety or fear, which the positive response to the test ampoule Anxiovita (as well as, later, the positive response to anxiety-eliminating therapy) confirms.

Not infrequently, the anxiety ampoule Anxiovita will also respond to various forms of addiction. For example, pathological alcohol consumption serves to cope with anxiety in the form of a not very efficient self-therapy. Understandably in anxiety cases, one should always begin by addressing the emotional cause, i.e. by administering Anxiovita, through anxiety-alleviating dialogues as well as the dissolution of emotional conflicts with PSE.

8.2 Nervous tension and overexcitement

For certain acute neural diseases such as multiple sclerosis, polyneuropathy, trigeminal neuralgia, as well as chronic pain such as migraine, neuralgia etc., Neurovita responds in the energetic remedy test (available in Switzerland as Melissa comp.). It has proven itself therapeutically as a general calmative and also for regeneration.

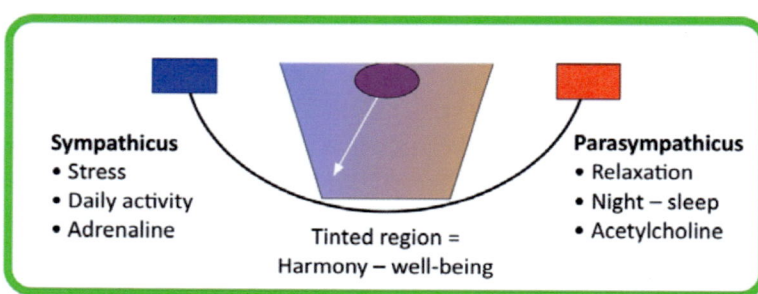

Fig. 8.1 – *The healthy autonomic nervous system avoids extremes and swings back and forth in a feel-good region (between sympathetic during the day and parasympathetic at night).*

8.2.1 Autonomic misregulation

The autonomic nervous system (ANS), somewhat like a home heating/cooling system, regulates central body functions such as sleep, skin temperature, digestion, metabolism and circulatory functions such as blood pressure and heart rate (cf. Fig. 8.1).

People with vegetative disorders complain of various symptoms such as cold hands, sweating, fast or slow digestive activity and many other feelings of ill health. Since the vegetative nervous system is responsible for our (sense of) well-being, those affected often feel permanently unwell.

It is important to distinguish between vegetative over- and under-function, because different therapeutic strategies are derived therefrom. Simvita reveals **sympathicotonic disorders**, which can be compared to an "overactive heating system" (with symptoms such as sweating, tachycardia, diarrhea, restlessness, weight loss). By contrast, Paravita addresses **parasympathicotonic dysfunctions**, comparable to an "underactive heating system" (with symptoms such as dry skin, freezing, bradycardia, tendency to faint, constipation and weight gain). Due to the functional counter-regulation of the vegetative nervous system, which can be both intact and disturbed at different levels, one should know that not all of the named symptoms appear, so that, in clinical practice, additional diagnostic signposts are needed.

With the aid of the kinesiological response of the Simvita or Paravita test ampoules (included in the Rubimed Basic Test Kit, Chapter 19.1), the corresponding dysfunctions can be detected and then treated with the same ampoules. Naturopathic therapy of the autonomic nervous system is a good idea if only because mainstream medicine has neither an objective diagnostic nor any therapy for autonomic dysfunction. Therefore, many such complaints are either misdiagnosed in daily practice, dismissed as psychogenic and often, from the viewpoint of those affected, unsatisfactorily treated. Due to the large subjective pressure of suffering, rapid therapeutic success is desirable, so Simvita or Paravita, at a dosage of 12 drops 2 to 3 times daily, often brings rapid relief (available in Switzerland as adrenaline or acetylcholine comp.).

The four PSE acute agents can be employed both purely symptomatically, based upon specific symptoms, as well as on energetic test results (including kinesiological remedy tests). They have proven themselves in daily naturopathically-oriented practice as fast-acting healing agents. With the vegetative action of the complexes Simvita and Paravita, the acute phases of a flu infection can often be arrested or cut short because, in this manner, it more quickly leads to autonomic adjustment and harmonization. Anxiovita aids in uncovering otherwise unidentified anxiety diseases and causally treating them.

9 Geopathy and Electrosmog

Nocturnal stress due to **geo-radiation** is a major factor in naturopathic medicine, from which the organism can only recover and once again react normally to therapeutic stimuli after the bed is shifted from a disrupted location to an unstressed one. This is why many people for whom therapy does not take very well turn out to be suffering from geopathic stress. Once they are sleeping in a stress-free area, their sleep is deeper, they wake up refreshed and generally feel more fresh and resilient. Many diseases and disorders directly related to geopathic stress – such as exhaustion and pain states, restlessness and tension, sleep disorders, nightmares and bedwetting – improve or disappear entirely. Experience has shown that the list of diseases and disorders related to geo-radiation can be extended indefinitely. Many people only get truly healthy again after they have had the geo-radiation accurately detected and then carefully eliminated by professionals, i.e. the bed has been relocated to a stress-free area.

The term *electrosmog* encompasses subjective stress due to cell-phone towers, radio and TV transmitters as well as disturbances from other radiofrequency and radar installations. In addition, there are household devices (homemade geo-radiation, so to speak) from cordless phones, Wi-Fi, as well as direct contact with many different devices and appliances that emit electromagnetic radiation, from clock radios at the head end of the bed to frequent cell phone use and wearing an active cell phone right next to the body. Since geo-radiation and electrosmog potentiate each other, I deal with them here together, even though they actually have nothing to do with each other.

9.1 Definition, physical proof and studies

Geo-radiation refers to local factors which, under prolonged exposure, develop unfavorable biological influences (called "geopathy" – literally "geo-radiation disease"). Those who sleep in a bed on a geopathically stress location will be energetically impregnated with it over time. They will sleep poorly, have nightmares, develop vegetative symptoms such as dizziness, feeling unwell, fatigue. Over the longer term, they may get seriously ill and develop cancer or other diseases. Farmers know specific spots in a barn where cows do not calve – and infertility is a consequence of geo-radiation in humans as well. Added to this are many more negative consequences which I'll get around to later, which are unfortunately attributed to other causes by many people (including therapists, sadly) out of sheer ignorance, but which actually originate from nocturnal geo-radiation stress. For the aforementioned symptoms, conventional physicians tend to think in terms of depression, poor sleep habits, marital problems and much more in the same vein – but never geo-radiation.

To this day, geo-radiation is **not physically detectable**, and it must also be said that they have not really been properly investigated either. Just as with other alternative-medicine issues, we are dealing here with scientific taboo topics, which serious scientists either do not investigate in the first place (since otherwise they would seriously damage their careers) or dismiss it from the outset as nonsense, thereby honoring the scientific creed according to which there is nothing to investigate in this area. These phenomena are evidently disharmonious information patterns which can, over time, disturb and disrupt biological systems (humans, animals and plants). If this is the case – and many thousands of tests and investigations into bedsite locations indicate that it well might be – then one can see why geo-radiation is not as yet detectable, because information makes a hard-to-measure qualitative difference that cannot be detected by physical measuring devices.

On beds located in geopathic stress zones, there are occasionally strong deviations of the Earth's magnetic field; there are also outer margins of water-runs, sometimes with clearly detectable changes in Earth-electricity, as well as possibly increased radioactivity or elevated cosmic daitation such as from solar radiation or similar factors injurious to cells. The latter would explain why shielding virtually always fails and why cancer continues to occur in shielded beds – namely, because solid particles penetrate the shielding and, over the long-term, fracture DNA molecules. And yet, despite all of these suppositions and individual observations, we unfortunately still do not know anything more specific.

The first large-scale **scientific investigation** of the topic of geo-radiation was carried out by the Austrian internist Otto Bergsmann [18]. He was able to demonstrate to a high degree of probability that geo-radiation exists. In particular, the erythrocyte sedimentation rate (ESR) was significantly altered in geopathic irritant regions. According to Bergsmann, this is an indication that irritant regions alter the surface tension of fluids. Since the human body consists mainly of water, its clear why geo-radiation changes the quality of the body's endogenous water. It also explains why irritant regions are harmful to the entire body, namely because all of the body's water is affected – regardless of whether one is lying with one's head or feet in geo-radiation. The serotonin level in the blood was the second highly significant altered parameter (of many others which were checked out such as heart rate, Schellong test, immunoglobulin etc.) which was altered by geo-radiation stress. Serotonin is the so-called "happiness hormone" and it has an influence on the quality of sleep. In addition, serotonin is involved in certain parasympathetic stress conditions which are particularly active at night. Since irritation regions provoke stress, that would explain the elevated serotonin consumption. A serotonin deficiency in irritation zones leads in turn to sleep disorders and depression.

The project "Geopathogenic Zones in the Home and Stress" (www.ezu.at/) was submitted in spring 2005 by the European Center For Environmental Medicine, approved and published in February 2007. The main results of the study are clear: the percentage of sleep disorders at sleeping locations classified as *geopathogenic* are significantly elevated. Very often, positive changes to the state of health of the test subjects when the bedside was moved were described. After these results, *geopathogenic zones* have to be regarded as an additional risk factor in the pathological process, just as had already been ascribed to lifestyle and individual and social factors.

9.2   Diagnosing geopathies

The big problem with the topic of geo-radiation is the great uncertainty when it comes to detection and, later, the reliable elimination of these disruptive influences. Patients often tell me, when I have determined geo-radiation stress in their case, that they already had three dowsers come by and all three had come up with different results. Many people therefore consider the topic to be extremely subjective and very critically dismiss it as superstition – which I think is going way too far, although it can be understood as an expression of understandable disappointment. It's clear that patients don't want to throw their money out the window; they expect trustworthy recommendations from their therapist, so that they'll get healthier. Then, later on, comes the great uncertainty as to how one eliminates geo-radiation and whether shielding would be enough. This too is a hotly contested area which has damaged the reputation of the entire subject.

Despite all the uncertainty, geo-radiation is an enormously important negative health factor whose elimination cannot be ignored. Any therapist who wants to run a truly responsible naturopathic practice must, despite all the uncertainty, find ways and means for correctly recognizing the problem and permanently solving it. My decades of experience as a physician, as well as that of my colleagues in the same field, show that geo-radiation can be reliably detected and just as reliably eliminated. In this next section, I'd like to describe how that happens in actual practice.

> **Procedure**
> The first thing is **reliable detection of geo-radiation stress**. In practice, this is done by querying about typical geo-radiation-related illnesses and symptoms or other anamnestic indications:
> - Sleep disorders, trouble staying asleep, nightmares, children lying cockeyed in the bed in the morning (fleeing the nest)
> - Tiredness, dizziness, feeling unwell
> - Cramps, rheumatic symptoms, pain states
> - Infertility
> - Lack of concentration, restlessness, nervousness, lack of resilience, bad mood, depression
> - Bedwetting in children, low grades in school, behavioral disorders
> - All chronic diseases, practically very often cancer (exception: some hormone-sensitive mammary tumors)
> - Therapy resistance, difficult patient (nothing helps)
> - Symptoms only began after patient had lived for a while in the current home
> - Noticeable improvement in symptoms while on vacation or after having lived for a longish time (more than 2-3 weeks) somewhere else

The problem with questioning is that many people do not feel anything directly from geo-radiation, either because they've become accustomed to it or they're too insensitive to feel it. One cannot therefore rely on the presence or absence of particular symptoms, just as there are many cases of sleep disorders and other geo-radiation-typical symptoms and diseases which have totally different causes. For many people, one can notice geo-radiation stress simply by their tired-looking facial expression from lack of sleep, but this too can be deceptive. Sometimes, an indication of geopathy is previous occupants who had also slept at that bedsite and become gravely ill.

For me, the surest way to detect geo-radiation is a positive response to certain test ampoules when performing energetic tests on the patient; if a test ampoule containing special homeopathics is introduced into the patient's energy field which vibrationally matches the geo-radiation, the organism responds with a positive test reaction. Basically, the message is that the organism already carries such stresses within itself and can only balance them out through a strenuous expenditure of energy when it is once again confronted with it.

Test ampoules which have proven useful here include Geovita, Silicea D60 or Polyxan blue, yellow and red. I have amassed decades of experience with Geovita. With a crosscheck from a good dowser, there is nearly 100% certainty that a significant geopathy is present.

In 1-2% of cases, Geovita does not test out even though the dowser found a geopathy. Thus, even Geovita, like any other diagnostic procedure, is not 100% reliable, but it still has a very high percentage track record which enables very confident declarations to be made. Sometimes, Geovita tests out at the second visit which takes place months later. It's possible that in some people the organism first has to become capable of reacting again, as for instance after one resolves emotional conflicts with Psychosomatic Energetics or stabilizes the organism in some other manner before Geovita responds.

If Geovita tests out, I always recommend consulting a reliable and experienced dowser to confirm my initial diagnosis and to then relocate the bed to a neutral spot. Generally, a bedsite examination last one to two hours, and calls for a great deal of attention to detail (**cf. Fig. 9.1**). Many patients want to save the money for the examination, but no other procedure has proven satisfactory. One possibility is randomly moving the bed to another location, which statistically works out about 70% of the time, but it's still a kind of health roulette.

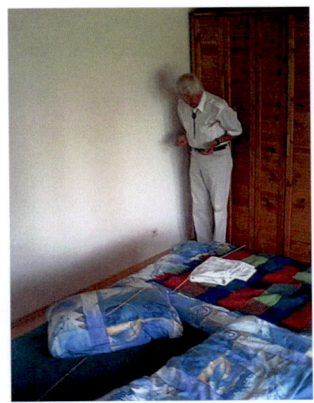

Fig. 9.1 – *The well-known dowser, qualified engineer Hans Zürn, examining a bedsite. On the bed, disturbance zones have been marked with rods.*

Shielding with cork, straw, silk and other inexpensive natural materials has only a short-term effect – almost never long-term – which is why I completely reject it, as do all responsible experienced dowsers that I know. One exception is temporary sleeping places such as guest beds, hotel beds etc., as long as one only sleeps there for a short time and the shielded geo-radiation-bed is not on top of a so-called "cancer zone" which cannot be shielded anyway. There is an entire shielding industry that lives off the cluelessness and laziness of many people, who want to have things stay the way they are. The more expensive the shielding mat, the more effective it should be, and in fact many geopathy-typical symptoms often disappear through their use, but the sick-making effect nevertheless remains. In my medical career, I have had at least several dozen desperate cancer patients sitting in front of me who in their ignorance slept in a shielded bed and consider themselves protected. Based on tests performed by good dowsers, practically all (!) shielding turns out to be worthless gadgetry. So, when it comes to geo-radiation, the only correct motto is: find a neutral spot and sleep there from now on.

Another problem is finding a **reliable dowser**. This is someone who reliably determines maximal zones in the bed which agree with the symptoms and ailments of the patient without the dowser having known about them beforehand. Patients are always very surprised, because they had not counted on such a high degree of certainty. My experience has been that there are not many in the dowser community who perform so reliably. As a therapist, therefore, one should check out which of them are capable of delivering such quality and only recommend those truly reliable dowsers.

9.3 Medications, relocation reaction, monitoring bedsite cleansing

Geovita as a medication, stinging nettle tea, formic acid embrocations, mistletoe tea and similar vegetable substances which flourish above geopathies can sometimes damp down the so-called *relocation reaction* which can appear for a few days when one sleeps in an unstressed bed location for the first time. One should not explicitly bring this to patients' attention, since it might deter them from relocating the bed and could trigger a "nocebo effect" (in other words, purely subjectively, they feel worse). In the case of some skeptical patients who improved after taking Geovita, I have been able to build up enough trust that in the end they agreed to a bedsite examination.

Empirically, it takes four weeks for Geovita to no longer respond in a follow-up test. If Geovita no longer tests positive, one may reliably assume that the geo-radiation stress has been permanently eliminated. Then, all the symptoms provoked by geo-radiation will improve. Previously not very effective therapies once again respond and the patient improves steadily.

Summing up, one can from this point on speak in terms of a successful bedsite cleansing. The long-term result generally persists, unless severe earthquakes, strong vibrations due to construction work and the like change the underground situation – but this happens very infrequently.

9.4 Conclusions concerning the topic of geo-radiation

My own medical experience of more than 30 years with thousands of patients, as well as that of other therapists doing similar work, has shown time and again that geo-radiation is an enormously important sick-making factor. Often, however, the actual problem is not correctly identified and inappropriately treated. Geo-radiation plays an important role for about one patient in three. In mountainous regions, as well as with many underground river flows, large tectonic faults and the like, there are many geopathies; in sandy regions with stable subterranean conditions, on the other hand, there are fewer of them. For cancer patients, one finds, in over 95% of cases, a strong geopathic zone which can be shown to coincide precisely with the cancerous location. I give every cancer patient the same advice given by the then world-famous surgeon Sauerbruch, to lie down to sleep in a bed other than the one in which he became sick.

Empirically, a bedside free of geo-radiation is extremely important if one is to get healthy and stay healthy over the long term. There are certain test ampoules (Geovita) which are helpful in the reliable detection of geopathy. A reliable dowser who can consistently and reliably detect maximal zones, does not use shielding, and in addition finds neutral locations, is recommended to the patient. The dowser checks out the suspicion of geo-radiation onsite and then recommends an undisturbed bed location. It takes four to find out whether the bed relocation was successful, because that's how long it takes for the organism's impregnation with geo-radiation to be extinguished. The Geovita test ampoule no longer responds and the patient is feeling markedly better as far as geo-radiation-related symptoms are concerned. Medical experience shows that a geo-radiation-free bed is just as important as physical activity and a healthy diet are to the maintenance of good health.

9.5   Reliably detecting electrosmog

Conclusive diagnostic indication of electrosmog stress is obtained with the test ampoule Phosphor D12 (available from Rubimed AG). The ampoule responds in approximately 1-2% of all cases. This tells us that electrosmog is relatively rare as the sole problem. Experienced dowsers who routinely examine houses and apartments have confirmed this: electrosmog is seldom the only problem; instead, additional disturbances are found such as geo-radiation and toxic building materials, radon and other environmental burdens such as noise and fine dust. Dowsers and organic consultants measure electrosmog with high- and low-frequency measuring devices (from the firms Biologa and Gigahertz). Often, no measuring device is needed: one right away sees large loudspeakers near the head end of the bed (magnetic field), reading lamps, electrically adjustable beds, electric blankets or heated waterbeds – all sources of electrical current, with no need for a measuring device.

Other disturbance sources include power lines built into the walls, with leakage currents emanating from defective power cable assemblies, metal beds which act as antennas, circuit breaker boxes directly on the rear wall of the head end of the bed in the neighboring room, as well as all kinds of electronic devices near the head end of the bed, or electrostatically active artificial fibers, for instance in stuffed animals in the kids' rooms. Added to this are electrically charged work tables, strongly radiating lamps in the vicinity of the head in the form of the biologically very unfavorable modern energy-saver lamps. In particular, high-frequency pulsed LEDs seem to be in some cases very harmful; this applies especially to the cheaper manufacturers. Sometimes the biologically very unfavorable current from nearby electrical light rail systems, as well as nearby cell phone towers, are the cause of the present electrosmog problem. Taking appropriate measures such as relocating the bed, electrical grounding, buying different lamps and special shielding precautions, can resolve most of the problems and effectively combat the electrosmog.

One possibility is a master disconnect switch for the bedroom, which – at least at night – ensures that no current flows in the sleeping area. The surest electrosmog protection is offered by a complete metal sheath, like an automobile with a metal hardtop. The principle of the Faraday Shield is the basis of many **shielding measures** (www.ezu.at/pdf/Abschirm-matten_Innenraumanalytik.pdf). In this context, once one realizes how strongly automobiles shield electrosmog, that obviously applies to the automobile interior space as well. Therefore, those who make cell phone calls in the car without using an external antenna force the cell phone to boost the transmitted signal strength, which makes the cell phone's harmful effect all the stronger. Cars also often have other electrosmog sources in their interior such as electrically heated seats and the like. Electrosmog in the home, such as from nearby cell phone towers, can be effectively shielded with a canopy which contains metal threads and thus acts as a Faraday Shield. Many writers recommend grounded aluminum foil on the exterior wall nearest to the cell phone tower. In these cases, I advise my patients to use competent specialists instead of trying to "whip up" something on their own, so as to have a professional installation with regular monitoring.

Interference suppressor chips installed in cell phones have no electromagnetic shielding effect: checking with measuring devices reveals that cell phones radiate just as strongly (or even stronger) after chip installation as before. These kinds of interference suppression methods nevertheless sometimes have a weak subtle-energy effect which can be shown using appropriate test instruments. When tested using the REBA Test Device, many suppressor chips improve the Vital and Emotional by about 10-20% – pretty meager results considering the horrendous prices of such chips. The energetic effect on the Aura is somewhat alleviated by suppressor chips, but they still do not totally negate the harmfulness of cell phones, making them yet another pseudo-solution. It is recommended to use cell phones as little as possible, and even then in speakerphone mode or using an earbud/microphone set. By the way, regarding cordless phones in the home there are now eco-mode models which turn themselves off when not being used.

9.6   Just how harmful is electrosmog?

Ultimately, if one asks how harmful electrosmog should be considered to be, in light of the increasing electrification of the modern world – which brightly illuminates the nocturnal cityscape, makes nearly every nook and cranny accessible to cell phones and links together nearly all cities, towns and villages with Internet, television and radio reception – it may be said from a naturopathic viewpoint that, for most people, the damage likely tends to be indirect. Electrosmog disrupts the subtle-energy system, which can, over the long-term, have negative metabolic effects. However, we still know very little about this, and if there are any effects, they are probably very weak.

Most of the studies on the topic of the harmfulness of electrosmog have turned up negative. But it must be said here that, because of the enormous economic consequences involved, industry and government have joined forces to suppress negative studies:

www.salzburg.gv.at/themen/gs/gesundheit/
landessanitaetsdirektion-2/gesundheitsschwerpunkte/umweltmedizin/
elektrosmog/elektrosmog_und_gesundheit/infoblaetter.htm

So, in Brussels (the seat of the European Union) there are two lobbyists for each parliamentarian, who see to it that the legal limits are set insanely high, or that senseless (but profitable) low-energy light bulbs are officially recommended. The same is likely true for North America. Thanks then to thoughtless regulations, a great many people are unnecessarily exposed to overly high levels of electromagnetic stress.

Based on my investigations using subtle-energy measuring devices, everything points to electrosmog being, above all, subjectively disruptive, dependent upon dosage as well as frequency. Electrosmog disturbs the subtle-energy system, which above all inflicts subjective suffering on its victims. Children and particularly sensitive adults are more strongly negatively influenced than "thick-skinned average guys". Experienced dowsers have told me that many children with behavioral disorders or learning deficits have totally electrified bedrooms. After cleansing these electrosmog-burdened sleeping areas, plus simple psychohygienic measures such as not watching TV before going to bed (which is known to diminish sleep quality), many complaints are often markedly improved or have vanished.

Basically, electrosmog in general seems to be a second-tier public health problem. Those who live a healthy lifestyle, sleep in a non-stressed bed location and maintain (or reestablish) psychoenergetic harmony, say through methods such as "Psychosomatic Energetics", autogenic training, Yoga and suchlike, will generally not be much affected by electrosmog as long as a certain intensity and disruptive quality is not exceeded. Nevertheless, electrosmog as described here should be avoided as much as possible, since too little is known about its long-term effects.

10 The Organ Test Kit

Psychosomatic Energetics works on three main testing areas, of which the first two have already been dealt with. The intent here is to uncover emotional conflicts, geopathies and functional organ stresses and/or chronic inflammation foci, which normally remain undiscovered but which experience has shown play significant roles in many health disorders (the necessary health kits for each are shown in parentheses):

1. Conflicts and Chakras (Basic and REBA Test Kits)
2. Geopathy/electrosmog (Basic and Supplementary Test Kits)
3. Organ Test Kit (Basic Test Kit, *Acidum lacticum* ampoule in REBA Test Kit)

The Organ Test Kit serves to uncover **functional organ stresses** such as intestinal flora dysbioses as well as **chronic inflammatory processes**, such as chronic sinusitis, which mesenchymally stress the entire body. There are many ailments that do not stress the body, such as intestinal polyps or a previous mild cardiac infarction in which the heart's pump functionality has not been impaired.

An estimated two thirds or more of all unhealthy organs do not respond to the Organ Test Kit because they do not mesenchymally impair the organism. This is quickly noticed when, for example, the diagnosis in the hospital discharge papers is compared with the Organ Test Kit results. The regular mainstream medicine diagnosis is needed because ailments not detectable by the Organ Test Kit might nevertheless have serious consequences. Therefore, one should **never perform normal organ diagnostics with the Organ Test Kit**, since this can lead one astray to misleading conclusions. The reason is (as has been said) that significant disturbances, such as a precancerous intestinal polyp, are often not testable.

The Organ Test Kit comes into its own at the moment that conventional medicine reaches a dead end. One then becomes a "disease detective", intent on tracking down and disposing of hidden disease causes. One searches for connective tissue stresses, i.e. concealed disease foci that burden the entire organism mesenchymally and can make it chronically ill. The following impressive case from my time as a Vegatest practitioner shows that this can mean:

- **Case study**

In the case of a young American woman, over a longish period of time there had appeared severely itching skin eruptions all over her body whose cause nobody could determine. Among other things, she had been very thoroughly examined at Harvard University and the Mayo Clinic, two of the most renowned clinics in the world, but no one was able to help her. Finally, in desperation, she came to see me in Germany – which was of course very flattering to the young doctor I was at the time. Using the Vegatest method, I discovered an inflamed appendix which tested out as a severe mesenchymal focus, but which was asymptomatic to her. A possible operation was thus based solely upon the energy test.

The examination in the hospital to which I referred her revealed that the appendix was slightly painful to the touch. The surgeon suspected chronic recidivating appendicitis and decided to operate. When the lower abdomen was opened up, the appendix was full of roundworms and chronically inflamed. After the operation, the patient was almost immediately completely symptom-free. During the discussion afterwards, she admitted to me that my colleague Helmut Schimmel and examined her in the US during a Vegatest seminar, where she, in desperation, had let herself be examined as a test patient. My colleague found the same cause that I had, namely the inflamed appendix – which, however, she had not told me – presumably because she didn't want to suggestively influence me. At the time, Dr. Schimmel had no free time on his schedule, or she otherwise would have gone to him. So the reality was that I was not the sought-after healer, but just her second choice. However, the agreement between my diagnosis and Dr. Schimmel's completely convinced her and encouraged her to undergo the operation.

As the above case makes clear, the Organ Test Kit is used when mesenchymal stress is present. For this patient, it was worms and an inflamed appendix which had evaded conventional diagnosis and provoked mesenchymal disorders, which were then testable. In such cases, the use of the Organ Test Kit is justified and often helps a skillful therapist along. The Organ Test Kit contains lightly potentiated basic tinctures (D1) from lamb (and also partly horse) organs, which are manufactured under sterile conditions for cell therapy. It contains all organs and functional organ systems such as the bile ducts which have proven to be mesenchymally disruptive. In this context, the decades of experience that I and my colleague Dr. H.W. Schimmel have had with the Vegatest method have turned out to be valuable in putting together the Organ Test

Kit. This applies both to the composition of the kit as well as to those organs which one should most frequently test (and hence prioritize), such as bile ducts, intestines and cranial foci (on which more later on).

10.1 Mesenchymal stress

Connective tissue is also known as *matrix, transit route, basic regulation* or *basal system à la Pischinger*. It is an archaic organizational system somewhat like subtle energy but, unlike the latter, materially (and thus substantially) verifiable. I refer to Chapter 1.4 (**The relationship of subtle energy to the mesenchyme, soma and Psyche**) in which the role of connective tissue (mesenchyme) has been summarized. The two regulatory systems are closely related; in this relationship subtle energy, as the superordinate system, influences the mesenchyme. However, it is sometimes necessary to address the mesenchyme directly: naturopathic procedures such as fasting, de-acidification and the like are meant to generally improve negative conditions – such as clogging, hyperacidity, "poor metabolism" (all of which are considered to be pre-disease conditions) – and stimulate self-healing powers.

How can connective tissue have such a great influence and yet be so unknown?

- Connective tissue pervades the entire organism as a kind of primordial sea in which the individual body cells swim. As a primitive somatic organizational system, it has a fairly early form of an immunological/nervous defensive/regulatory function, plus a very sluggish memory as well as a holistic manner of operation, all of which act regulatorily in striving to attain/maintain equilibrium (homeostasis) for the entire organism.
- Two researchers are deeply involved in exploring connective tissue: the Viennese University professor Alfred Pischinger and the German biologist and anatomist Hartmut Heine, who taught at Wittener University. These two researchers made the significant discovery that the mesenchyme is very difficult to detect (which is why it has been marginalized by conventional medicine) but nevertheless plays a very important role in health maintenance.

With patients, the mesenchyme can be likened to "poor soil" which is unhealthy for plants. In this context, darkfield microscopy has proven useful in my practice as a pilot diagnostic which I often perform prior to PSE testing, and which very well graphically represents the overall connective-tissue situation. In my experience, the examination lasts 15-20 minutes including explanations, and is a very worthwhile overview diagnostic for both patient and therapist in an all-inclusive assessment of the mesenchyme before going on to PSE and the Organ Test Kit to track down the precise causes of a poor mesenchyme.

10.2 Darkfield microscopy

Darkfield microscopy (short form "darkfield") refers to a special technique in which the objects in a drop of blood from a freshly taken blood sample show up brightly before a dark background, somewhat like the stars in the night sky. With this quickly learned easy-to-use method, blood can be observed virtually in its natural state. This has the great advantage that, in the unprocessed drop of blood, one sees pretty much exactly that which had been going on just before in the living organism. One sees, above all, erythrocytes and leukocytes, but also albumin and to some extent coagulation products (fibrin) as bright white objects before a black background.

Based on my roughly 10 years of clinical practice experience with darkfield microscopy on many hundreds of patients, it seems to very well reflect the overall metabolic situation. There is hardly any other method that can so well educate and persuade the patient when it comes to clearly and simply imparting naturopathic concepts! The darkfield can be viewed as an excellent translation aid enabling the patient to grasp the complex processes underlying the surface phenomena of the ailment. The patient can follow along on the TV monitor coupled via a camera to the darkfield microscope, and see whether the blood is "clumped up" or flows smoothly; whether it makes an overall "clean" impression or seems "clogged". Experience has shown that the darkfield usually looks precisely like the patient feels.

Most patients are quite amazed to discover such a universe in a pinhead-sized drop of blood from their own body. A darkfield diagnosis thus has a kind of magic that can enchant even the most down-to-earth contemporary – so I like to use it, particularly with skeptical patients who are reserved when it comes to naturopathy, as a preliminary diagnostic tool which, of course, is more persuasive than, say, abstract subtle-energy readings which, from the point of view of the critical patient, have little persuasive power. Instead of being confronted by a mainstream physician with virtually incomprehensible numerical results from lab tests, or examined with mysterious high-tech gadgets, darkfield diagnosis in a naturopathic practice provides the patient with something clear, vivid and directly graspable. The patient immediately gets what it's about and assesses the images precisely as they really are – i.e., this is a largely self-explanatory diagnostic method. Now of course the therapist has to explain certain circumstances, such as the significance of disturbed erythrocytes etc., but most of it the patient can see for himself or evaluates it as it really is.

The biggest downsides to darkfield are high susceptibility to external interference and a lack of standardization – but with enough experience and observance of a few ground rules, one can largely get the hang of it. Still, one should be clear that darkfield diagnostics definitely involves a certain subjective factor; how large this is remains to be determined by future research. Moreover, it seems to me that darkfield has a fairly coarse-grained resolution. There is no way that it can replace necessary conventional medicine diagnostics or a differentiating naturopathic diagnostics. In short, it is a rough pilot diagnostic method that only allows a general overview.

- **Assessment**

In assessing darkfield microscopy, four criteria stand out:
1. Considerable rouleau formation or large erythrocyte adhesion generally indicate a poor vascular and metabolic situation.
2. Also indicating a poor vascular and metabolic situation is a deficiency of blood proteins (in particular albumin), of which there are normally a great number dancing about in Brownian motion in the microscope image field. If these are reduced in numbers, and there are only a few dozen or 100 in the field of view (instead of many thousands), then this also indicates a poor overall metabolic situation. Coarse clumping of normally finely fluffy albumin molecules is likewise a sign of a poor overall metabolic situation.
3. Fibrin threads due to overly rapid coagulation (markedly less than 4-5 minutes) can also be a sign of stress, such as carcinomas, thrombosis tendency etc.
4. Aging, worn-out erythrocytes (recognizable by ring formation in the cell membrane, as well as inclusions in the cellular nucleus) also indicate a poor overall metabolic situation. Empirically in this situation, there is often as well a deficiency of B vitamins and folic acid (inadequate supply, or intestinal flora).

• **Case study**
Mr. S., 52, businessman, suffers from great occupational stress, is overweight and has essential hypertension that is kept under control with medication. He constantly feels tired, complains of dizziness and feeling unwell, but no reason can be found. PSE testing reveals reduced Vital and Emotional readings of 30%, geopathy in the head region, plus considerable large-intestine dysbiosis and a large conflict in the sixth Chakra with the theme "Restlessness".

After calling in an experienced dowser, the bed is relocated, Mutaflor and Kanne Brottrunk (bread drink) is prescribed for the dysbiosis, and Emvita 22/Chavita 6 for conflict resolution, for about four months. The first darkfield shows considerable "slagging" (**cf. Fig. 10.1**). Four months later, at the follow-up examination, the patient reports feeling well and refreshed; blood pressure is greatly improved, he is better able to cope with stress; although he is still just as overweight, he is considering a fasting cure. PSE testing returned normal Vital and Emotional readings of 100%; the darkfield now shows a flawless image with healthy singly separated erythrocytes and a wealth of well-dispersed dancing protein molecules.

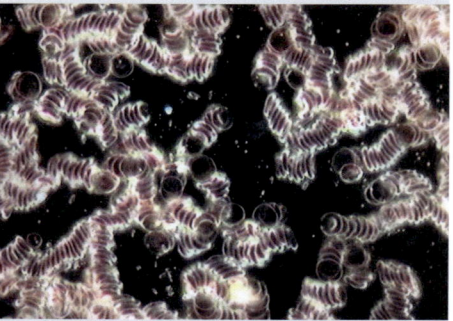

Fig. 10.1 – *Typical rouleau formation and relative absence of fine flocculent, dancing proteins, instead of which some coarsely clumped forms.*

• **Assessment**
There are three additional parameters in the darkfield which, unlike the aforementioned nonspecific signs, provide indications of specific disorders:
1. Leukocytes normally are mobile on their own, moving about independently like amoebas, and have a normal size and structure. Rigid or burst leukocytes point to a weakened (cellular) defensive system, often seen in cases of carcinoma and other severe chronic diseases. Therapy consists of immune stimulation, i.e. with zinc, selenium, thymus, SANUM agent (Utilin S), or Horvi snake toxins, homeopathicized substances of the citric acid cycle (Ubiquinone comp.).

2. Metabolic disorders often manifest murky veils (cholesterol) as well as fatty acid crystals (triglycerides) – here, the recommendation is dietary counseling, liver/gallbladder therapy, dietetic walnuts, red wine, green tea, Mediterranean diet.
3. Erythrocyte disorders in the form of poikilocytosis or pale anemic erythrocytes usually indicate – for a normal hemogram (should be prepared for differential-diagnostic reasons!) – Intestinally-conditioned deficiency situations (dysbiosis); therapy with B vitamins, folic acid.

At the next consultation, most patients spontaneously express a desire for a follow-up darkfield, so that they can observe the changes. This tells one how well-motivated the patients have become: they can see with our own eyes whether or not the therapy has accomplished anything. By the way, I would just like to add that virtually every effective biological healing procedure results in an improved darkfield, in other words, one is by no means constrained by it to a particular methodology.

10.3 Acidum lacticum ampoules

To check whether the Organ Test Kit should be used, one can employ lactic acid ampoules of various potentiations from the REBA Test Kit. Lactic acid is generated in the intracellular space when metabolic combustion is impaired, which in turn is caused by mesenchymal stress. Like an oven which is not drawing well, glucose is not properly "burned" when the organism is stressed by inflammation foci and other mesenchymal stresses.

Therefore, low potentiations of lactic acid signify poor aerobic combustion, i.e. the lower potentiations of a suitable optical D1 or D6 then test positive. Once the metabolism improves, the higher potentiations such as LM 6 (level 0) or D60 (level 1) will respond:

> • **Lactic acid potentiations for mesenchymal diagnostics**
> *Acidum lacticum* LM6, D60, D30, D15 D6, D1 (LM 6 undisturbed mesenchymal functions (level 0), D60 mild (level 1), D30 (level 2) and D15 moderate (level 3), D6 strong (level 4) and D1 (level 5) very severely disturbed)

In my experience, either a particularly poor level will respond (*Acid. Lact.* D1 or D6) or the normal range (LM6 or D60). For stresses in the moderate to severe range, one should utilize the Organ Test Kit to look for mesenchymal disorders.

10.4   The Organ Test Kit

The Organ Test Kit contains 35 organ test ampoules which can be subdivided into various categories. The first group comprises **functional organ disorders** which have to do with a complex functional disruption of one or more organs and organ systems. One example is disturbed intestinal flora (dysbiosis), which affects various organs such as the large and small intestines, as well as touching on various specialty areas such as infectology and immunology, and more recently clinical molecular biology. A highly complex, objectively difficult to verify ecosystem in the intestinal tract with myriads of bacteria is out of equilibrium for a longish time and is stressing the organism. Here, what actually happens pathophysiologically in the body – and this applies to all functional organ disorders – has been very little investigated as yet. We in naturopathy are treating what is virtually unknown territory to mainstream medicine.

> • Note
> The following are some of the functional organ disorders (frequency in percent):
> - Colonic/jejunum and ileum – indication of intestinal flora disorder (dysbiosis, 40-50%)
> - Gallbladder (including bile ducts) – indication of biliary drainage disorder (30-40%)
> - Pancreas – indication of pancreas function disorder (10%)

Another important mesenchymal stress is **chronic inflammation**, which the body cannot heal up on its own by means of regeneration and secretion processes. Like a simmering fire blight, a constant inflammatory process guarantees enormous mesenchymal, immunological and hormonal/neural stress. One example is chronic sinusitis, which can persist for years and even decades, and can lead to severe exhaustion states, chronic bronchitis and/or bronchial asthma, immunological overshoot reactions such as urticaria, neurodermitis attacks etc.

> • Note
> The chronic inflammation foci include head and abdominal foci (frequency in percent):
> - Sinuses (5-10%)
> - Dental/mandibular (2-3%)
> - Tonsils (1%)
> - Appendix (1%)
> - Ovaries/uterus/prostate (2-4%)

Then there are the **systemically active organs** which, in severe degenerative disease cases such as advanced cardiac insufficiency, breast cancer, cirrhosis of the liver, renal insufficiency etc., can all have mesenchymal repercussions throughout the entire organism. A severe organ disease disrupts the entire body, acting in a sense as a focus. Also lymphoma, Helicobacter-pylori-induced gastritis and similar disease pictures potentially weaken the entire body, which one can ascertain with the aid of the ampoules listed below. The list of systemically active organs is actually considerably longer, but most of these ampoules are seldom needed, so I have omitted them (available as Large Organ Test Kit from Wala Eckwälden).

> • Note
> The organ test ampoules with systemic effect include (frequency in percent distinctly less than 1% in each case):
> - Brain
> - Thyroid
> - Heart
> - Bronchia/lungs
> - Thymus
> - Mammaries
> - Liver
> - Stomach/duodenum
> - Spleen
> - Kidneys
> - Adrenal gland
> - Testicles

Finally, there are ampoules that serve as **filters** in the remedy test. They are used as a reference for assessing whether certain chosen therapy combinations, placed in the pelvic Yin region, lead to an improvement in the REBA Test readings. For example, one can see whether therapy with Chavita/Emvita plus bedsite cleansing, simulated with Geovita (placed in the Yin zone) has a positive effect on rheumatoid arthritis (organ ampoule "Bones/joints"), in that the latter ampoule no longer responds. Beforehand – i.e. before placing the Geovita etc. ampoule in the Yin zone – the "Joints" ampoule placed in the REBA Test honeycomb responded; afterwards, it no longer does. This means that the chosen combination in the Yin region is therapeutically quite promising and energetically compensates the rheumatoid arthritis. Sometimes, "filter ampoules" also make sense, in cases of severe systemic disease, for detecting causalities in organ stresses: which organ influences which when, say, sinusitis triggers chronic bronchitis. Therapeutically, in the case of a patient with a severe skin disease, one can test what does in the most good energetically. I describe how this is done in the *Filtering* chapter (Chapter 10.7).

> • Note
> **Organ ampoules for filtering include (frequency less than 1%):**
> - **Bones/joints**
> - **Nerves (peripheral)**
> - **Connective tissue**
> - **Fat**
> - **Lymph nodes**
> - **Arteries**
> - **Veins**
> - **Musculature**
> - **Skin**

When using the Organ Test Kit, it is important to test the most frequently occurring organ test ampoules first, i.e. intestines, gallbladder, pancreas, sinuses etc. – unless the anamnesis has yielded a definite preliminary suspicion. As for the number of tested ampoules, one should keep this **as low as possible**! Experience has shown that it is only one or two (rarely three) organ test ampoules which stress the mesenchyme. Anyone who gropes around randomly in the Organ Test Kit doesn't understand the testing principle: ultimately, one seeks out *the* particular organ that strongly stresses the mesenchyme – and that will very rarely be a motley mixture of disturbances, but rather, as a rule, one, two or three stress sources, where most times one of the responding organ test ampoules will dominate.

> • **Note**
> **There are certain ailments and questions for which there are often special ampoules which are then tested first:**
> - Infection-prone teenager: tonsils, colon/jejunum
> - Woman with migraine, dizziness: gallbladder? Sinuses? Liver?
> - Overweight patient, flatulence: intestinal fungi?
> - Asthma, chronic bronchitis: sinuses?
> - Immune disorder: head foci, appendix, pelvic foci?
> - Older man after apoplexy: prostate?
> - Eczema patient = gallbladder, pancreas, kidneys, intestinal tract

10.5 Functional organ disorders

The most important test ampoules in the Organ Test Kit have to do with functional disturbances of the intestines, bile ducts and pancreas. These include intestinal flora disturbances, bile flow disturbances and pancreatic functional disturbances. Because of their importance, they should always be tested first. How to proceed in this context, how to seek out the best therapy and how to best explain the entire complex topic to the patient is described in the chapters that follow.

10.5.1 Intestinal dysbiosis

The most important milieu stress is intestinal dysbiosis. In contrast to healthy intestinal flora (eubiosis), what we here have is disrupted intestinal flora (dysbiosis), and this includes, strictly speaking, the oral pharyngeal flora including the gums and their bacterial colonization. Accordingly, whoever has disrupted intestinal flora automatically has disrupted pharyngeal and gingival flora as well. One can recognize this when one has diarrhea plus a sticky and very furry tongue. In the case of patients with therapy-resistant periodontal bleeding (periodontitis), I have had complete success with intestinal flora cleansing, even when the patients in question had previously undergone local dental treatment for years to no avail.

Of all the organs, the intestinal flora is the most frequently disturbed – and indeed for practically all conceivable clinical pictures. Decades of observation in naturopathic practice has made it clear that the intestinal flora is in very poor state for many patients, and that many ailments improve when the intestinal flora is improved. Influencing intestinal flora through fasting, enemas, lactic-acid drinks, probiotics etc. has been a central part of naturopathic practice for ages, and in this context, the melodramatic sounding (yet basically correct) slogan "Death lurks in the intestines" has been a formative influence. Long derided in mainstream-medicine circles, it has lately undergone some rethinking there, with the realization that there might be something to this slogan after all. The nearly miraculous total recovery of a seriously ill ulcerative colitis patient on the brink of death after her intestinal tract had been completely cleansed and then administered a small sample of her husband's stool has made many gastroenterologists very thoughtful.

The intestinal flora is very hard to investigate in part because the bulk of the bacteria are anaerobic and thus immediately die upon leaving the intestines. Now however, genetic analyses can portray the intestinal flora quite well [111]. It has been determined that overweight patients have a markedly different flora than slender patients. The poorest intestinal flora have been found in autistics. Based on Michael Gershon's investigations into the "belly brain", we now know that a major part of the neurotransmitters are created in the intestines. Modern research has found indications that specific types of disturbed intestinal flora are typical for depression, and possibly linked to them. We in PSE have known that for quite a while, and can easily confirm it through filtering, for example. Placing the jejunum/ileum or colon test ampoules in the Yin region causes the Emotional readings on the REBA Test Device to shoot up from e.g. 20% to 100% in many depressive patients. Their mood lightens up when their intestinal flora situation improves, whereby their serotonin levels rise.

The intestinal flora consists of good and bad bacteria; they comprise a highly complex system which plays a large role in the immune system (mucosa associated lymphoid tissue = MALT) [20]. Infants come into the world sterile. If they are inoculated a few weeks after birth with good bacteria (Mutaflor Suspension, a few drops per day orally for a few weeks has proven beneficial and is well documented by studies; may be ordered from Ardeypharm), one will note markedly fewer allergies, infections and the like. The intestinal flora make up ten times as many bacteria as body cells, and they assist the body in the uptake of vitamins, minerals and other dietary components. Many people with poor intestinal flora have an instinctive tendency toward extreme diets to supply the missing substances, but they simply make the situation even worse in the process. One must begin with the intestinal flora, and then supplying a lot of orthomolecular substances won't be necessary. Mere dietary change does not usually improve poor intestinal flora; clearly and lastingly improving the patient's flora calls for specialized professional support.

For at least every 2nd to 3rd patient, disturbed intestinal flora significantly predominates in the entire disease process. It is of course true that overall energetic conditions play an additional important role, since energy blocks disrupt the autonomously regulated intestinal peristalsis, such that fecal impaction increases and the intestine-associated defensive system suffers from it. Regarding the defensive system, it should be added that, quantitatively, the greater part of the lymphatic tissue is found in the intestinal walls.

Typical external signs of **dysbiosis** include the widespread bloated and hanging bellies which F.X. Mayr (the developer of the intestinal cleansing cure named after him) discovered nearly 100 years ago, a greasily-coated tongue (particularly in the rear third [colon field]) and, with fungi, a fairly light greasy-yellowish coating of the tongue. The inflamed cecal root is a deep region painful to palpate about 1 to 2 fingerbreadths below the navel. People with disturbed intestinal flora often having an unhealthy appearance, unclean skin, mouth odor and complain of reduced resilience, fatigue, feeling unwell, dizziness and other nonspecific symptoms.

The folding of the intestinal villi results in an enormous total area the size of a football field. In this gigantic resorption area, intestinal toxins clearly will have immense repercussions, and it has been calculated that, even in healthy persons, the total amount of intestinal toxins would be three times a fatal dose were they to get into the bloodstream, which the intestinal flora, acting as a barrier, naturally prevent. Now if the toxin level increases under pathological conditions, then at some point the barrier will collapse and the toxic consequences of dysbiosis will be set in play.

An intestinal tract made porous by toxins (bacteria, fungi) represents a significant cause for many of the diseases of civilization, from overweight, homocysteine deficiency, arteriosclerosis on up to allergies. Virtually every disease and every symptomatology can be related to an ailing intestinal tract. Atypical, extremely troublesome and hard-to-eliminate symptoms such as hypoglycemic attacks, periodontosis, flatulence, unclean skin and "head in a fog" disappear much of the time once the ailing intestine (the actual cause) has been cured.

My recommendations for dysbiosis therapy are based upon three different test diagnoses:

1. **Regular intestinal flora dysbiosis** – testable with the "Colon" organ test ampoule, and a positive response to dysbiosis agents such as Mutaflor. Here, the optimal therapy consists of Mutaflor 100 S. 1 capsule 2-3 times a week and Hylak forte 1 mL in parallel (alternatively to Hylak, Kanne Brottrunk (bread drink) can be used); duration of therapy is about 6-10 weeks. Other E. coli strains such as Colibiogen, Omniflora and Symbioflor II should be tested on a case-by-case basis. In cases of regular colonic dysbiosis, inoculation with about 4 billion units of an extremely health-promoting E. coli strain (trade name Mutaflor) is administered. Mutaflor was isolated in World War I by the Freiburg hygiene professor Nissle from the stool of a medical orderly who had remained healthy in the midst of a severe diarrhea epidemic. It later turned out that Mutaflor acts somewhat like an antibiotic against diarrhea pathogens. It has an overall immune-stimulating effect, and so, for instance, it elevates the immunoglobulin A level in the throat – indispensable for an intact immune defense – by a factor of ten, thus having a very positive effect in children and teenagers who are susceptible to infection.

   In Germany, Mutaflor may be prescribed by health-plan doctors if the standard medications for ulcers colitis fail – i.e. it also has an anti-inflammatory effect. A 20-pack is generally enough to reestablish a healthy intestinal flora (the enteracoated capsules must be swallowed whole). It is important to also administer eubiotically active agents in order to at least temporarily simulate a healthy intestinal flora, so that the fastidious Mutaflor bacterium has a chance of getting a foothold. The best therapy consists in parallel administration of Hylak plus. For financially strapped patients, Kanne Brottrunk (bread drink) and/or bio-yogurt (less effective) from a health food store can be prescribed. It is sometimes necessary to repeat the therapy after three or six months. By the way, Mutaflor cannot be stored in the refrigerator and it loses about 1% of its active bacteria per year when stored at room temperature. For small children, Mutaflor is available in suspension form.

2. **Overgrowth syndrome** (synonym: leaky gut syndrome) – recognizable by the organ test ampoule "Colon" or (if the case is more serious and the pathogens are situated in the sensitive absorbent part of the small intestine) the organ test ampoule "Jejunum/ileum" and the positive response to dysbiosis agents such as *Saccharomyces cervesiae* (Perenterol). The optimal therapy consists of *Saccharomyces boulardi* (Perenterol, Perocur, 2 capsules daily) and natural disinfectants such as garlic (3-4 cloves pressed into a glass of milk with honey). In severe cases one can, in the initial phase, administer a week of Metronidazol 25 g (Clont, Trichex, 2 x 1). Sulfredox is also quite effective. In some stubborn cases, I noted surprising improvement after enteroscopy, which evidently can be traced back to the preceding radical cleansing. I therefore occasionally prescribe preparations such as X-Prep with good results, or use colonic hydrotherapy. Also, swelling substances such as Indian flea seed (psyllium) (Mucofalk) from and cleansing agents such as Luvos-Heilerde (healing soil) are often very useful. For all kinds of ailments, members of primitive tribes eat silicate-containing and clayey soil.

    If the test ampoule *Saccharomyces boulardii* responds, that usually indicates the presence of a predominantly toxic anaerobic organism (e.g. Pseudomonas, clostridium etc.) which makes the intestinal walls permeable, making it easier for intestinal toxins to get into the intestinal tract. Even a normal intestine contains enough toxins to kill a number of persons. A healthy intestinal wall can see to it that these toxins do no damage. Administering *Saccharomyces boulardii* can markedly reduce the number of toxic anaerobes. This substance was discovered at the beginning of the previous century in Southeast Asia by an expedition. It was given to ailing expedition members by a local medicine man, originally in the form of a beer-like liquid served in a gourd. Expedition leader Hansen was so impressed by the therapeutic effect that he brought the dried liquid back to Europe and had it produced commercially. Today, it is a standard remedy the world over for infant diarrhea, but is also very effective for patients with a permeable intestine. These are very often patients who have had symptoms for decades whom nobody had been able to help so far. This is easily understandable, since the toxic anaerobes don't disappear on their own. Along with *Saccharomyces boulardii*, one can also administer Hylak plus. I have also recommended milk-fermented sauerkraut (health food store) as well as copious amounts of garlic. Often after treatment of a porous intestine (leaky gut), intestinal flora need to be built up again with Mutaflor at the next therapy session.

3. **Fungal infestation**, particularly by mucous-membrane-invasive pathogens, recognizable with the organ test ampoule "Colon" and a positive response to Nystatin or – in the case of an invading pathogen – by systemic anti-mycotics. Unlike the conventional wisdom, it seems to me that the pathology often does not result from supposed surface mucous-membrane colonization, but rather conditioned above all by the mucous-membrane invasiveness of the pathogen. In these cases, the fungi sit in the mucous membrane and from there disrupt the entire milieu. Based on patient histories the actual causes of the invasion of the mucous membrane are times of exhaustion and increased stress (cortisone secretion!). Once the fungi have gotten into the mucous membrane, one normally can no longer get rid of them.

Patients with intestinal fungal infestations are usually long-term beset by paralyzing weariness and also often have hypoglycemic attacks provoked by the sugar-stealing fungi. Many patients complain, regarding their weight, of "blowing up like yeast dough" even though they hardly eat anything – which is understandable because of the disrupted barrier of the intestinal wall. Also typical is hypersensitivity to alcohol due to constant overstress on the liver, which is burdened by the overproduction of intestinal toxins. Added to this is a general hyperacidity triggered by histamine release in the inflamed intestines. All in all, these patients suffer severe hyperacidity of the entire metabolic system, along with complaints of tension and, revealingly, often a yellowish-greasy coating on the rearmost third of the tongue (colon reflex field).

Oral Amphotericin lozenges have proven themselves therapeutically, also adding 2-3 weeks of Nystatin with Kanne Brottrunk (bread drink) (1 full shot glass twice daily). The patient should eat few sweets, but not totally eliminate them, since otherwise the fungi, in their search for sugar, will turn into mucous-membrane invasive pathogens! In moderate to severe cases (about 70-80% of patients) I briefly administer one week of systemic antimycotics such as itraconazole (Tempera or Sporanox, 1x1) and then after four weeks an additional week so as to prevent recidivism from spores (e.g., recognizable due to the fact that itraconazole tests out excellently and brings the Vital readings up to 100% as long as the corresponding symptoms are there). After that, the intestinal flora should be built up to restore good mucous-membrane protection (as described under Point 1).

Because of the tight coupling between **intestinal peristalsis** and the autonomous nervous system, adjuvant PSE therapy has proven to be highly beneficial, as the following case shows.

> **• Case study**
> A 68-year-old woman has suffered from constipation since childhood. Sometimes she goes an entire week without a bowel movement, and she then feels (in her own words) "miserable as a dog"; at such times she reaches desperately for laxatives even though she knows that they don't do her any good. She has undergone thorough internal examinations a number of times without anything having been found outside of some diverticulum. In an energy test using the REBA Test Device, I get low Vital and Emotional readings of around 30% (normal is 100%). A conflict is found in the second energy center with the theme "Hectic". She confirms that, despite her outward serenity, she is constantly restless and driven inside. Besides the appropriate Emvita 5 and Chavita 2 drops, I recommend stool-softening milk sugar (lactose, several teaspoons of Eugalan Töpfer, say, in muesli) as well as mechanically-acting Glycilax suppositories for emergencies. In exchange for this, she must for her part promise to stay away from the laxatives and to eat enough apricots to offset the loss of potassium. In the organ test, the bile ducts also respond – a finding more common in constipation sufferers (bile acts as as a laxative, backed-up bile as a constipator). For this I prescribe liver-gallbladder drops from Cosmochema and recommend a bitter spicy high-fat diet (such as olive oil, eggs more often etc.).
> I see her again four months later; her constipation is better, but not gone. Now, a conflict with the theme "Tense" responds in the sixth energy Center. In the organ test, the ampoule jejunum/ileum responds as the expression of disturbed intestinal flora and is compensated by Mutaflor in the remedy test. Once again, it takes an additional four months of homeopathic remedies to eliminate the conflict. She then reports that, for the first time in her life, the constipation is permanently gone (follow-up observation time: 24 months).

In cases of **dietary intolerance**, one very often finds disturbed intestinal flora, and when these get better, dietary intolerance is often reduced and sometimes even eliminated. To the patient, the pathological process can be likened to a sunburn, where even the light touch of a shirt on the skin is unpleasant. An irritated intestinal wall reacts in a comparably sensitive manner to all kinds of dietary components, just as the sunburned skin does – which, however, has nothing to do with the diet itself, but rather primarily with the irritated intestinal wall.

Often, a widespread mild gluten sensitivity, lactose intolerance or intolerance to wheat-germ lectin (found in the outer layer of wheat kernels, i.e. in whole wheat) is taken by some naturopathically-oriented colleagues as a reason to categorically ban milk and wheat, simply because they had previously responded in the remedy test. In these cases, the actual causes are often overlooked, namely intestinal flora dysbioses and energy blocks triggered by emotional conflicts and, for instance, geopathy. Once the actual disturbance sources are eliminated, most of the dairy products such as yogurt and buttermilk, and wheat (which has been ground, and is therefore lower in lectin) are then tolerated with no problem.

One comes to the realization that there is a gradation of the significance of disturbance factors which one absolutely must be aware of in order not to be misled into error. Unfortunately, this is much harder to do in naturopathic medicine than in mainstream medicine, because one is dealing with significantly more complex harmful factors. Nevertheless, naturopathic medicine has primary causal and less important secondary disease causes, which need to be kept apart in order not to be misled and give patients bad advice.

At this point, I would like to mention the AutoColi vaccine (additional information available at http://sym-biovaccin.de or www.amt-herborn.de cash) which, although it does not directly influence the intestinal flora, nevertheless has something to do with it. The indications are recurring urinary tract infections whose colonization often takes place via endogenous E. coli bacteria. Inoculation with endogenous E. coli bacteria has a high success rate of over 90%. A nasal spray bottle has recently become available.

10.5.2 Bile duct dysfunction

The gallbladder test ampoule contains both the extrahepatic and intrahepatic biliary tracts. The ampoule responds for roughly every third patient and is therefore, alongside intestinal-flora dysbiosis, the commonest disorder among the functional stresses. In mainstream medicine, the disease picture of disturbed bile flow is virtually unknown and is considered to be historically passé – which I believe is a very big mistake. To be clear: this has nothing to do with physically stressful gallstones or the like.

This has to do with functional disturbances of intrahepatic bile flow, in which congestions and small concretions turn out to be disruptive; this then negatively affects the liver cells, which can be considered to be the organism's big chemical factory, which explains the very broad effect of disrupted bile flow. In addition, bile flow disruptions result in parasympathetic dysfunctions such as vertigo, susceptibility to cramps, e.g. in the form of migraines, spastic constipation, cold extremities, feeling unwell and suchlike. Added to this are negative repercussions for digestion as well as cholesterol and hormonal metabolism in general, but also lipid digestion and mineral metabolism.

A popular saying gets it right when it says that "good medicine is bitter medicine", because bitter substances stimulate bile flow. In folk medicine, bile-stimulating substances such as Swedish bitters and bitter dietary aperitifs such as Campari, Aperol and the like have established themselves. Morning coffee with the breakfast eggs, like stomach bitters after lunch are proven choleretics intended to stimulate bile flow in the biliary system. However, in many cases these home remedies are not enough, and so more effective medications are needed.

Humoral medicine (the ancient medicine of Galen) represents buried medical treasure in the European Occident; in it, the gallbladder plays a central role. It is no accident that this ancient medicine talks about Melancholics and Cholerics (from Greek *chol*, gall or bile). Compared with Asiatic ancient medicine (TCM, Ayurveda), humoral medicine may be considered to be of equal rank, but unfortunately has to date been totally overlooked by Europeans and Americans. In this context, I'd like to call attention to the highly readable books of the well-known Viennese gynecologist Bernhardt Aschner [4]. He was the great rediscoverer of the old European humoral medicine who, during and after World War II, enjoyed great success in his New York practice with these old procedures, particularly with respect to bile flow and metabolic stimulation.

In my experience, disrupted bile plays a role in about half of migraine cases, numerous shoulder and neck tensions as well as hip problems and numerous other disturbances such as many forms of low blood pressure and stubborn cases of ill humor. Pathophysiologically dependent on the bile ducts are: cholesterol and steroid synthesis, the parasympathetic system, above all of course the liver as the organism's largest chemical factory, as well as numerous lipophilic vitamins and minerals, plus energetically the gall meridian – all of which makes understandable the broad-spectrum of disease effects.

For me, a simple yet effective bile-duct therapy continues to be an unsolved problem: the bile capriciously demands ever new cholagogic plant tinctures and homeopathic complexes which promote bile flow. Some simple recipes include Legapas drops in a sub-threshold non-laxative dosage (e.g. 5 drops in the morning diluted in some water), plus liver-gall drops from Cosmochema (10 drops twice daily). One should check out various bitter-substance drugs and homeopathic complexes to find out which mixture works best (which often changes after a few months). The highly-advertised therapies of the biologist Hulda Clark or the naturopath Andreas Moritz sound very promising, but I've had little experience with them. Besides, a few of Clark's patients continue to exhibit bile duct disorders in the energy test despite administration of their agents.

10.5.3 Pancreatic functional disorder

Despite its tucked-away location and frequent lack of symptomatology, the pancreas is enormously significant in many chronic ailments and metabolic disorders. First of all, it has to do with a disturbed pacemaker function for the digestive complex, and additionally a trigger function for acid-base metabolism. it is no accident that the two liters daily of pancreatic juice have a high bicarbonate content. In addition, the pancreas has an interesting relationship to the skin, presumably because skin and pancreatic enzymatic functions proceed in a very similar manner. Many eczema patients exhibit an energetically disturbed pancreas, and as soon as normal pancreatic function is restored, the eczema amazingly disappears as well. Added to this is a close relationship to the vegetative nervous system, which can be seen in the fact that the vagus nerve directly influences the pancreas. Therefore, patients with disrupted pancreatic function often have a disturbed vegetative system – for instance, neurodermitis patients.

As with the gallbladder, there are for the pancreas no simple prescription recommendations, which means that you have to look at the products of companies such as Pascoe, Heel, Nestmann, Madaus etc. for mixtures that work. Among the botanical agents, one might consider Harongan as well as enzymes such as Wobenzym, Enzym-Harogan etc.

10.6 Chronic foci

Chronic inflammatory processes are known as "Foci". A distinction is made between **cranial and pelvic foci**, of which the former includes paranasal sinuses, teeth and tonsils, and the latter the appendix as well as the prostate and adnexa. The consequences of foci are so dramatic that they cannot be assessed highly enough. For instance, the well-known biologically-oriented oncologist Josef Issels once observed the immediate disappearance of cancerous metastases after removal of a severe tonsillar focus [170]. The naturopathic dentist Ernesto Adler [1] reported sudden miraculous cures to dental cleansing, such as extremely psychotic psychiatric patients, hospitalized for many years, normalizing from one hour to the next, or wheelchair-bound paralytic persons being able to leave their wheelchair standing in the corner. I can testify to similar results, and have seen it for some patients after dental cleansing, although it occurs relatively seldom.

Many focal cleansers report modest success – which brings me to the sore point when it comes to focal cleansing. Because it is predominantly an "art" (i.e. a skill), at least in the area of dentistry, success and failure often lie close together. Many dentists have tried to attack the problem with radical exodontia ("Everything comes out!"), but this comes to grief due to the fact that cleansing often takes place all around the focus but not the focus itself. Basically, the rule of thumb is that, for serious chronic ailments such as MS-focalized teeth, they more likely should be radically removed, whereas in milder cases, as well as for younger persons (less than 50 years old), a more conservative cleansing and a gentler approach such as root resection, is recommended. PSE therapists should therefore be particularly choosy in selecting dental "focal cleansers"; the professional associations of biological dentists would be the first places to look.

10.6.1 Chronic sinusitis

Chronic sinusitis is often not noticed at all, though it can last for years and even decades. At some point, the patient gets an antibiotic prescription for acute sinusitis, but follow-up checks are skipped or bungled and the inflammation turns chronic. A shadowy area in the sinus X-rayss, noticed by chance, is often not followed up on – mostly because chronic sinusitis generates few symptoms, and specific complaints such as pressure in the head, stopped-up nose, hyposmia, purulent discharge and the like are lacking. Typical overall symptoms, often not associated with sinusitis, include long-term fatigue, cervical spine tension, heightened allergy susceptibility, manifold immunological disorders, worsening of pulmonary ailments such as asthma or chronic bronchitis. Ultimately, there is hardly any disease that is not made worse by chronic sinusitis and can also be influenced thereby.

Indications of chronic sinusitis include some well-known clinical findings such as pain on percussion of division II of the trigeminal nerve and a purulent mucus trail in the throat, but these are often not present. Often, chronic sinusitis is also responsible for persistent exhaustion states and lowered resistance. When chronic bronchitis or bronchial asthma is present, one should always consider sinusitis (sinobronchitis) because of the uniform reaction of the mucus-membrane/pulmonary tract any bacteria that might wander in! A response from the test ampoule "Sinuses" then confirms the sinusitis hypothesis. If the X-ray findings are unremarkable for the maxillary and frontal sinuses, one should look into the concealed decidual-membrane and sphenoidal sinuses, which are often overlooked.

Besides sometimes indispensable antibiotics, acute sinusitis can be handled very well with essential oils such as Gelomyrtol, Japanese Healing Plant Oil, as well as Sinupret and Sinuselect. Inhalation and sniffing with isotonic saline solution has also proven very useful ("nasal shower"). The best human results that I've seen in the majority of chronic sinusitis cases have been with the loofah sponge (Chapter 19.4), which should be applied once a week for four weeks. The loofah cucumber, a South American folk remedy, was discovered after World War II by a German naturopath. The plant contains essential oils which, due to their high volatility, are released when boiled, thereby artificially inducing sniffles, which stops the chronic inflammatory process of sinusitis – almost always long-term successfully.

> **• Using the loofah sponge**
> On Saturday or Sunday morning (during the day, one can then have sniffles for the entire day!), steep 1/4 of a *Loofah purgans* in a quarter cup of boiling hot water. Strain and let sit for a while. Using a cotton swab, sniff up the liquid into both nostrils, making sure that no loofah drops get into the throat or esophagus, because they could cause an unpleasant irritation there.

The loofah cure has a high success rate of over 95% (as published in the *German Journal of General Medicine*). The loofah cure is of course ineffective in cases of allergic rhinitis because that involves a different pathological mechanism. In my opinion, there are no alternative therapeutic options when it comes to efficacy, for instance homeopathic loofah, which is largely ineffective. Loofah is very reasonably priced, besides which using this therapy supports the Indios in South America who harvest these plants (reference: www.loofah.de/). One quarter of the sponge is used and briefly brewed in some liquid. Sniffing up the cooled liquid artificially induces cleansing sniffles which last a few hours. Afterwards, the sinusitis goes away, often for years; if necessary, the loofah cure and be repeated at any time with no problem. Still, one should wait a little while (about 6 to 8 weeks) before repeating it, so as not, in an extreme case, to provoke iatrogenic sinusitis.

10.6.2 Dental foci

The most important dental focus is **chronic mandibular ostitis**, which mostly appears after a root resection, and occasionally after tooth extraction and as chronically inflamed mandibles in the 8th region as a problem of the retained tooth. Ostitis is most common after a root canal operation. Since, when removing the root, the finely-branched vessels of the nerve root cannot be completely removed since this is anatomically quite impossible, this triggers bacterial decomposition processes in what remains of the dead nerve. The toxic byproducts thereof then run down the root canal, ultimately leading to chronic ostitis in the surrounding bone tissue. The crux of the matter is an incorrect radiological depiction of the chronic mandibular inflammation, which, thanks to leukocytes containing heavy metals, often simulates normal density (according to Dr. Johannes Lechner) and is therefore frequently overlooked.

> • Note
> **Chronic mandibular ostitis**
> Sometimes also known as NICO (Neuralgia Inducing Cavitational Osteonecrosis). In patients with trigeminal neuralgia who have died, pathologists have found osteonecrosis of the mandible, which is said to have irritated the trigeminal nerve. According to Haley of the University of Kentucky, the bacteria of mandibular ostitis are thought to generate extremely poisonous toxins: "Some of the most toxic substances known to man." (cited from [86])

Therefore, complementary-medicine energetic test procedures are utilized to arrive at a correct diagnosis, starting with the ostitis nosode of electroacupuncture and going on to the organ test ampoule "Tooth" (which by the way, also specifically contains mandibular bone in addition to tooth bone). Since further clarification is not possible in a general-medicine practice, such patients should be referred to a holistically oriented dentist who has the proper specialist knowledge (addresses available at www.gzm org). One machine-aided option is the ultrasound device Cavitat, which can image osteolytic necrotic regions. When correctly cleansed, the test ampoule "Tooth" in the energy test no longer responds, and the patient's corresponding complaints have improved or entirely disappeared.

10.6.3 Chronic tonsillitis

The tonsils are an additional important focus in the cranial region. Because there are so many tonsil abscesses in poorly vascularized regions, the organism is unable to rid itself of them through self-healing processes. In my experience, chronic tonsillitis almost always leads, due to the inflammatory reaction, to small tonsils, meaning that large, easily movable tonsils are seldom focalized. From the outside, tonsil foci often look quite normal.

Recurring throat and tonsil inflammations, as well as deeply pressure-sensitive areas of the angle of the mandible in the tonsil region, provide further indications. An elevated Streptolysin titer and elevated C-reactive protein, as well as being symptom-free after a neural-therapeutic spray of the tonsillar poles, are additional indications. Chronically inflamed tonsils should almost always be removed and can very seldom be rescued. Lymphatic agents such as Lymphomyosot, Lymphdiaral and embrocations of the lymph nodes in the neck with Unguentum lymphaticum are very useful, but only as pre- and post-treatment. Also demonstrably useful are the stimulating influences of seaside climate as well as all kinds of thermal fortifying (sauna, Kneipp).

10.6.4 Chronic appendicitis

In the introductory chapter about the Organ Test Kit, I described an impressive but atypical case of chronic appendicitis. It mostly has to do with a chronic appendix inflammation, usually based on severe dysbiosis complicated by deposited coproliths, mechanical constrictions and chronic infections. For an estimated 7% of those who sometime in their life suffer from appendicitis, one should expect that about 1.5-2% of them will have chronic appendicitis, which corresponds in Germany to the population of a middle-sized town. Many of these people have focally-conditioned symptoms having to do with various ailments such as exhaustion, feeling unwell, skin eczema, constipation, headaches etc. Very few patients have recurring pains in the right lower abdomen, which means that most patients are therefore not diagnosed at all or are misdiagnosed. Experience tells us that a chronically inflamed appendix is among the most severe foci there are, which makes the entire situation downright tragic: often it is only nontraditional methods such as PSE which help to show the correct hypothesis and how to tackle the problem in a causal manner.

As a counter-reaction to the appendectomy rage of earlier times, the diagnosis of chronic appendicitis has fallen into disrepute, and it takes an open-minded surgeon – or a patient who can credibly tell the surgeon about recurring appendicitis attacks – for the diagnosis to be made. Before considering the operation, one should first try dysbiosis therapy and PSE, since both have proven quite effective. In addition, Belladonna Similiaplex 20 drops twice daily (OP Pascoe) is very helpful in trying to possibly rescue the inflamed appendix – and, of course, something with a draining effect such as Lymphomyosot 20 drops twice daily (OP Heel) as well.

If the test ampoule Appendix responds, then it might sometimes be a case of inflamed diverticulitis instead of appendicitis, which occurs particularly among older persons. Since chronically inflamed diverticulitis calls for a different procedure, one should be aware of this differential diagnosis, so as not to take the wrong path or mention the differential diagnosis on the referral form.

10.6.5 Pelvic foci (ovaries/uterus/prostate)

One big problem for men is **chronic prostatitis** – mostly on the basis of prostate hypertrophy and dysbiosis – in which the pelvic diaphragm acts as a sludge trap for intestinal toxins. Unfortunately, the prostate exerts a remote effect on the entire organism, in particular via the above/below coupling in the cranial region. (Examples include stroke susceptibility, eye ailments and headaches.) Therefore, in every case involving apoplexy or TIA, one should first take a look at the prostate. In apoplexy or TIA cases, I strongly favor Phenprocoumon long-term therapy (Marcu-Mar), which brings the recidivism risk down to nearly nil. Phytotherapy with saw palmetto, pumpkin and rye pollen has proven effective in prostatitis cases, e.g. Cernilton 2x2 and Talso Uno 1x1 for six months. In cases of bacterial colonization of the prostate, there's nothing like a 10- to 20-day Ciprofloxacin cure at a high dosage of 500 mg twice daily, with Metronidazol to ward off anaerobic co-infection.

In younger females, the problems are **chronic adnexitis** (warning: Chlamydia) and endometriosis; for older females, they are prolapse of the uterus and enlarged *Uterus myomatosus*. In these cases, the organ test ampoules "Ovary" or "**Uterus**" respond. In this context, the uterus is not an inflammation focus, but rather mostly a mechanical problem which stresses the energetic bad-weather area of the abdominal region. As we know, so-called "kundalini energy" is located in the first Chakra, and anyone who subjectively suffers from an oversized and/or displaced uterus often has consequent effects as well in the form of chronic exhaustion and similar psychoenergetic sequelae.

Since therapy must be precisely tailored to each individual, there can be no general therapy recommendations. The following have proven their worth: Agnolyt, Lamioflur, Gynaecoheel, Aletris Similiaplex, and Horvi and Sanum agents. Sometimes "Ovary" also responds in cases of severe hormonal deficiency. Although menopausal complaints in the majority of females are not only hormonally conditioned and very often have emotional causes as well, about 10% need a multi-month course of hormonal support, for example with Presomen, a biological hormone from pregnant mares, or locally applied estrogen salves (Linoladiol etc.). Women with a need for hormonal replacement can be identified by the fact that they react with radical mood improvement to the administration of hormones; evidently, their brain has an unusually high hormonal sensitivity.

10.7 Filtering

Filtering is a test technique originally developed by HW Schimmel for the Vegatest method.

The basic principle of filtering is simple:

Step 1: two ampoules independently test positive (for example, they both trigger a difference in the kinesiological arm-length test). This applies to ampoules with diagnostic or therapeutic significance.

Step 2: if one now places one of the ampoules in the Yin region (as if the organ were healthy, as if the remedy were taken), the second ampoule above, placed in the REBA Test Device, no longer tests out.

Step 3: there is a diagnostic or therapeutic statement depending upon the specific ampoule in question.

Diagnostic filtering with organ ampoules can detect causal linkages and derive therefrom prognoses for the respective ailment. Filtering should be logical, i.e. that disturbed intestinal flora or chronic inflammation such as dental foci, tonsils, sinuses exacerbate chronic bronchitis or asthma, whereas the inverted sequence makes absolutely no pathophysiological sense and therefore should not be tested for.

With the organ ampoule in the Yin region, one proceeds as if the disturbance in question were already gone. One can then, from

- the non-response of a previously positive organ test ampoule,
- the improvement of the *Acidum lacticum* ampoule and
- the improvement of the test values from the REBA Test Device

determine how strong the disturbance is.

In therapeutic filtering, a remedy is placed in the Yin region, where it acts as if it had been taken. When a particular organ thereupon no longer tests out in the REBA Test Device, then the remedy is empirically strong enough to be effective. Therapeutic filtering can evaluate whether an already tested-out PSE therapy is enough by itself to markedly improve a particular organ, or whether one has to add additional therapies. For many ailments, a number of different remedies are administered together to make a "drug cocktail", i.e. in cases of cardiac insufficiency digitalis, beta blockers as well as calcium antagonist etc. One then places all the remedies together in the Yin zone: if then the organ Heart no longer tests out, then the drug cocktail will be enough; however, if it continues to respond, it is necessary to keep on looking.

10.7.1 Filtering with organ ampoules

There are certain ampoules such as Joints, Skin, Kidneys etc. that are meant only for filtering. For instance, for a patient X, one can place a specific combination in the Yin region, say a particular Emvita and Chavita which test positive on the patient, adding Geovita for geo-radiation stress (which also responded) and for suspicion of a dental focus (represented by the Oregon test ampoule "Tooth"). Next, one can check whether the aforementioned combination (or parts of it) energetically compensates a particular organ such as skin for an eczema patient: if so, then the Skin organ test ampoule previously placed in the REBA Test Device would no longer respond, meaning the eczema would be energetically compensated. In this manner, one can determine which optimal therapy and procedural method are needed for a particular disease picture. Experience has shown that complete energetic compensation means that the self-healing powers will often be strong enough to make healing possible.

In a comparable manner – i.e. by means of a precisely-tailored remedy test – I have:

- For patients with *Helicobacter pylori* infestation, several years before publication of the famous French system involving Omeprazol, Clarithromycin and Amoxicillin I tested my patients with an identical scheme which I had found through the energy test alone. I simply had to place the Stomach ampoule in the device, which had previously tested positive and served as indicator. I then had to search through various antibiotic combinations until the Stomach ampoule no longer responded;
- for a patient on dialysis, who for years had had double to triple the normal creatinine value, I was able to completely normalize his kidney results in a few months solely with a perfectly testing Spenglersan D;

- for a female patient confined to a wheelchair for years due to severe rheumatic pain, dental cleansing made it possible for her to leave the wheelchair and walk, pain-free, on her own two feet through her Alpine village.

There are many such examples which at times seem like biblical miracles, and that make it clear that energy tests are indispensable when posing many kinds of questions. One can see here that energy tests can help therapists along even in conventional medicine, regardless of whether one is looking for an appropriate contraceptive pill, appropriate chemotherapy or whatever. Now of course testing is not enough, and it calls for the necessary medical expertise, which is then, so to speak, potentiated by testing as a curative agent, as one gains new insights. Yet at the same time, one should guard against overvaluing the remedy test and thereby giving patients unwarranted hope. The diagnostic and therapeutic potential of the remedy test is sizeable but, as with any medical procedure, there are no guarantees.

10.8   Therapy conclusion

From the standpoint of testing, mesenchymal therapy with the Organ Test Kit is finished when only high potentiations of *Acidum lacticum* and no organ ampoules respond anymore, the Vital and Emotional REBA Test Device readings are at 100% and, last but not least, the patient no longer has any bothersome symptoms. In the darkfield microscope one sees a normal picture and the patient feels normal. If, at the follow-up check, the *Acidum lacticum* ampoule responds at level 0 or level I, this means that the milieu is normal again and that the treatment has come to a successful end. To be doubly sure, one can recheck the previously tested organ test ampoule to see whether any post-treatment might be necessary.

Naturally, the patient's symptoms also play a role in the evaluation – but for me, the test result is the deciding factor. For example, if a patient with irritable colon still has residual symptoms even though the test ampoule "Colon" no longer responds, then it will usually be because of vegetative/energetic causes rather than genuine dysbiosis. One can then reassure the patient and assure him that he has already got successfully past a sizeable hurdle on the road to healing. As a rule, then, any residual symptoms can be banished by psychoenergetic post-treatment such as conflict dissolution, as well as an intestine-friendly lifestyle with lots of activity, Mediterranean diet etc.

Part 3
Clinical practice

11   Using Psychosomatic Energetics Correctly

In the following chapter, I describe the practical application of Psychosomatic Energetics (PSE), its advantages and disadvantages, and how the tester should work with it. In the chapter on the historical development of PSE, I had already described the most important components of the method, and I will expand on that here, which inevitably entails a certain amount of repetition. In what follows, I would also like to give some practical recommendations for applying the method in everyday clinical practice, introduce the Chavita plus agents and answer the most important questions from users. Added to this are some proven method-independent therapeutic strategies from naturopathic practice.

11.1   Test site prerequisites

Energy testing calls for an undisturbed tester's energy field. As was shown in Fig. 3.1, a tester tests a patient's energy field (Aura) with the aid of their own energy field. Logically, the tester's energy field should be as neutral and uninfluenced as possible, so that it may serve as a true mirror for the patient's energetic reactions. Since it is such an important point, I hereby repeat that the tester needs to be free of conflicts and other energy blocks.

The energy fields of all persons involved – patient as well as therapist – is massively disrupted by geo-radiation, so the testing site should absolutely be free of geo-radiation. I advise leaving this important work to a good dowser, who can also keep a lookout for electrosmog, which is alsp disruptive. Regarding electrosmog, this also includes the testing site being free of electrosmog-radiating cell phones, laptops, tablets or PCs, all of which should be at least 4 to 6 feet away from the testing site. Wi-Fis and other transmitters should as much as possible be 30 feet away or more, and the overall geo-radiation-stress should be as low as possible.

At the testing site, noise and strangers with their energy field are likewise undesirable; in the case of children, the mother can sit 4 to 6 feet away, maintaining eye contact, which is trouble-free even for two-year-olds. Unfamiliar surroundings, commotion and time pressure are also enemies of good test results – testing should be done at a familiar and well-known location, where one can be relaxed and in a neutral mood, whereby a clear and alert yet meditative temperament is best. The test site should be clean, orderly, well-lit and pleasant, without too many medications and other energetically disruptive devices in the immediate vicinity.

11.2   Patient prerequisites

Patients do not need to heed any particular instructions before PSE testing. Since the energy readings are pretty stable, a stressful drive to the examination, for instance, does not lead to any significant alteration of the results. Medications can be taken at the usual time. It is a good idea to bring regularly taken medications to the examination, so that they may be tested. During the examination, cell phones should be turned off and kept at least 6 feet away from the examination site. Most jewelry is energetically neutral, but amber necklaces or bracelets might occasionally have an energetically weakening effect. The same applies for jewelry that has energetically effective symbols: jewelry is taken off and tested prior to testing and then tested when it is put back on again at the Vital and Emotional levels at the end of the session. Piercings can sometimes be very energetically disruptive, which can be seen if one briefly removes them and then retests the energy readings.

11.3   Tester prerequisites

Testing ability in energy-medicine tests depends on innate talent: a third of the people may be considered to be good to very talented, another third are average and trainable, a quarter are little talented and about 1 in 10 are not suitable. One can find this out fairly easily, for instance at a kinesiology weekend course or during the practical work at PSE courses, and in the event of a lack of talent, one should use other methods. Within limits, testing ability can be trained and improved. In this process, it is important to gauge one's testing relative to objectively verifiable facts as well as other good and reliable testers, plus constantly refining and learning. One often sees the greatest deviations particularly when it comes to the Mental and Causal values (personal as well as conflict values), presumably because the higher frequencies are harder to test. In this case, it is recommended to use good testers as a gauge and to learn from their test results.

Using Psychosomatic Energetics Correctly

> In my experience, basically all people can do energy testing, because it deals with a universal language in which our organism constantly reacts to stimuli, but not everyone can express it equally well. Universal triggers can be internal stimuli such as an unpleasant thought which makes us shudder, or external stimuli in the form of water-runs which, for example, can cause many a driver to jerk the steering wheel, such that certain stretches of highway accumulate accidents. Almost everyone reacts to strong geopathic disturbance zones; one can see this in bar patrons who have unwittingly sat down on geopathogenic zones – sometimes such persons gradually become pale and nervous, seem distracted or shift their barstool back and forth. In classes at school, the Austrian dowser Käthe Bachler has had the experience time and again that inattentive students are often seated on geopathic zones (cases of this kind are found in the books authored by the primary-schoolteacher Käthe Bachler [5] [6]). The examples can be extended at will.

Good testing calls for constant training as well as the ability to gather one's thoughts, as well as mental and physical self-discipline, living a healthy and well-balanced life in order to be in a good energetic state. People who have little energy and energy blocks of their own do worse at testing; conversely, the better their energy system, the smaller empirically the errors. Those who subscribe to crude ideological theories or are emotionally labile are seldom good testers: testers should be generally "well-grounded", psychologically and emotionally normal and be capable of clear thinking. There's a good reason why the best radiesthetes at the beginning of the 19th century were military or priests – both professions which characteristically call for discipline and concentration on the matter at hand.

Testers who naïvely trust their results are lacking necessary distance and tend to believe everything sight unseen. All testers make mistakes once in a while, and yet oddly enough some will believe that they are not among the fallible – which of course cannot possibly be right from a purely logical standpoint alone. Therefore one should, as a matter of principle, not just believe everything that one tests and critically question it, especially if peculiar and inconsistent results arise. On the other hand, those who are too suspicious from the outset and internally have not been able to build up any trust in their own testing ability will be unable to muster the necessary relaxed nature and psychoenergetic openness which good testers also have to have. How does one know that one is testing well? By having things turn out to be true that one had not known at the time of testing, or by having a patient bring in test results, from another tester, which have found out the same things.

Light-colored clothing made from natural fibers (cotton, linen, silk etc.) is more suitable for testing than dark colors or synthetics (because white has an energetically shielding effect, and natural fibers are generally more energetically positive). Testing is a meditative act calling for the right mixture of mental clarity and alertness along with a loose, relaxed attitude. In addition, testing calls for creative intelligence, the ability to think logically, a dash of intuition and a spiritual mindset. For example, when testing, one can call upon higher spiritual powers if one believes in such, or implement certain rituals – e.g. cleansing oneself energetically after every patient by washing one's hands in running water and/or brief phases of meditative relaxation.

In actual daily clinical practice, Psychosomatic Energetics is more demanding than it might seem at a casual glance, which is why nonverbally learning certain testing tricks and procedural approaches is indispensable. For instance, I have learned more in a few days of auditing famous colleagues such as Helmut W Schimmel than I could have learned from years of reading books. Like good cooks' "magic touch", it's the little incidentals, minor matters which, just like the overall psychoenergetic outlook of the role model, which can hardly be imparted verbally. Like every craft, therefore, Psychosomatic Energetics should be learned as a skill and then later exercised practically.

Imparting PSE results calls for a great deal of professional experience and a sure instinct on the part of the therapist, so it is no wonder that PSE is so highly regarded by my more experienced professional colleagues. The therapist needs a full measure of life experience, but also a certain psychological knack, in order to manage PSE with the assured touch of a master. PSE holds up to the patient an unvarnished mirror which makes negative personality traits visible, and this is not always a pleasant sight. For instance, overweight patients with a depressive exhaustion symptomatology find out that they have an unconscious conflict with the theme "Frustration". Not every patient is emotionally mature and open enough to recognize his own role in his destiny and then to make constructive use of this insight. Therefore, PSE is not suitable for all patients and it can represent an emotional challenge for many people.

11.4   Step one – patient questioning and examination

Before making use of special examination techniques such as PSE in a general-medicine practice, one talks with the patient for the anamnesis, what course the symptoms have taken and what their current status is, what meds are being taken (it's a good idea to have the meds brought in so that they may be tested at the end), what diagnoses have been arrived at and what is in the works from any others who are also administering treatment in parallel. Many patients have their medical papers with them, which makes things much easier. In short, one draws up a comprehensive representation of the entire clinical picture, and of course the patient's biography is part of this. If one is using PSE in as a special method in mainstream clinical practice, then the aforementioned preliminaries and pre-examinations have already been done – i.e. the patient is already well documented by conventional-medicine protocols and can be given a special PSE appointment.

The aforementioned pre-examination is important for two reasons: first, for general-medicine and formal-legal reasons, since, in order to continue to treat a patient correctly, it is necessary to know their current status and what is desired. Patients who have not had a mainstream-medicine pre-examination should be informed that PSE does not replace a conventional medicine consultation. Therefore, if a patient has had abdominal pains with weight loss for five years, he should be told that this should be cleared up using current mainstream-medical methods parallel to PSE, instead of treating him with alternative methods for years and then, as a complementary therapist, at some point possibly looking foolish and morally vulnerable because something crucial was overlooked. In short, PSE complements and supplements mainstream medicine, but does not fully replace it, and this should be communicated to the patient specifically and practically.

The second reason for a pre-examination is the subliminal influence on my test results – but also the conscious search for particular problems, to the extent that I have then learned what I would fail to do if I had known nothing about it. Let's start with the first point: every tester is subliminally influenced by patients and their case history. Critics will object that we only test what we expect anyway, but that just isn't so. One often gets unexpected test results which later turn out to be correct, for instance they agree with control checks involving clinical, X-Ray etc. findings. If everything were just a put-up job, then there could not be such a statistically unlikely pile-up of confirmatory data. Nevertheless, I maintain that every tester is influenced by patients and their case history, i.e. even so, the critics are a little right. But such suggestions can also be viewed positively and made productive use of, since the more I know about patients, the better I'll be able to test them.

11.5 Step two – testing the energy levels

Testing the energy levels can be designated as "**taking the energetic blood pressure**". As the blood pressure measurement reflects the heart/circulatory situation, the energy-level tests yield a good picture of the overall physical and psychoenergetic situation. Psyche, Soma and subtle energy thereby form a unified whole: whoever is emotionally sick – long-term unhappy and neurotic, say – is going to have poor energy readings. Whoever has a serious physical illness – advanced cardiac insufficiency, say – will likewise have poor energy readings. And whoever is energetically disturbed – is under severe stress from geo-radiation, say – will also have poor energy readings, will also feel bad (possibly irritable, tired) and can become long-term physically ill. It is then the task of the PSE therapist, above all to find out the energetic and emotional cause of the poor energy readings in order to then improve them through therapy.

As I said, the energy readings are relatively stable; I'd like to illustrate this with an example. An Australian colleague was tested by a female colleague at a seminar in Europe. When he took out his old seminar notes at the end of the day, he noted to his great surprise that the current results, including the conflict and its values, as well as the associated Chakra, agreed 100%, down to the fractional part, with the readings obtained exactly 12 months ago at a PSE seminar in Australia! He had not treated the conflict at that time for lack of proper medication. When the Australian colleague – who, as a scientifically trained physician could assess the full import of these results – became aware of the dizzying "coincidence", he was so agitated that he couldn't sleep for half the night.

> As a statistical check whether the Australian colleague's two sets of test results might be a mere coincidence, one multiplies together the ten 10% scales of the 4 Aura levels (10 x 10 x 10 x 10), then the 7 Chakras and 28 conflicts, and finally the 4 Aura levels of the conflict (10 x 10 x 10 x 10) resulting in the figure 19,600,000, which corresponds statistically to the number of experiments one would have to run to get the same results again by pure chance. One would have to test forever,

and measure the current world population three times over to come up with a comparable value through random chance.

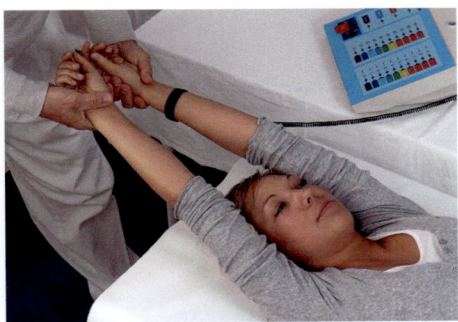

Fig. 11.1 – Typical PSE test situation: recumbent kinesiological arm-length test to test out the four subtle-energy levels; in the background the REBA® Test Device and the Test Kits.

PSE, as a naturopathic diagnostic and therapeutic procedure, serves to quantitatively test a patient's subtle-energy system, initially with the aid of the REBA Test Device (**cf. Fig. 11.1**). Man has four subtle-energy levels whose charge – like a battery's charge – serves as a reliable indicator of overall well-being and health (Chapter 3). Those with a lot of energy do and are well, those with little energy are or will become sick. As in Yoga and Traditional Chinese Medicine, PSE considers harmonious and vigorous life energy to be central to the maintenance of health. Sick and emotionally/physically weakened persons as a rule have diminished energy values, while healthy persons exhibit normal energy values.

From the standpoint of PSE, the cause of low energy values is mainly unconscious emotional conflicts which act as energy thieves. They can be tracked down with specific homeopathic compound agents (Emvita) and then eliminated by administration of the tested-out agents (Chapter 5). The normalization of energy values which this initiates then triggers emotional/physical self-healing processes. Briefly put, PSE can be designated as "psychotherapy with homeopathic drops", but besides their emotional effect, they can also have a positive effect on physical ailments.

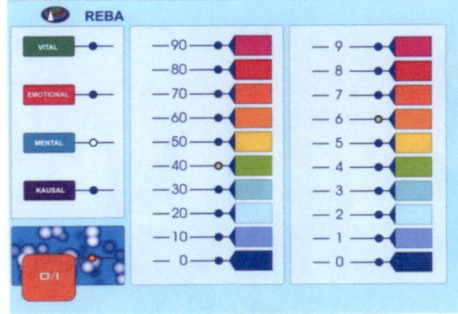

Fig. 11.2 – Front panel of the REBA® Test Device.

The REBA Test Device has four preselect switches for Vital, Emotional, Mental and Causal, which are tested out in sequence (**cf. Fig. 11.2**). There are two value ranges of 10% steps and 1% steps. One begins at zero and tests the 10% scale upward, at each step checking the patient's reaction, for instance whether, in the kinesiological arm-length test the position of the thumbs varies. If the difference in position is not just slight, but rather clearly evident (about 1-2 cm or more), this corresponds to the energy value on the current level. If there is no response at the 90% level, then testing continues on the 1% scale, and if there is no response at the top of this one, then the test has ended at 99% (rounded up to 100%). When all four levels have been tested, the test switches for Vital, Emotional, Mental and Causal are pressed once more to store the values, so they can be called back up in sequence and entered into a test protocol form. Any PSE therapist can understand the values entered into the protocol form, so that even if one goes to another therapist, the continuity of treatment is preserved.

The **normal values** are 100% Vital, 100% Emotional, 100% Mental and 40% Causal. This applies to healthy young to middle-aged persons who feel normal. Due to the age-dependent multi-morbidity of older persons of ca. 70-80 years of age, the normal values could well be be lower. Sometimes healthy patients come in to the practice, say at the wife's urging or out of curiosity, and ask to be tested with PSE. As a rule, one finds normal values for them, no disturbed energy center nor any conflict and no geopathy. Consequently, there is nothing for a therapist to do here and the PSE treatment is over.

> • **Note**
> In medicine, it's customary to use more extensive spot checks to pin down normal values and thereby validate them. This has so far only been possible for PSE with a very small spot check. As part of a doctoral dissertation involving 19 novices of the Zug ice hockey club, in 2008 Mr. H. P. Häfligeri Buchrain (Switzerland) had the opportunity to measure the average values of healthy persons (or at least the test subjects said they were healthy). The Vital reading was 92, the Emotional 84, Mental was 90 and the Causal value 57. One remark here: the investigator noticed, before testing began, that a number of these young men had very sweaty hands – a nonspecific sign of vegetative dysfunction. One might therefore well wonder whether all of the test subjects could be considered to be healthy.

By the way, the accuracy of PSE in distinguishing between sick and healthy persons seems to be quite good. In a non-selected average population one can expect that about 30-40% of those examined will have poor energy values (i.e. Vital or Emotional below 70% or less). In surveys taken by opinion research institutions, about 60-70% of the respondents feel well, which Psychosomatic Energetics can fully confirm from its examination results. I mention this because there are more than a few naturopathic diagnostic procedures according to which everybody is sick (Reminding one of the jocular adage that everyone is sick at some point if the doctor simply keeps on looking long enough.). I once heard from the inventor of electroacupuncture, Reinhard Voll, that he had only ever tested out fully normal values in some villagers in the Pyrenees Mountains who led very healthy lives, and that otherwise everybody he examined was sick to some degree. It seems to me that a diagnostic scheme that sensitive is too finely meshed if everybody tested gets caught up in it. On the other hand, other methods such as the usual mainstream-medicine investigative procedures (lab tests, X-Ray etc.) are too coarse, so that many people are declared a healthy even though they feel sick. The diagnostic "mesh size" of PSE, on the other hand, realistically reflects the subjective feelings of illness or health of many persons.

11.6 Step three – testing geopathy, Chakras and conflicts

After testing the four energy levels, the device is switched to 0.0 (usually Causal, since it was the last tested or whose value was retrieved.

One then tests whether the patient has geo-radiation stress, whether an energy center is disturbed, and if so, which emotional conflict is responsible. If an ampoule tests positive, it is put aside to be tested again at the end, so as to be sure. If an ampoule does not test out, it is put back in the test kit.

> **• Instructions**
> If a tester has a bad day or is a beginner, one can set the test device on the Vital or Emotional level 10-20% lower instead of zero/zero. To do this, the level at which the patient had previously exhibited the lower reading is selected – i.e. for Vital 70% and Emotional 30%, the device is set to Emotional 10%. This way, the patient is "shot at" with a slightly dissonance-inducing frequency and thereby rendered labile, which makes testing the ampoules easier (the way it is easier to tip a standing person over who is already unsteady).

Using the Basic Test Kit, one first checks whether

- the patient exhibits a test reaction to Geovita. This is the case in about 25-30% of patients, and even almost 100% for those with malignant diseases. In **Geopathy and Electrosmog** (Chapter 9), I described what one does in such a case. the ampoule Geovita will respond for geo-radiation or, if electrosmog is suspected, the test ampoule Phosphor D12 (in the Supplementary Test Kit) will respond.
- One then checks whether the patient has a disturbed energy center (Chakra); regarding this, see **Chakras as conflict storage** (Chapter 2.4) and **The seven chakras** (Chapter 4). Usually, only a single Chakra will respond.
- Finally, one checks which conflict tests positive. Since each energy center is associated with a specific list of conflicts (**cf. Fig. 2.11**), this reduces the number of possible conflicts, so only those conflicts need to be checked which belong to the Chakra in question: for instance, if Chakra 5 tests positive, only the Emotional remedies 17 and 18 are checked for a test reaction.

> - **Instructions**
> Those who test a lot and have no test device available (with built-in honeycomb) can get a simple chrome kidney dish (from any medical supply business) and attach a cable to it with an alligator clip; the other end of the cable can be mounted with an EKG hand electrode of the type that clamps to the wrist. Many EAV manufacturers also offer hand electrodes with attached honeycomb (second possibility). The actual reason for doing this is possible contamination of the test ampoules by the patient – fingerprints and the like – which can lead to imprecise test results. The experienced testing physician Dr. Dieter Aschoff therefore recommends regular cleaning of test ampoules with 70% ethanol. I would like to add my recommendation to replace frequently used test kits with new ones after a while, because it has been my experience that unavoidable pollution can lead to imprecise results.

Many testers test out the ampoules sequentially, while others feel that this influences them and so test them in random order. Each tester needs to find out which way feels best for them.

Practically all patients will turn out to have a disturbed Chakra and an associated conflict. The next testing step checks whether the found Chakra and Emotional remedies (possibly Geovita as well, if it tests positive) improve the energy readings. For this, the ampoules are placed in the Yin zone of the patient's pelvis (e.g. for males in the opening of a trouser pocket), which simulates taking the remedy. If there is a positive reaction to Geovita, this simulates the elimination of geopathic stress rather than taking a remedy. After the ampoules have been placed in the Yin region, the Vital and Emotional values are retested using the REBA Test Device; for males with low Mental readings possibly this energy level as well: if, after placement of the tested-out remedies, the readings markedly improve or even return to normal – which is usually the case – one can be confident that the tested remedies will be helpful.

11.6.1 Acute agents and masked anxiety disease

If the Vital and Emotional values at the location are not yet optimally compensated, the search can continue with the acute agents. The acute agents are used when corresponding symptoms are present – anxiety, neurological complaints, autonomous dysfunction – or when it is suspected that a masked anxiety disease might be present. This is more often the case than one might think, e.g. in cases of addiction as self-therapy, but also for many complaints which are not normally associated with anxiety disease.

With the passage of time, it has become increasingly evident that many patients with chronic exhaustion syndrome, pronounced vegetative dysfunctions such as irritable colon, sweating, cardiac arrhythmia as well as people with chronic pain likewise have anxiety disease, i.e. they respond to Anxiovita. When afterwards I query these patients more closely about fears and anxieties, they mostly tell me about generalized worries or apprehensions which are sociably acceptable, but hardly ever about specific anxieties. They have a feeling of being constantly driven and of tension, as well as pains and overall unwellness, whereas the underlying fears are often repressed and no longer perceived. However, if one keeps on asking more precisely, even here they will often tell of exaggerated fears and worries.

> • **Case study**
> **Generalized anxiety disease**
> Ms. S., a single 48-year-old secretary, has suffered for years from chronic exhaustion with vegetative complaints in the form of irritable colon and dizziness. She will not take psychotropic drugs, which don't really help anyway, and a course of treatment at a psychosomatic clinic yielded no improvement. Low Vital readings of 30% and Emotional 20% in psychoenergetic testing; the 6th Chakra responds with

> the conflict "Restless", Anxiovita tests positive. She says she often worries about losing her job and in general has trouble "switching off" and relaxing. After four months of therapy with the homeopathic compound agents Chavita 6, Emvita 22 and Anxiovita she feels considerably better, has more vitality, does things on her own in the evenings because she no longer comes home from the office so exhausted. According to her coworkers, she is more confident and assertive, and no longer worries about losing her job.

Children with Attention-Deficit/Hyperactivity Disorder (ADHD), learning disorders and diminished self-confidence often suffer from anxiety disease as well, as the following case history shows.

> **• Case study**
> 12-year-old Sara seems markedly younger than her actual age. According to the mother, she has had a handwriting deficiency since second grade, she cannot concentrate and gets words mixed up, and also complains often of headaches. Striking also is her extreme shyness in public, though she is completely normal at home. Therapy with the school psychologist has not changed anything. The psychoenergetic test reveals a strikingly low Emotional value of 30%. The conflict "Rushed" in the 5th Chakra responds, as does Anxiovita. In a conversation, she says that she is very afraid of exams, which evidently was not previously known, since the mother seemed very surprised. Prescribed Chavita 5, Emvita 18 and, initially, Anxiovita. At the follow-up check six months later, the mother reports that Sara is much more self-confident, her grades have improved and the headaches have gone away.

Fear has a psychoenergetically crippling effect which is exhausting over the longer term; it weakens self-confidence and the ability to concentrate the mind for very long and remain centered. Fear also has a great vegetative disruptive effect and evidently also elevates the pain threshold. Fear is a big energy thief and, in the background, successfully neutralizes all individual attempts to regain footing and self-regenerate. Many people unconsciously develop a denial strategy in which they refuse to believe or accept their fears, recasting them into socially acceptable feelings such as being worried.

Psychoenergetic testing shows that anxiety ailments turn up more frequently in clinical practice than is generally known. One often finds hidden anxiety disease particularly with problem patients who have disorders which are hard to treat, such as chronic vegetative exhaustion and pain states. The same goes for children and teenagers with learning and behavioral disorders. The discussion which is triggered by psychoenergetic testing often seems to act as a mini-psychotherapy and have a markedly unburdening function. In like manner, the dissolution of the underlying emotional conflicts with the aid of homeopathic compound agents (emotional remedies) is often very helpful. Based on experience to date with many hundreds of patients, the results seem to be sustained.

11.6.2 Remedy test

The remedy test simulates future healing and causes the organism to energetically behave as if the tested-out agents had already been taken. This is because, below the diaphragm – ideally in the pelvic region – applied test ampoules and remedies are energetically completely "resorbed" by the organism, as if the patient had already taken them. To do this, one places on the patient the found Geovita, Emvita etc. ampoules (in the side trouser pocket for men, waistband or skirt belt for women). Tell the patient what you're doing first, so as not to startle him or her. The energy values for the patient are then tested out, for example (Vital/Emotional/Mental/Causal in percent):

- Before 10/30/100/70 – with Geovita 100/100/100/70 = severe geopathy (which must be cleansed)
- Before 10/30/100/70 – with Geovita 30/50/100/70 = moderate geopathy (which doesn't have be cleansed immediately)
Or:
- Before 10/30/100/70 – with Emvita 9 100/100/100/70 = large conflict (which must be treated)
- Before 10/30/100/70 – with Emvita 9 30/50/100/70 = small conflict (which doesn't have to be treated immediately)

These examples make it clear that testers are normally only satisfied with significant healing affects. "Scratching together" tiny healing effects, Sisyphus-style, in order to thereby manage to garner larger effects – which I did for years on end as a Vegatest practitioner, back when testing was truly backbreaking work – is now, in light of the aforementioned procedure, a thing of the past. Because Psychosomatic Energetics almost always deals with large conflicts and strong geopathic effects, one obtains large, often downright fantastic effects with the remedy test. When the patient comes back for follow-up checking, one can thus very often determine that the remedy test enables one to make extraordinarily reliable "precision landings" – because the patient has almost always attained the targeted values (as long as no new conflicts have turned up)!

11.6.3   Organ Test Kit

For a patient with a long-term chronic ailment, one commonly uses the Organ Test Kit to look for hidden inflammation foci and functional organ stresses. Even when – using the remedy test with placement of the tested-out Emvita, Chavita etc. – no optimum compensation is attained and/or one gets the impression that the Organ Test Kit should be used for other reasons (such as a possible focus), one first checks with the lactic acid ampoules to see whether deep potentiations respond. If they do, then the most frequent organs are tested first: if, for example, Colon is found, one checks whether additional placement in the Yin region leads to Vital and Emotional norm values of 100%. The rest of the procedure has already been described in the Organ Test Kit chapter (10.4).

11.6.4   Testing other medications

As a matter of principle, PSE tries to make do with as few medications as possible because, among other things, experience has shown that patient compliance diminishes directly as the number of prescribed medications increases. Since most patients also take allopathic medications such as hypertension agents etc., one should really limit oneself to those few truly important points. This includes dissolution of the currently active conflict, elimination of geopathy, deactivation of chronic inflammatory foci and functional organ stresses. This procedure is successful for an estimated 98-99% of patients and promises good self-healing processes.

   It is fairly seldom necessary to go hunting for other medications. Detoxification of supposed deposits of heavy metals, parasites and the like, so often recommended by complementary doctors, has proven to be unnecessary in PSE. Therapists are of course free to go their own way, but the experiences of independent PSE therapists with thousands of patients have shown that the normal PSE procedural system is almost always sufficient; necessary detoxification processes take place on their own, so that one should limit oneself to the procedure described above.

Many patients come in with their pockets full of medications. It is a good idea to test them at the end of the PSE session: take them one at a time (for pills that are shrink-wrapped in aluminum foil, press the point out to make them testable) and place them in the test honeycomb of the REBA Test Device. To prevent the pills from falling down the shaft of the device, one can use a piece of notepaper as a covering. Medications which elicit no test reaction are empirically ineffective therapeutically and can be set aside. In most cases, of 20-30 dietary supplements, vitamins and various medications taken, only 2-3 preparations will respond. These are next placed in the Yin zone and checked to see how much they improve the Vital and Emotional readings. There are three therapeutic strengths (assuming the patient has a Vital and/or Emotional reading of 10-20%):

- Mild for 10-20% improvement
- Moderate for 30-40% improvement
- Severe for 50-90% improvement

When the energy readings are pretty good, it's hard to test for therapeutic strength because the improvement is so small – e.g. if the patient's readings are at 80%, then the improvement is perforce limited to a maximum of 20% before it hits the 100% reference value. Now, if the difference is so slight then, logically, one cannot know whether one is dealing with a weakly or strongly effective therapeutic agent. Hence one unfortunately cannot differentiate between various agents, but this does not empirically crop up very often. Well-tested PSE agents usually exhibit strong improvements, as does Geovita when indicating geo-radiation stress.

Most of the **vitamins and dietary supplements** which are taken for a long time turn out to be energetically ineffective and are thus, empirically, ineffective therapeutically. The organism quickly adapts to the supply by excreting surplus vitamins. I advise doing without them and, if necessary, to take them at intervals: after a three-week pause, take for one week, another three-week pause and so forth. Personally, I tend to be fundamentally opposed to orthomolecular medications, with the exception of selenium for carcinoma, folic acid during pregnancy, vitamin D during colder times (somewhere between 2000 and 4000 IU) as well as low-dosage iodide in areas of iodine deficiency (say as iodide 100-200 µg per day).

Allopathic medications test out exactly like homeopathics, i.e. the more effective, the better the resulting energy values. In this manner, one can test out many medications and their combinations. When conventional medications test out neutral or positive, then of course they can continue to be taken during PSE therapy. Allopathic agents that test out poorly, but which the patient needs, such as anti-epileptics or chemotherapeutics, are a tricky issue. One needs to proceed cautiously here, and possibly manage to get the energetically unfavorable therapy modified by the colleagues treating the patient. Experience has shown that energetic test results are not a very good argument with mainstream-medical colleagues, since they consider that sort of thing to be impossible, which means that one should instead emphasize possible side effects.

Speaking from nearly 40 years of experience with the remedy test, I'm able to sum up that, generally, sensible energy medicine without the remedy test, and moreover without the qualitative differentiation made possible by the REBA Test Device, seems totally impossible. I can also distill out some elementary rules which have general validity. Thus, good allopathics are on a par with naturopathic agents, and one of the ineradicable prejudices is that chemical agents are worse than biologicals. This often simply does not apply in such an extreme formulation, quite aside from the fact that there are indications for which allopathics are simply indispensable, such as in the area of hypertension treatment.

In the spirit of the principle of *primum nihil nocere* (first of all, do no harm), homeopathics are naturally usually freer of side effects because they only contain the healing vibration, and none of the associated substance. Nevertheless, there are many harmful homeopathics whose healing vibration the patient is no longer able to tolerate after a while. By definition, homeopathics are harmful vibrations whose healing effect is checked on healthy persons thereby, that they provoke a clinical picture from disease symptoms. This immediately sounds totally reasonable, but in reality it is often ignored when patients take the same homeopathic for years. We should not be surprised if they at some point develop symptoms and the corresponding clinical picture! By the way, this also applies to the biochemical agents of Schüßler, which likewise contain homeopathicized substances.

Keep the following in mind for patients who take medications over longer spans of time: just as you get so used to the pictures on the four walls of your home that you only notice them again after returning from a long vacation trip, so too does the body seem to become energetically downright insensitive to a constant onslaught of many healing stimuli. But there is yet another rule that says that one does not get accustomed to <u>important</u> stimuli. Anyone who has a genuine Picasso hanging on the wall will probably overlook it much less than the monthly picture on the complimentary supermarket calendar. Thus, important agents never test out neutral even after having been taken for a long time! This is why as a therapist, I almost never prescribe substances which test out neutral for most patients. I thus learn a lot from these remedy tests, and learn in particular to keep the size of my collection of valuable medications within reasonable limits.

What the organism is saying with a positive test reaction is: "That changes me energetically!" However, the test reaction does not reveal whether the change is for better or for worse! This important point is overlooked by many testers, who subscribe to the misconception that any test reaction amounts to approval. Testers must be absolutely clear about the fact that negative substances also provoke test reactions. My task as tester is to check out, with the aid of the REBA Test Device, whether the positively tested medications actually have good or bad effects. For this, I place the medications one at a time (or, if pressed for time, all at once) in the patient's pelvic region and then test the Vital and Emotional levels. As was mentioned earlier, the medications which the patient is to take in future are then placed in the pelvic region in order to check out their therapeutic effect. Since this region is a strong Yin zone, the remedy test simulates the artificial circumstance "as if the agent had already been taken". Thus, one can thereby very simply and elegantly check out the energetic therapeutic effects of a medication.

11.7   Step four – conflict size

Conflict size is tested next, using the testing agent (from the REBA test kit) corresponding to the tested-out conflict. For instance, for emotional remedy number 9, one places test substance number 9 in the REBA Test Device and then measures the four levels Vital, Emotional, Mental and Causal. The test substance acts as an energetic "magnifying glass" which for a brief moment of testing enormously magnifies the conflict (cf. **Fig. 11.3**). In this manner, the size of the conflict can be measured with the aid of the test substance. This yields four values, except in this case they relate to the conflict rather than the patient. These values are then recorded in the testing form. Average conflicts have sizes ranging from 60/60/10/60 to 80/80/10/80; very large conflicts such as a Central Conflict from 90-100/100/10/90.

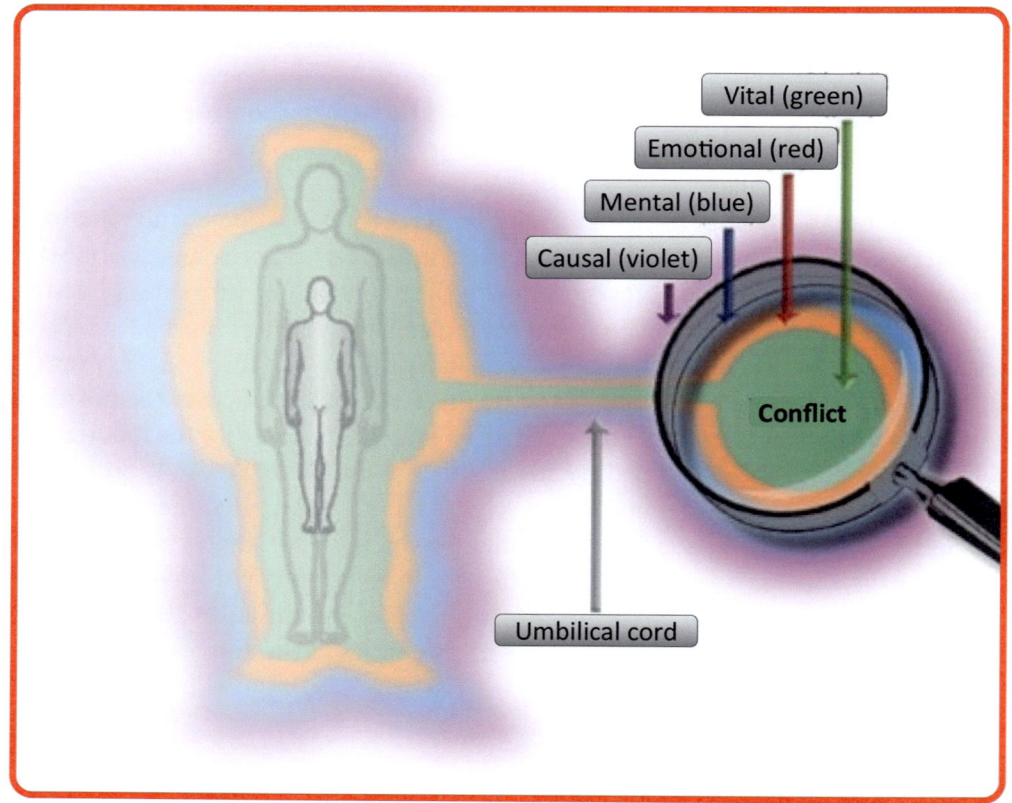

Fig. 11.3 – *The conflict is enlarged by the test substance acting as a kind of magnifying glass, while the patient energetically fades into the background.*

The **Vital and Emotional value** of the conflict indicates how much energy the conflict has stolen from the conflict host. Since, quantitatively, the conflict not the same size as the conflict host, these values cannot be equated, but instead are just used as a rough idea to explain the benefit of conflict elimination to the patient. For example, if the conflict values are 80% Vital and Emotional, then one is dealing with a large conflict whose elimination would be particularly beneficial. The **Mental value** indicates the degree of awareness of the conflict and usually ranges between 5-25% with a median of 10%. Since by definition conflicts are always unconscious – they wouldn't be conflicts otherwise – the Mental value cannot really be any higher. Finally, the **Causal value** is usually between 50-90% with a median value of 70-80%. It corresponds to the age of the conflict and the stubbornness with which it resists dissolution, but also the duration of therapy: every 20% Causal reading translates to 4-5 weeks of therapy, i.e. an averagely large conflict of 80% will need to be treated for about 4 months.

Determining the exact size of the conflict also enables monitoring the course of treatment, something which is not possible to this degree of precision with comparable procedures – for instance, even during treatment lasting months, one can clearly determine whether the patient is taking the prescribed meds on a regular basis, or whether they have any therapeutic effect at all. Sometimes, homeopathic agents are not correctly stored by the patient, e.g. in the vicinity of strong magnetic fields which quickly render them useless. Testing can determine this quickly and reliably, instead of continuing with months of possibly ineffective therapy.

If, after a few weeks or months of therapy, the patient wants to know whether the tested-out agents are the right ones, they can be checked for a positive reaction, i.e. one first places the prescribed Emvita and Chavita in the test honeycomb and checks whether the patient responds, which can be seen in a difference in thumb position in the kinesiological arm-length test. One can then be sure that the agents have been correctly tested. Next, they are placed in the Yin zone of the pelvis to see whether the Vital and Emotional values rise, which indicates satisfactory effectiveness. Finally, a diminishing Causal value of the conflict says that the meds have indeed been taken and are working.

11.7.1 Therapy recommendation

The "emotional remedies" (available as Emvita from Rubimed or as notified complexes in Switzerland) are used to eliminate conflicts. These are 28 different homeopathic compound agents which I have developed over the years. A thorough exposition of how these emotional remedies came to be can be found in my book *Healing through Energy Medicine* [8].

There are 50 mL dropper vials in blue glass (which preserves high homeopathic potentiations better) with liquida, as well as globuli – the latter are recommended for children, recovering alcoholics and people who reject alcohol for ideological reasons. Because of the higher active-substance content, the liquid forms are recommended as standard therapy.

For nearly all patients, the corresponding "Chakra remedy" (Chavita, Rubimed) is also prescribed. In this context, I am guided by the idea that the conflict is melted away by the emotional remedy, while the Chakra remedy expands the conflict's birth canal, thereby easing conflict dissolution. Conflicts provoke segmental autonomic dysregulation, which is eliminated by the Chakra remedy. In a very small number of cases (<0.1%), only the Emotional or Chakra remedy will be needed – mostly for extremely hypersensitive persons with particularly large conflicts which first need to be made "birthable".

Dosage
Standard prescription
Emvita 9 OP Rubimed (3-4 vials)
S. 2x12 drops on the tongue
Chavita 3 OP Rubimed (3-4 vials)
S. 2x12 drops on the tongue

Prescribing only an emotional remedy is a good idea when trying to completely eliminate the last vestiges of an almost completely cured conflict (Example: conflict readings of 10/20/20/20). In the aforementioned example, one vial of the corresponding emotional remedy would be prescribed.

When a large conflict has been tested out which has a Causal value of 70% or more, then the initial prescription should be enough to cover 3 to 5 months (this means 3 to 4 vials, i.e. 1 vial per 20% of Causal value) and the patient is advised to faithfully take the remedy at the prescribed interval. The **standard dosage** for adults and children over the age of 6 is 12 drops twice daily (below that 6 drops twice daily, for very small children 1 drop per year of age). This dosage of 24 drops per day should not be arbitrarily modified, as it has proven itself with countless patients over more than a decade; raising or lowering the dose has proven to be unnecessary: if more is taken, it does not accelerate the healing process, but on the other hand if less is taken, it delays conflict dissolution.

> Many therapists test the dosage mentally, but this has not proven effective, quite aside from the fact that mental testing is very error-prone (more on this later).

For **sensitive individuals**, I recommend taking the corresponding daily dose of e.g. 2x12 drops of Emvita and 2x12 drops of Chavita diluted in water, for example sipping from a water bottle throughout the day (**bottle method**). This avoids strong initial reactions or worsening, which then virtually never crops up while still guaranteeing conflict healing. By "sensitive individuals" I mean those with known strong reactions to energy-treatment methods (such as homeopathy) as well as those with a Causal reading above 70%.

The method described reliably prevents the otherwise so annoying "**drop neurosis**" – by which I mean the overanxious reduction of the daily drop amount, initiated either by the therapist or from that point in time at which side effects or worsening crop up. This can be a problem particularly during the first couple of weeks, and does not occur very often, but only now and then. Not infrequently, a reduction of this sort can sooner or later lead to discontinuing therapy, which does nobody any good, because at some point the patient reacts very frightened and panicky. However, with the aforementioned "bottle method", that will then hardly ever be the case.

Often, overanxious therapists become (erroneously) convinced right at the outset that Emvita is too strong for a patient. If that is the case, they will often get falsely negative test results which will then mislead them into reducing the drop count or possibly testing them mentally in order to find out how much the patient presumably can still tolerate – a cardinal error on the part of therapists that is very hard to eradicate, which

- induces drop neurosis in the patient (the so-called "nocebo" effect, i.e. a nervous therapist produces negative therapy effects in the patient, who then expects frightening things to happen if he takes more – which then turns into a self-fulfilling prophecy),
- also misleads to false test results, because mental testing nearly always yields false test results (e.g. for 2x2 drops for an adult to test out as appropriate is nearly always wrong!),
- in addition delays conflict healing, which extends to extremely long timespans (24 months at 2x2 drops for large conflicts, which nobody in his right mind would put up with!!),

- is therefore often brought by therapists, via conflict uncoupling, to an apparent but insufficient end (Therapist to patient: "The drops are taking too long, but I have something better for you" – and the therapist then applies conflict uncoupling, whereby conflict dissolution does not take place, but healing is only apparent).

Not infrequently, therapy is then also simply broken off with no results. Drop neurosis is therefore a big problem in PSE and should absolutely be avoided. It arises from a mixture of ignorance as to what is right in PSE along with unwarranted therapeutic nervousness and a foolish attitude on the part of the therapist, who pretends to find out what is right and individually suitable for the hypersensitive patient by means of mental testing. Summing up, this kind of thing brings PSE into disrepute and leads to unsatisfactory conflict healing.

On the other hand, those who
- recommend the side-effect-free bottle method,
- test out conflicts correctly (which reliably prevents medication pictures) and
- confidently recommend the standard dosage of 2x12 drops

will have many satisfied patients with good therapeutic results.

At the end of the session, I tell patients that they can contact me if they have any questions. I also make sure to mention that normally there are no questions and that the healing process almost always proceeds gently and imperceptibly. Normally, the only **side effects** noted are vivid dreams, which relatively many patients experience (probably as an expression of the unconscious self-healing processes, of which I make explicit mention). I don't usually mention any other side effects to patients, first of all because there usually are none, and secondly so as not to provoke self-fulfilling prophecies (known as "Nocebo"). However, for children with behavioral disorders there will occasionally be some initial worsening in the first week or two, which the parents should be made aware of.

Normal medications can continue to be taken with no problem during PSE therapy. Strong sedatives (such as benzodiazepine abuse) are a problem and can, in the worst case, neutralize the effects of PSE therapy. Fast-acting parallel therapies such as Bach Flowers, some phytotherapeutics, EMDR and Energy Psychology (tapping) have proven effective. Psychotherapists report being able to "get to the point more quickly" with the aid of PSE therapy, and the same applies to hypnotic and other regressive procedures.

In closing, I would like to address the question as to whether other medications and therapies besides the Emotional and Chakra remedies can eliminate conflicts. I worked for many years with Edward Bach's flower essences and with homeopathic high and top potentiations, yet never achieved the long-lasting deep-rooted results I had been hoping for. The same applies for all the other therapies which either I myself tried out or colleagues of mine made use of. This does not, however, mean that I categorically reject possible alternatives. I am grateful for all constructive suggestions from colleagues which help accelerate and intensify the dissolution of conflicts – but so far I know of nothing else which, in this context, has led to comparable, reproducible results (by independent colleagues) besides PSE.

Some experiments with higher dosages of the Emotional and Chakra remedies, or resonating with other media (artificial or radionic homeopathy) have not lived up to their promise; on the contrary, the knowledge gained tended to the negative. Evidently, each conflict needs a certain amount of time (healing phase) as well as a certain amount of specific medications (the Emotional and Chakra remedies) before it will dissolve. Added to which, experience has shown that any kind of **resonating and copying** that uses bioresonance devices does not work, presumably due to the overtone qualities of the Emotional remedies, which contain very high potentiations. Basically, what I have observed is that therapeutic procedures other than PSE have been mostly unable to energetically eliminate conflicts. One possible exception might be strongly catalytic therapies which trigger genuine emotional upheaval and reorientation, as well as the administration of very high-vibration healing energies. Very few or no conflicts have often been observed in people who have undergone such experiences.

11.7.2   Testing with the Basic Test Kit

At first, many PSE novices use only the Basic Test Kit, which is considerably more affordable than the REBA Test Device. However, they must then do without testing of the energy values of both the patients and the conflicts, nor will they know how effective the agents will be in the remedy test. Yet despite these limitations, many therapists have had good results with the Basic Test Kit, and there are just a few things to keep in mind:

- Because it is not known how large a conflict is, treatment with the corresponding Emvita and Chavita can only run for about 4-5 weeks (prescribing one vial). Particularly in the first few weeks, the prescribed PSE medications often have an energetically strong compensatory effect, which can make retesting somewhat difficult.
- After 4-5 weeks, one should absolutely always first test the Emvita and Chavita which had been prescribed, by placing them in the patient's Yang energy field above the navel, for instance in a money bag worn around the neck into which the remedies are placed.
- Since most conflicts have a Causal value of 80% (sometimes 50-60%), often – at the second visit at least – the correspondingly prescribed Emvita and Chavita are still indicated, and indeed quite often at times even at the third visit.
- In an estimated 95% of cases, the previously prescribed Emvita and Chavita still test positive, and so they are simply prescribed for another 4-5 weeks until, after 3-4 prescriptions, the old agent no longer responds. The conflict has then been eliminated and the search for a new conflict can begin.

If these procedural guidelines are not adhered to, there is a risk that follow-up checks will constantly test out new conflicts which are then treated, even though the old conflicts have not yet been eliminated: understandably, the patient will only get worse and worse when subjected to such treatment. Therefore, working with the Basic Test Kit calls for particular care and conscientiousness.

11.7.3   The course of therapy

The usual experience in the majority of cases is that, at the first visit, the patient has an active conflict which is eliminated on average within four months. After just a few weeks, most patients notice a clear improvement. As the months go by, there will usually be some mild relapses as soon as, after 3-4 months, a new conflict becomes active. This new conflict will also take an average of four months to be eliminated, until once again a new conflict arises. In most cases, only after three or four conflicts have been eliminated does it lead to clear and enduring improvement or even a complete cure (cf. Fig. 11.4).

Because patients undergoing PSE therapy feel noticeably better as time goes by, patient management is usually not a problem. To be sure, patients need to be

Using Psychosomatic Energetics Correctly

informed of the ups and downs of the therapy so that they remain cooperative and understand the basis as to why new conflicts keep cropping up. These can be likened it to bulky refuse pickup, which the organism sees as an opportunity to get rid of old ballast. The patient's higher-frequency vibrations during the course of PSE therapy keep on activating lower-frequency conflicts. Many also talk in terms of "onion-peel layers" by which the body rids itself of old psychoenergetic husks which had once served as defensive bastions and instruments of repression of unpleasant feelings, but which now only tie up unusable energy. If it is made clear to the patient that eradicated conflicts do not return, i.e. that they are permanently rid of them and thereby are getting back a lot of blocked energy, this will provide the motivation for them to stay the course.

After thousands of patients had been treated by many different testers, a typical course of healing became discernible (**cf. Fig. 11.4**). Because of the large number of patients and good agreement among independent therapists, we are dealing here with universally applicable regularities and patterns. Patients should be told right from the beginning what is expected of them in terms of personal effort. They should know what they are letting themselves in for and should have a good idea what they need to invest in time and money. For over 90% of patients, the healing process can be likened to a roller coaster if the symptoms are correlated with the elapsed time.

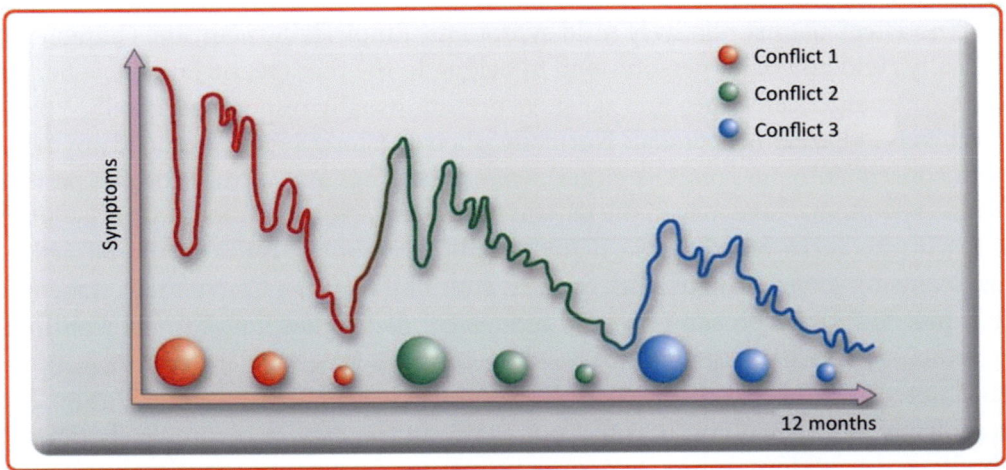

Fig. 11.4 – *Usual course of PSE therapy for most patients.*

> For three visits at €80-180 [$90-200] (naturopath or physician) +10 vials of Emvita and can files of Chavita at €12-16 [$13-18] each adds up to an annual cost of €480-860 [$535-955]. Added to this is the time spent in taking the remedies every day and sticking to the schedule as closely as possible.

One should also keep in mind that the symptoms of most patients are made up of a potpourri of multifarious complaints. If a patient comes in with a migraine headache, it might be that he reports little improvement after a few months – but if one queries more closely, it turns out, for example, that the long-standing lower back pain, which had also been plaguing the patient, has disappeared. So, one should make a note of all major symptoms and ask about them in sequence. If certain symptoms disappear for good, that's a sign of success even if the predominant symptom continues on for a while.

In about 10% of patients, only a single conflict is found and eliminated before achieving a good permanent condition. Afterwards, a follow-up check finds not a single additional active conflict. In most cases, the person is either very simply structured or spiritually very advanced. In about 20% of patients, there is unfortunately no improvement in their symptoms even after a year: in about 5% of these cases one then sees, after additional conflict treatments, a good effect after all, but this can drag on at times for two or three years. About 15% of patients are therapy recalcitrant for unknown reasons – sometimes there is success with the severest clinical pictures but then no effect against relatively mild symptoms. Empirically, neurotic, characterologically rigid and older persons tend to belong to the therapeutic failures, whereas younger, energetically open and sensitive persons usually respond very well.

When is PSE treatment ended? Normally when no Chakra agents respond anymore (and consequently no conflicts either), energy readings are normal and the patient has no symptoms. One may, if the patient so desires, arrange for follow-up checks at 1-2 year intervals – or, of course, if any symptoms reappear. If the patient nevertheless wants to go on being treated, one can continue with the Chavita plus remedies (Chapter 11.7.4), which can ferret out hidden conflicts. How long can one continue treatment with PSE? Usually until no more conflicts are testable; sometimes, up to 20 different conflicts can surface one after the other, but it is extremely rare that completely eliminated conflicts test out again. In the case of incompletely purged conflicts, this seldom occurs, but it might, say, for current conflict contents which reactivate an older conflict.

11.7.4 Chavita plus agent

So-called "miasmatic" conflicts probably play a role in therapy resistance, and residual symptoms of patients categorized as hopeless cases. Such deep unconscious conflicts are for the most part passive and so normally not testable. Sometimes, incompletely dispersed conflicts can also be a problem. These conflicts can be tracked down and treated with a mixture of special high potentiations which are classified with the seven Chakras and also contain nosodes of the miasmas. Many therapists have reported impressive healing results even with decades-long therapy-resistant patients.

For this testing, there is a special test kit containing 7 Chavita plus and 1 Miasma BB ampoule (a mixture of all 7 Chavita plus agents). First, the Miasma BB ampoule is placed in the patient's Yin zone and then testing is done in sequence corresponding to the 7 Chavita plus agents. After that, the Emvita which corresponds to the Chakra which responded (e.g. for Chavita plus 5, Emvita 17 and 18) is tested. Usually, only one conflict is found, but sometimes there are several, which might be earlier conflicts that were not completely dispersed. These conflicts often make a lot of sense depth-psychologically and biographically. Using the accompanying test agents, one tests for conflict size in the customary PSE manner and then treats accordingly by prescribing the appropriate Emvita as well as the associated Chavita plus. To monitor therapy, the found Chavita plus agent and the positively tested conflict are placed in the patient's Yin zone. All the values should improve noticeably.

The recommended therapy is 5 globuli of the tested Chavita plus per day, as well as a daily dose of 12 drops twice daily of the respective Emvita. As always, duration of treatment depends upon the conflict's Causal reading (20% = ca. 4-5 weeks). Occasionally, Chavita plus can provoke intense initial reactions, so it is recommended to dilute the daily dose in a small water bottle to be sipped throughout the day; this makes the agents considerably easier to tolerate.

11.8 Step five – explaining the test procedure to the patient

When explaining the results of PSE testing, many patients ask me about PSE methodology; these are mostly curious, critical, conscientious and/or technology-interested persons who want to know how testing actually works. Since the underpinnings of the PSE testing technique have so far not been explained in detail, the following explanations are also aimed at therapists. I tell patients that the REBA Test Device is a stressor with which the four levels of their energy fields are placed under escalating levels of stress. The more they can endure, the healthier they're considered to be. I explain to those with some scientific knowledge that it places a stress or load on the human Aura, thereby indirectly measuring life energy. Since this is a standardized procedure working with precisely defined frequencies, one obtains – unlike other techniques such as Aura photography – reproducible and meaningful test results. The frequency mixture emitted by the REBA Test Device enters into resonance with the four known **brain-wave** (EEG) frequency regions of the patient's brain, namely

- Delta (deep sleep),
- Theta (dreaming),
- Alpha (awake) and
- Beta (stress) frequencies.

In the same sequence, these four EEG regions correspond to the four Aura regions of Yoga tradition:

- Vital field (Delta)
- Emotional field (Theta)
- Mental field (Alpha)
- Causal field (Beta).

Empirically, it turns out that the more a patient can tolerate a particular frequency mixture before exhibiting signs of energetic stress in a kinesiologically test reaction, the healthier and more "charged up" in the associated Aura field the patient can be considered to be. For example, if a patient can tolerate the entire Delta frequency spectrum (REBA test value of 100% Vital) before triggering an energetic test reaction, then this is a sign of strong Vital energy, i.e. the patient is full of life force.

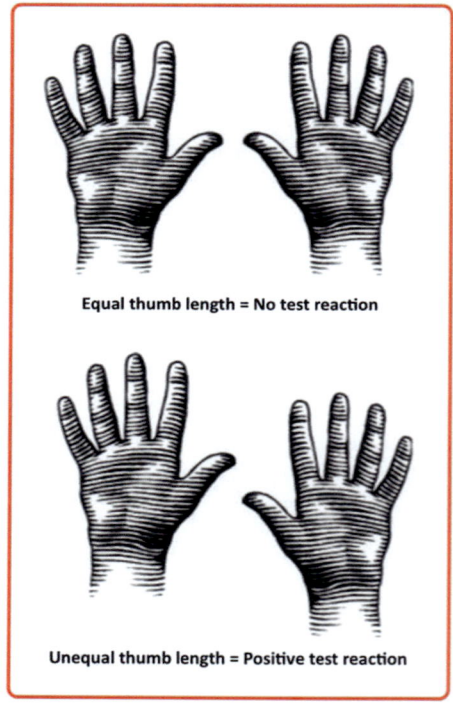

Fig. 11.5 – *Kinesiological arm-length reflex test with neutral and positive test reaction.*

In PSE, the energy test used is the **kinesiological arm-length test**, because it is easy to learn and fairly insensitive to interference. I show patients the effect at a Vital reading of, say, 20% (assuming they have such a reading). At 0%, I bring their arms together without pulling, then at 10%, where they already see a slight difference in the thumb positions, until at 20% the thumbs deviate noticeably from each other (cf. Fig. 11.5). Most patients are very surprised at this phenomenon. I explain that it is a stress reaction which disrupts the interplay of muscles between the left and right sides of the body, comparable to the back hairs of a cat standing on end. The delicate balance between the left and right sides of the body is upset and the thumbs are no longer parallel to each other. For patients whose arms are not parallel to each other even at the outset, the arms are pulled into a parallel position. It's just a matter of a clearly noticeable difference of 1-2 cm (or more) between the right and left thumb, regardless of whether the arms are straight or not. In the case of a paralyzed arm, it is used as an indication instrument; for those with no arms, the legs are used.

By the way, the arm-length test can also be done as a **self-test** which one can perform on oneself if necessary by placing the ampoules in sequence into one's breast pocket. Since it is very difficult to maintain a neutral attitude toward oneself, only very good experienced testers, who are able to empty themselves out completely internally, should perform the self-test.

The stress on the brain immediately irritates the coordination of the left and right lobes of the brain – respectively, the muscle tension between the left and right sides of the body. The image I have here – to go visual – is of a coachman trying to direct two horses, one with the left and the other with the right arm, who, due to a disturbance of some kind – say a mosquito bite or a greeting from a passerby – all of a sudden no longer has a steady hold on the reins, just as the arms seem to have a different length after the muscle tension on the two sides of the body has been altered. With the coachman, the result will be that the horses begin to curve to the left or right rather than going straight. This applies not just to left and right arms as in dowsing or the arm-length test, but also to unilateral tests such as pendulum swinging, one-hand dowsing or EAV testing, because the arm under test also has agonists and antagonists whose interplay is disturbed during the test, thereby leading to a positive test reaction.

11.9 Step six – interpreting the test results

One is most deeply affected by those truths which one would rather have not known. (Friedl Beutelrock)

The hardest part of Psychosomatic Energetics turns out to be explaining the test results. This is primarily due to time pressure, the brevity of the actual findings, the causes of the ailment, plus explaining the life-dynamics of character and on top of it all drawing up a therapy plan. The energy test itself often lasts just a few minutes and makes many a patient ask incredulously it is already done. Testing itself is not a lot of work for me, although even here the experience can vary widely – with many patients, the test proceeds effortlessly, but with others it can degenerate into a downright wrestling match. On the other hand, experience has shown that explaining the test results takes up most of the session time, but is the part that the patient benefits most from.

In the patient's language, it should be explained what it is that is psychoenergetically disturbed and what this disturbance signifies. The trick is to make the explanation so clearly understandable and easy to relate to that the patient can see himself in it and, ideally, has an "Aha!" Experience. The aim is to fetch the patient from the "train platform" on which he finds himself. One speaks differently with a less educated person than one does with a university professor, and one deals differently with a depressive character than with a schizoid. After many years of professional experience as a naturopath and physician, I've developed a conversational routine which I like to call the Golden Mean.

An important part of this process is the therapist's personal authenticity, something that patients appreciate and which comes across to them as honesty and willingness to make an effort. Unlike my early years, when I was still fighting for every patient and made many compromises, I express myself these days bluntly and forthrightly when it comes to crucial issues such as the absolute necessity of geopathic cleansing or the rejection of nonsensical adjuvant therapies. I get the impression that patients appreciate fatherly authority and forthright clarity, and find it comforting because they know where they stand and also sense the doctor's strong fatherly guidance. However, turning it around, the patient must likewise have an opportunity to express his concerns and thereby feel accepted as a person. It is thus not a power struggle, but rather a cooperative effort. In the ideal case, therapist and patient become a close-knit team, fighting enthusiastically for the common cause of healing.

The first thing I do is explain the test results by drawing a sketch on a blank piece of paper (one can also use a preprinted graphic) (**cf. Fig. 11.1**).

In the case at hand, my explanation is as follows: "You have low Vital and Emotional values, and such low Vital values – which relate to life energy – with readings of 20% are usually associated with a feeling of permanent exhaustion. The Emotional reading of 40% – which relates to moods and feelings – as a rule points to a grumpy mood in which one often feels joyless and doesn't really have much desire to do anything. The low Mental reading – associated with rational activity and thinking – at 70% usually is associated with concentration, thinking and memory disorders. The Causal reading has to do with intuition and spiritual openness. Its high value here signifies that you're a sensitive person."

With few exceptions, most patients confirm my explanation by telling me it agrees perfectly with the way they feel. Nevertheless, the testing process is always good for the occasional surprise, as the following report from an experienced colleague shows.

	Normal	**Value on 3/13/2000**
Vital	100	20
Emotional	100	40
Mental	100	70
Causal	40	70

***Tab. 11.1** – Test results.*

• Case study

As a matter of fact, I sometimes see some amazing things during the REBA test. A while back, I had a female patient with a somatic problem which did not seem to be particularly emotional and in fact nothing of this nature came out. The REBA test said that her Vital reading was not bad, yet the Emotional reading was 20! When I showed her that, it all came tumbling out: considerable emotional stress due to family problems along with an older incest episode involving her. This surprised me no little bit since, after 29 years of general practice, I can usually sense when something is amiss in the psychic-emotional area, but not this time. (Email from Dr. Harry Bodde, general practitioner from Rotterdam)

Because of factors such as habituation, repression and social conformity, the energy values are often more truthful than that which the patient says about himself.

In the REBA test, certain specific combinations of circumstances are indicative of particular clinical syndromes and of characteristic symptoms (cf. **Fig. 11.2**).

The next thing I do is draw a picture of the conflict for the patient, making the affected segment the starting point of the conflict balloon. This is a simple and quickly-drawn ballpoint sketch that aims to make it easier for the patient to understand, along the lines of "a picture is worth a thousand words". Then I write down the main theme of the conflict such as "Rage" or "Wrong thinking" and jot down the conflict values, for instance 78/80/10/70. I explain these values to the patient with the following words: "Your conflict has to do with suppressed rage, which you probably experienced in early childhood did not dare to express at that time. This led to the formation of a kind of energy bubble enclosing the Rage theme. This Rage now constantly sucks energy out of you, namely 70% of your vitality, and what's more steals 80% of your *joie de vivre*. At 10%, you are relatively unaware of the conflict, and at 70% it is a stubborn structure that will take at least three months (i.e. three vials of Emvita 9) to resolve. Once the conflict has been resolved, then it is almost always gone forever, and you get back your life energy and *joie de vivre* which had been trapped inside it."

There are characteristic REBA test results for both patient and conflict (cf. **Fig. 11.3**).

Rebatest values	Possible diagnoses
10/10/100/60	Depression with initiative inhibition, e.g.
90/20/100/70	Depression without initiative inhibition, e.g.
10/40/100/50	In cases of focal stress, an energy-sapping organ ailment or geopathy, e.g.
40/10/30/60	Geopathy with severe energetic head block and depressive initiative inhibition, e.g.
80/30/10/70	Psychosis with depressive tinge, e.g.
30/40/90/80	In cases of active Central Conflict, e.g.
20/30/100/90	Hyperactive child (ADHD), e.g.

Tab. 11.2

Rebatest values	Conflict size
30/50/5/40	Medium-sized subconscious conflict which drains off a good deal of emotional energy
80/90/10/80	Typical large conflict; such values obtain with a +HO% difference in 80–90% of conflicts

70/80/30/40	Large conflict, relatively high degree of awareness (30%) which is in the process of dissolution (instead of 70%, Causal is down to 40%)
80/100/10/90	Typical Central Conflict

Tab. 11.3

> Whenever a therapist tests out atypical conflict values in his patients – e.g. 30/20/60/40 (such high Mental values are extremely unusual), or 100/100/100/100 (such values are vanishingly rare) or 10/10/10/10 (conflicts this small are more the exception) – in all likelihood has an internal problem as therapist. This can either be unprocessed conflicts or partly mental testing, with which one constantly "sabotages" the test results unawares. In such cases, my advice is to undergo thorough self-therapy for the conflicts with the aid of an experienced colleague. Self-therapy is now a compulsory part of the training to become a certified energy therapist, just like practicing in small groups under the leadership of an experienced colleague, so as to get used to the correct manner of testing right from the beginning.

There is a general rule of thumb according to which high conflict values are bad and low values better, since a large conflict inflicts more harm on a patient than a small one. Therapists have the task of melting away the conflict like a block of ice, so that the bound-up energy is once more available to the patient. High Vital or Emotional values for the conflict indicate how much life energy and good mood it is constantly stealing from the patient. The **Conflict Causal Value** is the guide value for the amount of melting away, since it is only increasing conflict healing that brings the Causal values down closer to zero. It has proven to be important to melt away conflicts down to a Causal value of zero because a residual conflict can continue to block patient energy, added to which incompletely dissolved conflicts can, in rare cases, begin growing again.

The **Mental value** can be viewed as yet another measure of conflict healing, since the more conscious the patient becomes of the conflict, the sooner it will dissolve. Normal conflict values range from nearly zero to 10-20%, which might rise slightly during the course of treatment (usually to 20-30%). A rising awareness of the conflict usually manifests itself in the form of vivid dreams, although less frequently in the patient consciously thinking about the conflict contents. In my opinion, this is precisely what a therapist should not bring about! It is a fundamental tenet of PSE to avoid emotionally provocative therapy, since this just supplies the conflict with more attention and energy.

I was thus able to determine, after deeply touching Family Constellations sessions, that the participants' conflicts were markedly larger than before. For those not undergoing treatment, the situation persisted afterwards for a good long time, while the patients being treated with Emotional remedies soon had smaller conflicts, which went hand-in-hand with a feeling of improvement and healing. In like manner, one can often detect, in psychoanalyst clients, large conflicts which are constantly being "pushed" by the therapeutic situation and thereby made larger. Yet the right way would be the exact opposite, namely disarming the drama of the conflict by offering a good and emotionally pacifying solution. In fact, it seems to be precisely this that is the secret of good psychotherapist: keeping in mind the positive end result.

When discussing the **conflict contents**, it's a good idea to mention only one or two keywords which succinctly summarize the conflict contents. In some cases, one might need additional formulations which are more comprehensible to the patient, e.g. instead of "Rushed" (Emotional remedy #18) an alternative might be "Driven, crowded, restless". I have made it a habit to draw a circle around the found conflict in the Patient Advisory ("Patient Informational Brochure") and give it to the patient to read. Basically, I talk about the conflict contents as little as possible in order, as it were, to provide only an initial impetus. The patient can come up with his own ideas about the conflict at home, say by reading books about Psychosomatic Energetics or talking over childhood experiences with his parents. After all, I as therapist am also an important information source for the patient's subconscious, economically and restrainedly conveying during the conflict discussion not to "take it so seriously anymore, it's all in the past now!"

11.10 Step seven – discussing character

I take more time when discussing character because it is a central topic. When the Central Conflict is active, I also talk about character, for the most part. Exceptions to this rule of thumb include children, emotionally very labile adults (example: active psychosis, borderline etc.) and persons who categorically reject emotional/psychic topics; in those cases, I do not talk about character type, or if I do, then only with close relatives, such as a child's mother or father concerning upbringing or educational problems (but not in the child's presence).

Character is an integral part of everyday consciousness and an unavoidable fact of normal daily life. Unlike a conflict, character is not any kind of psychic scar anchored in the deep unconscious, but rather involves omnipresent personality traits. It is thus not a matter of waking "sleeping dogs", but rather doing active life counseling. Discussing character facilitates self-discovery, emotional reorientation and the integration of the darker aspects of a person's being. At the same time, it helps patients in their daily social interaction by better learning the character of others and thus how better to get along with them.

Character traits are a "mixed bag", i.e. we distinguish between good and bad ones. Religious terminology sees them in terms of virtues and vices, while psychologists talk about neurosis, antisocial behavior, insecurity etc. and on the other hand about positive social abilities, empathy, stable self-esteem etc. It is desirable to have many good and few bad character traits if one aspires to be a contented and cultivated person, emotionally at ease and able to work well with others.

Negative character traits are decisively involved with the Central Conflict. Thanks to the insinuations and blandishments coming from the Central Conflict, people are mainly, so to speak, "not in their right minds", "not all there" and behave "off the mark" or at least not how they would really like to. For example, I might tell a patient: "You have a fixed character which influences your mind and your metabolism and thus also your health. Your particular character was described in ancient times as 'Choleric', a type which swallows everything without complaint, but at some point explodes. Characters of this sort believe that, above all, other people must be doing well before they can think of themselves. Unfortunately, you thereby expose yourself to being easily manipulated. You need to learn how to say No when you mean No, and not to just put up with everything. You are not always dependent upon other people in order to get by, and you can also live well when acting in your own interests."

It is usually not advisable to tell patients too much about their truly negative dark sides, because this can open up old wounds and simply strengthen the Central Conflict. As near as I can recall, I have yet to offend a Depressive type with the embarrassing revelation that, deep inside, he is tormented by nagging frustration and is always and everywhere finding a "hair in the soup" – or that a Schizoid type is, deep in his heart an arrogant know-it-all who needlessly alienates others; or that a Hysteric type is a mean-spirited pest who enjoys the suffering of others and who, deep inside, is actually an extremely insecure person; or that an Obsessive-compulsive type is an internally rigid nitpicker who sucks up to others to camouflage his overdone fastidiousness.

As far as atmosphere is concerned, it seems to be enough for me to know about patients' dark sides – and, of course, that the patients also know about them, since ultimately they know themselves well enough, even if nobody says a word about it. The crucial strength needed for positive character change and maturation comes from the dissolution of the conflict. Most people change for the better as soon as they have resolved the large conflicts which had heretofore made them internally frustrated, irritable, envious and aggressive. Evidently, their self-image is refreshed and reinforced with positive light energy, so that they no longer feel it necessary to plead for the approval of others, to say nothing of demanding it forcefully. Instead, a healthy self-image makes the patients much calmer than before and much more relaxed inside.

11.11 Step eight – relationship topics

Finally, I'd like to address the ticklish topic of partner choice (Chapter 6.7). In the broader sense, this has to do with all close interpersonal contacts, whether at work or within other social groups. The topic integral to any discussion concerning the active Central Conflict, because then the associated character type is out in the open, but there are also patients whose symptoms have directly to do with a partner or relationship problem. When it comes to the discussion question of interpersonal compatibility, of getting along well or poorly together, I make use of the aforementioned scheme of character types that are well, less well or badly suitable with each other (**cf. Fig. 6.7**). In this process, I retreat to the standpoint of the purely factual and do not act as referee.

Neither the Hysteric nor the Schizoid, as precisely neither the Depressive nor the Obsessive-compulsive are to be blamed for the fact that they normally so frequently get in each other's hair and permanently misunderstand each other. Antipodal people should simply not live too closely together in a common living space. Sometimes there's nothing that can be done about it, such as when it involves incompatible family members. However, one can make it easier for the patient by explaining the secret and unknown (but of course nevertheless always valid) "instruction manual" of the other character type. The main thrust of my explanatory attempts goes in the direction of "Martians after all have their own rules and customs". Much has already been achieved if the strategies of the incompatible types are recognized, not as personal failings and weaknesses, but rather as characteristic features. If (to stay with the image) the patient accepts that Martians mean no harm in sprouting antennas from their heads, but rather that this is quite normal Martian behavior, then this opens up the way to a better understanding.

11.12 Step nine – karmic interpretation of the Central Conflict

Another very demanding topic of PSE interpretation has to do with the possibility of a karmic origin to large emotional conflicts (Chapter 7). Since this is a highly speculative area which is furthermore ideologically charged (mosaic religions such as Christianity, Judaism, Islam completely reject it, as do also scientifically-oriented persons), this ticklish topic should be approached very cautiously with patients, say along the lines of: "Can you conceive the possibility of something like personal reincarnation?" If patients answer in the negative, I abandon this approach and shift over to a more conventional explanatory model. One can also see, in the dramatic aspects of a conflict, fairytale archetypes that correspond to universal depth-psychological processes, and so my explanations then proceed in this generally accepted direction.

On the other hand, the topic of personal reincarnation is often very appreciated among spiritually advanced and very open persons. Unlike hypnotic diagnosis, which is suggestible and failure prone, PSE has in my eyes the advantage of supplying clear insights. In my book *Healing through Energy Medicine* [8], I have outlined possible scenarios for the origin of Central Conflicts. If one opens oneself up to this view of things, it thereby reveals a completely new view of the individual soul which, traversing many incarnations, undergoes a maturation process, in which the Central Conflict is a central formative element, by means of which – and only by means of which – the individual consciousness can develop.

Basically, what I do is, for instance explain the karmic aspect of Central Conflict #4 (theme: "Self-control") to the patient as follows: "I can give you some suggestions for your problem which correspond with the experiences of people in a trance, clairvoyants and spiritual teachers. This entire thing is a model which I can offer you as an explanatory aid. According to this, sometime long, long ago you had an existentially threatening experience which had to do with the theme of your Central Conflict. You faced a deadly threat and then in fact died an agonizing death, even though you tried to prevent it with a show of self-control. The psychic posture of being in control led to the formation of a Melancholic character …" (At this point, I insert the aforementioned part concerning the significance of Central Conflict and character.) "You adopt a predominantly rational and in-control posture, but dream of being allowed to live out your hidden yearnings and emotional side. The Central Conflict, once created, thereafter puts its stamp upon your entire emotional life, and you see everything through the tint of its glasses. In your subsequent reincarnations, you've always chosen families and existences in which the theme of self-control is addressed. Therefore, like layers of onionskin, one similar injury follows another. You always unconsciously try to restage your conflict even though your true inner being absolutely does not want to."

For most patients, this image is a revelation which opens up to them completely new vistas. Most times, I learn from such patients that they, amazingly, have had very similar suppositions, because certain dreams and premonitions revolved around these themes. Or I will hear, to my surprise, that quite a while ago a medium told them the same thing, or that a book describing similar historical topics had deeply moved them. For many patients, however, it is a new and unaccustomed image, which I then do not enlarge too much upon, especially if I get the uneasy feeling that I might be overtaxing the patient. If the whole thing looks like it might be degenerating into fairytale time – which does happen now and then – then the limits of the tolerable have definitely been crossed, and I change the subject immediately.

The valuable core of the image of the karmically "wandering" Central Conflict often only reveals itself at second glance. As a therapist, one must grow into this image and become familiar with it – but then it will become an indispensable aid to emotional diagnosis and psychic healing! When the Central Conflict for millennia molds the entire life of the individual Psyche, then we are dealing with psychic evolution which enfolds the individual into the overall development of creation. No one is then a lost creature which once and only once, namely in this single life, briefly dwells upon this earth and is afterwards dead for the rest of eternity – in accordance with the usual bleak picture of the modern enlightened scientific worldview. On the contrary, the model of a reincarnating soul imparts a reassuring image of an eternal and immortal individual consciousness.

Along the path of spiritual maturation, the individual proceeds from one incarnation to the next, accompanied by well-known and beloved fellow humans – as well as, of course, by enemies and a Central Conflict (the largest and at the same time completely secret enemy). Paradoxically, our worst enemies often turn out to be our biggest benefactors, because they impart lessons that are, to be sure, painful yet necessary, lessons which would have gone unlearned had it not been for their actions. And it seems also to be precisely the case here, so that the Central Conflict becomes the staff up which our individual psychic development can climb like a grapevine.

11.12.1 Patient resistance and therapist conflicts

Really, every person should strive to get rid of his or her emotional problems as quickly as possible. However, that is surprisingly not the case. For the most part, resistance to conflict dissolution via PSE manifests as perceived excessive side effects which supposedly coerce into breaking off therapy. However, the aforementioned "bottle method" almost always succeeds in elegantly navigating around this obstacle (mix the daily dosage in a bottle of water and sip at it throughout the day).

Sometimes, in the first few weeks of therapy, patients will come forward with objections, misgivings, basic questions indicating a desire to break off therapy. Experience so far suggests that this is based upon an unconscious inclination on the part of the conflict, which is fighting for survival. But if the therapist stands firm and encourages patients to stick it out during the turbulent initial phase of therapy, which only lasts a few days or weeks, then the problems almost always go away without further ado.

The therapist is powerless against another frequently-used form of conflict resistance; it manifests itself as deficient compliance and ultimately interruption of therapy. I frequently see this in emotionally very labile persons, such as those with personality disorders (borderline), pronounced addiction with in part self-destructive tendencies (gambling addiction), manic-depressives and psychotics. In these cases, it is a good idea from the very beginning to bring in a trustworthy relative as co-therapist, who will see to it that the PSE medications are taken regularly as prescribed.

There's an old saying according to which the shoemaker's children go barefoot. It is well known that therapists have many disorders, shown statistically in elevated addiction tendency, various psychological problems, behavioral disorders etc. Since in the past few years I've been able, at seminars and individual testing sessions, to examine many therapists using PSE, it quickly came to my attention that they have certain specific conflicts at a higher than average rate. In what follows, I'd like to describe some typical individual cases – first, because it can be useful to the reader as self-insight, and second, because the same themes also play a role with many patients.

The emotional remedies #10 ("Always wanting more, constantly dissatisfied, powermad") and #11 ("Deeply dissatisfied, creating good feelings, addiction") have tested out on various therapists. Interestingly, conflict #10 often turns up in cultivated and educated persons as a thirst for learning, for instance in the form of a constant round of seminar visits, an oversized personal library, pronounced spiritual and intellectual craving for recognition and obsessive possessiveness etc. – often not, however, in the form of increased food intake (adiposity) or craving for conventional possessions (house, automobile), as with the average patient. With conflict #11, there is an agonizing feeling of unconscious frustration which has to be kept in check and compensated for with all kinds of maneuvers. One way this is done is via the socially acceptable form of workaholism, or else other socially scorned addictions such as alcoholism, anorexia etc. One finds in these cases that the conflict is realized in such a manner that the therapist cultivates a downright symbiotic chumminess with the patient, in order to get attention and affection by way of the exaggeratedly intimate therapeutic alliance.

Remarkably often, therapists exhibit conflicts having to do with anxiety and isolation. Quite a few of the classic symptoms of helper syndrome (compassion fatigue) are seen mirrored here:

- Fear of failure and not being good enough, but also
- Escaping one's own isolation through closeness to the patient.

It seems paradoxical that therapists – whose job is supposed to be to have a calming and reassuring effect on patients – often themselves unconsciously suffer from anxiety and nervousness. It seems equally odd to find a conflict with a theme of isolation in a person who had chosen such a highly social profession as that of Doctor. However, the fluctuating relationship between closeness and distance is an essential part of a physician's toolkit: anyone who cannot observe patients from a properly critical distance, and who empathizes too strongly, will either misdiagnose and choose inappropriate therapies, or the necessary emotional distance will be lacking such that suffering along with the patient will also injure the therapist.

Occupations and hobbies involving anxiety or fear, such as racecar driver, stuntman or extreme mountain climbing, are frequently chosen by people with large anxiety conflicts. As we know, there's hardly any other social situation that is as daunting as a doctor or dentist appointment. The highest intensity of this anxiety is reached with emergency doctors who, with the red emergency light blinking, fight for every second with death always staring them in the face, struggling for another person's sake with the fear to end all fears – the fear of death – often thereby unconsciously carrying it about within themselves. When a doctor is in the role of Lord over Life and Death, unconscious feelings of power and powerlessness play a major supporting role, known to have a background effect in all conflicts.

Therapists, along with their own unconscious emotional dynamics, are ensnared in the doctor-patient relationship and, basically, often practice a form of inadequate self-therapy as they indulge their unconscious negative conflicts by performing therapy. The net result from testing many colleagues was that, behind the flawless façade of the medical profession there not infrequently lay dormant a latently baneful psychodynamics which – although it worked to the patient's benefit via compensation mechanisms such as self-sacrifice, putting in long hours of hard work, friendliness etc. – over the long term was very harmful to the therapists themselves. The therapists' subconscious dynamics led to them no longer being able to properly recognize their own most basic needs, such as knowing when to stop working so as to avoid burnout.

Yet another conflict theme among therapists is "Restless, mentally hyperactive" (Emvita 22). This conflict is found in those who work with their mind, those who, through mental structuring and systematizing programs, frequently treat their own organism worse than they would, say, their pet dog. The hyper-intellectuality of many mental workers also leads to energetic disharmony because the mental apparatus is overdriven and thereby overvalued. In the case of the conflict theme "Helpless, at the mercy of" (Emvita 3), the practice of medicine, with its great power and omnipotence, leads to compensation of the unconscious emotional themes in which doctors actually feel "completely helpless".

Finally, I'd like to discuss the conflict theme "Wrong thinking" (Emvita 28), which is pretty hard to explain using simple terminology. It is found fairly often among those who make a living through mental activity. I see this theme as a distrust conflict due to karmic disappointments, in which for those affected, in an earlier life had a traumatic experience that caused their entire worldview to disintegrate. Back then, the person had indeed thought wrong and bet on the wrong horse – or at least that was the unconscious dying fantasy which was taken into the next life and which goes something like this: "If I had not believed in Jesus, I, an early Christian, would not have been nailed to a cross." Those with this kind of unconscious belief topics afterwards have disrupted basic trust which often manifests itself either in an unconscious search for ultimate truth or else in a particularly cynical and rationalistic attitude along the lines of "I'll never ever let myself be fooled again like that. From now on, I'm not going to believe anything whatsoever!"

In closing, I'd like to report what happened to the colleagues who resolved their emotional conflicts with the aid of PSE. The driving force behind the pursuit of their career was no longer led astray by false neurotic impulses, but rather determined by the spontaneous love of their calling and the primordial human pleasure at being able to help others. Many of these colleagues have reported a changed attitude toward their work, as they pay more attention to themselves and their needs, and are for the first time able to say No, which had previously been enormously hard for them. In so doing, many therapists only then discover how important a full private life can be as a compensatory balance to their professional life.

12   Useful Information about Energy Testing

In an earlier chapter, I went into the historical development of Voll's Electroacupuncture (EAV) and its further evolution into Psychosomatic Energetics (PSE). Because of the central significance of the energy test for PSE, but also due to the many error possibilities and pitfalls, I'd like to readdress this area in a special new chapter. I would like also to explain why energy tests often fail when subjected to scientific scrutiny, while still getting good empirical results in clinical practice. It is important to know this, for example, when dealing with skeptical patients who need to be persuaded with a good and cogent argument.

By **energy testing**, I mean all procedures in which extremely weak energetic-psychic alterations are amplified enough to make them visible and perceptible. The methods include dowsing, pendulums, kinesiology, Voll's Electroacupuncture or Nogier's Auriculocardial Reflex (RAC). For many particularly sensitive persons, testing is unnecessary because they perceive the test results internally, either as a kind of tingling of the palms, an uprising feeling of Yes or No, or an inner image. Animals react very directly to energy fields and modify their behavior accordingly, i.e. wild animals will follow subterranean watercourses to the source.

Many people are good energy testers without knowing it. For instance, I once heard, from enthusiastic patients, of the outstanding successes of a strictly orthodox-medicine senior physician. When I used the Vegatest to check out his prescriptions for patients that we had in common, I was surprised at the result: complete energetic compensation. These were standard commercial allopathic medications which my colleague had so perfectly chosen intuitively that the patients responded very well to them. This good response was in turn an expression of the excellent energetic compensation which this highly intuitive internist had achieved with his prescriptions for our common patients without having consciously been aware of his talent as a tester. One can only appreciate how amazing this result is if you know that a good Vegatester normally needs nearly an hour with a patient, and has to test out a number of medications, in order to attain a comparably excellent result.

12.1 Disturbance due to external influences

As I've said, energy tests should always be done in geo-radiation-free zones, since otherwise the results will be distorted. The simplest check for geopathy can be done with a muscular person stretching out an arm at a 90° angle to the side, and maintain it in a horizontal position as another person tries to force the arm down. That is a basic kinesiological test that can be done very easily. Having the tested person then sit for 5 minutes in a geopathic disturbance zone will have such an energetically weakening effect that the arm will then be easy to force down afterwards. However, if the outstretched arm remains strong then the area is neutral. (Note: during the 5-minute sit, the arm should of course not continue to be held outstretched, sitting still will be quite enough.) By the way, the same test can easily be used to check whether a bed is geopathy-free or not, by having the test person simply lie down on it for 5 minutes, testing muscle strength before and after. Basically, I recommend consulting an experienced dowser (rather than resorting to the interference-prone self-test) and also measuring the level of electrosmog.

I have already mentioned the influence of electrosmog (active cell phones). The testing room should be calm and quiet so as to enable working in a relaxed manner. The energy fields of other people present in the room can also be a disturbance factor, especially if they are close to therapist and patient (closer than about 6 inches). Energetically active devices such as salt-crystal lamps, pyramids, medication packets lying around loose and the like can also be a source of disturbance. It goes without saying that the testing site should be clean and tidy. It is also important to always test in the same familiar place, since one is then working in a familiar setting. Therapists who travel around making house calls have a markedly harder time of it due to new and unaccustomed stimuli, and their results are not as reliable. That also applies, by the way, to testing practice at PSE seminars, where one should not take the results all too seriously, and perhaps get retested by a good tester once one has returned home.

Because of the disruptive effect of energetically contaminated fingerprints, I never let patients directly touch the test ampoules. When I hold the ampoules, that seems not to matter much, evidently because testers learn to fade themselves out energetically. Testers should take a little rest after each test, before examining the next patient, so as to "recharge the inner batteries". Testing always entails the loss of a good bit of life energy. This can be felt at the latest as exhaustion in the evening of a day in which one has energetically tested too many patients. I therefore test no more than six patients per day, taking one hour per test, and I still often feel drained afterwards. Since our energy systems work best in the morning and early afternoon, test appointments should be scheduled within this timeframe (for example 8 AM to 1 PM and 2 PM to 5 PM). I absolutely do not test after 5 PM because the test results are usually too imprecise.

It has been shown to be beneficial to briefly rinse one's hands in running water after testing – soap doesn't have to be used every time, instead a hefty spritz of 70% isopropyl alcohol is enough if one is also interested in a disinfectant effect. As we know, physicians' hands are some of the greatest sources of infection, and I think that this extends to the energetic aspect, since therapists contaminate themselves through dirty hands. Many colleagues find that it is a good pick-me-up to rest a couple of minutes or drink some clear mineral water in the interval between patients. Many meditate and have a softly burbling fountain installed to help them center and feel well, or they listen to some music. Testers need to each find their own way to best gather strength for the next patient.

12.2 Disturbances due to unconscious mental stress and doubt

When energy tests are scientifically investigated, the results are (apart from a few exceptions) very often catastrophic, in the random region. Critics conclude from this that one might as well throw a pair of dice as use a dowsing rod, kinesiology or EAV, and insinuate that the users are guilty at least of naïve self-deception. The thing is that the critics have a great deal of trouble understanding that the problem lies with themselves. Energy tests react extremely sensitively to any form of mental stress, such as when an energy tester's testing ability is blocked by emotional stress brought on by the presence of critical persons in the room. The tester is often completely unaware of the stress, but it seems to be present in many testers when a checking situation arises which is coupled to the test results.

> • **Note**
> One of the few **positive studies** of kinesiology was titled "Individual prognosis of the effectiveness of a therapeutic measure through the pre-therapeutically applied kinesiological muscle test". Study head Waxenegger and his colleagues

have a positive attitude towards kinesiology and thus had good self-confidence in the study, so they obtained good results (Source: *The Scientific World Journal*, September 2007).

I myself – with a similarly positive attitude as the Waxenegger team – in a small pilot study involving about 14 children in the Heidelberg University Clinic in 1979, correctly identified nine out of ten cancer patients using the Vegatest method and, with the test ampoule *Carcinomum comp.* as a marker for malignancy, had a 90% hit rate (I erroneously assigned one of the four healthy children to the cancer group). The healthy patients included an identical twin brother of a leukemia patient: the disease was not evident in either of the children. None of the children had any kind of cancer-specific symptoms such as alopecia etc. Unfortunately, when it came to the sub- differentiation with disease nosodes (e.g. lymphatic leukemia etc.), I was only able to get a 60% correct classification rate, which the (highly critical) medical director in charge dismissed as sheer chance, and although his statistician thought otherwise, his negative opinion of any form of alternative medicine unfortunately continued rock solid.

Typical example of a **negative study**: R. Pothmann: "Evaluation of clinically applied physiology to treat juvenile food intolerance". In: *Forsch Komplementarmedizin Klass Naturheilkunde* [Complementary-Medicine Research – Classical Naturopathy]. 2001.

Similarly devastating results can be found in numerous Wikipedia articles on kinesiology, Voll's Electroacupuncture and the like.

Any skepticism regarding the test itself becomes the occasion for a self-fulfilling prophecy, since energy test results get worse the more one doubts them. Now, as we all know, reasonable doubt is one of a scientist's most important tools. Scientists who stop being skeptical end up in the undesirable territory of speculation and belief. At this point, they would need to get a hold of themselves and adopt an unscientific, objective and positively-oriented attitude. Yet energy testers also constantly confront the problem of either believing their test results (and this attitude is reinforced by good test results) or doubting the correctness of their test results and thereby frequently producing nothing but unreliable results.

One often finds obsessive-compulsive characters among those testers whose doubt has led them to a permanent break with energy testing, for instance because they are too skeptical and for them everything has to be 100% correct. Such self-doubters need to learn how to differentiate between the important and the trivial, and also to loosen up a bit. Testers with a Schizoid or Depressive character structure seem to make the naturally best testers, while those of a Hysteric nature often tend towards the chaotic and to constant checking out of anything new (as per the misconception that anything new must be fundamentally better). Going this way, one can never become really good at anything, because good testers, like classical violinists, need years of practicing the same techniques and methods in order to perform masterfully and consistently.

As soon as any kind of doubt surfaces regarding energy testing, the error rate rises dramatically. The mere announcement of a scientific scrutiny hinders good results for nearly all test subjects. I, along with other experienced and well-known test physicians, have taken part in double-blind experiments in a hospital in which anonymized test ampoules – filled with various homeopathic cancer nosodes – were to be administered to anonymized patients. These experiments produced devastating results in the range of random chance. The bottom line of many such experiments is basically that energy tests are not scientifically verifiable as soon as doubt of any kind enters the picture. Even a tester's uneasy feeling ("Am I going to maybe make a fool of myself? I sure hope I test it right!") is enough to completely sabotage testing ability.

Despite these negative experiences, energy test procedures in daily practice do work, and in fact to an astonishingly precise degree! The Stuttgart EAV dentist Dr. Fritz, from whom we have the well-known EAV dental scheme which assigns the odontomas in each case to particular organs and functions, once assured me in a personal conversation that he, in more than 30 years' practice, always got test results that corresponded with the subsequent operation findings and the histology. I myself have made focal diagnoses on hundreds of patients which were confirmed by specialists in virtually all cases. I have had similarly good experience with energy-medicine testing, which sometimes even gives some support for making further progress using conventional methods such as surgery. Herewith an example from my practice.

• Case study

A 50-year-old female patient has had very severe lower back pain, day and night, radiating into both legs, for several years now. The patient has no more strength left. Various different examinations in the neurological and orthopedic departments of a university clinic, including computer tomography (CT) of the lumbar spine, failed to reveal any pathological findings.

> In my energy-medicine testing, the test ampoule for the spinal cord marrow (*Medulla spinalis*) responds as disturbed organ. At my suggestion, the patient requests a nuclear-spin tomography to display the soft tissue in the pelvic region. This very expensive examination had previously been rejected because a CT had already been performed, but the patient points to my tentative diagnosis and ultimately gets her way. To my colleagues' astonishment, the tomography reveals a large spinal cyst exerting mechanical pressure on the spinal column which is probably the actual source of the pain. After surgical removal of the cyst, the patient was permanently free from pain. During some shop talk with a neurologist acquaintance of mine, I later found out that cysts of this kind are often only found by chance, and that the usual radiological examination methods often overlook them. Without my energy testing, it is highly likely that the cyst would have remained undiscovered for a long time.

Not only objective findings agree with PSE test results, but above all, also the patient's impression, who will spontaneously say to me: "That's exactly how I feel!" Likewise, the PSE test results of conflicts are confirmed by the following typical statement from patients: "The trauma that you detected is one that my psychoanalyst has already been dealing with." At the PSE seminars one can regularly see that different testers working in different rooms (i.e. could not have secretly been peeking) always come up with the same test results. Statements from patients such as "My naturopath tested out this conflict in me a month ago!" I hear so frequently that it has become the rule rather than the exception. Consequently, testing provides very reliable results in daily practice – but above all, it almost always confirms to the patient that the testing was done correctly.

There are exceptions, for instance, if the conflict is part of an unconscious defensive strategy or a self-fulfilling negative attitude. Then, the conflict will often be denied at first, because the person doesn't want to believe it. For example, people with the conflict "Rage" claim that they never get angry. However, they suppress their aggressions instead of letting them out, or at least saying No at the proper time, while beneath the surface a hidden rage builds up. Many of those with the conflict "Mistrust" maintain that they are not mistrustful but, quite the contrary, all too trusting. Very often, it must laboriously be made clear to them that, unbeknownst to them, this makes it easier for other people to pull the wool over their eyes, thereby confirming their unconscious mistrust, of course.

Energy testers should make sure to exclude overly skeptical patients – and, of course doubting relatives – from energy tests, since nobody benefits when these testing procedures lead to unreliable results. I'd like to say that I, as a physician, find myself predominantly in an area of broad approval and the trust of all those present during energy testing. The patient wants to know what is wrong energetically, and above all would like to get healthy. This positive consent of the patient's, and my own desire to help, is the basis of my energy tests functioning and producing reliable results.

For many people, skepticism and a gnawing mistrust is simply part of their character. As long as I, as tester, don't let myself get "infected" by such feelings, then things are okay. The following is a clear example of this.

- **Case study**
  During a seminar, a large conflict with the theme "Mistrust" was detected in one of the therapists present. When asked whether the conflict meant anything to him, the test subject, surprisingly, did not want to say anything in public. It was an awkward situation, since the quality of the test result could not be clearly established. I began to wonder whether the test might possibly have gone wrong, and I spoke to the person privately during the break. He surprised me with the admission that the test result was right on the money, it's just that he didn't want to say that publicly because he was always having bad experiences with some other therapists (who were in the room), because these people, at his seminars (he was a recognized authority in certain areas) would steal important results and later pass them off as their own. Thus, his mistrust gave rise to his need for secrecy, which made understandable his desire not to talk about his emotional theme in front of the group. If his thieving colleagues were to learn about his "intellectual property" through his admission that he was wise to their tricks, then that would have been even more humiliating for him.

Evidently, this therapist with the theme "Mistrust" had a very real problem with mistrust, and the point is that his public silence originated precisely from this mistrust! I have seldom experienced a more perfectly clear example of a conflict during test demonstrations. It's just a shame that, because of his private admission during the break, I was the only one who was allowed to savor, privately, the diagnostic triumph of Psychosomatic Energetics.

Yet I also experience such curiosities time and again in other forms. For instance, many new patients surprise me by saying that they don't want to tell me anything for the patient history since, after all, diagnosis is my job, if you please. I then regularly bring something like "Mistrust" to the surface. As long as one doesn't let oneself be affected by this kind of aggression (because that's exactly what such attacks are), but rather stays calm and in a good mood, there's not much that can happen to the tester in such provocative situations; to a certain extent, it is a mild and amusing form of skepticism which, unlike scientific scrutiny, does not disturb the test results.

12.3 Pitfalls of mental testing and training good testers

One needs to distinguish between mental and physical testing. **Physical testing** means working with actual persons and actual test ampoules, such as testing the geopathy ampoule (Geovita) in the patient's energy field. **Mental testing** means asking the patient to make a visual image of the bed at home, as if lying in it, and then testing energetically whether and where a geopathy is found, such as by asking: "Is there a a geopathy?" The answer, via kinesiological test, is Yes or No; then: "Is it in the head region?" Answer Yes or No and so on. Mental testing means mentally asking oneself all the questions and naïvely assuming that the wisdom of one's own organism and that of the patient is enough to reveal the truth. But that is very often a fateful error! When mental testing is compared to the results of a good dowser physically testing on-site, they very often disagree. The same applies to many other findings which, with physical testing, usually agree very well – e.g. testing with the REBA Test Device, but not with mental testing.

Very few testers are at all capable of performing good mental testing. These few outstanding mental testers are often those who have developed a method such as kinesiology and teach it as well. On the other hand, for the other 99% normal mortals, mental testing is often too great a hurdle leading mostly to regrettable testing errors. Since the tests fundamentally are mostly located in a virtual realm which is very hard to verify, testing errors only come to the notice of the well-informed, e.g. if one, as a good tester, double-checks colleagues' results.

Most testers should be clever and critical enough to use a testing device such as the REBA Test Device, which emits defined physical frequencies that make reliable testing possible. Moreover, the REBA Test Device has the advantage of being able to evaluate the resulting test findings on the very important Vital as well as Emotional levels. Thus, one sees immediately whether a test finding more influences life force (Vital level) or the emotions (Emotional level), and to what percentage degree it does so. In this manner – besides the aforementioned extremely reliable test consistency – the tester receives an ideal assessment as to which harmful factor is how strong and on which energetic level it is most enervating, and which remedy will best heal, how strongly and on which energetic level. All who use kinesiology should therefore check their test results with a test device which emits an objective signal and sorts out their significance.

Because mental stress is so toxic to good energy testing, all forms of mental testing should be absolutely avoided! In my experience, energy testers who are blessed with particularly good results are those who can turn off their thinking and empty themselves completely. If I, as a tester, have the inner thought: "This patient definitely has conflict XYZ!" or "I hope the geopathy ampoule does not respond!", then I'm subject to a modest yet definite mental stress which downright sabotages an unprejudiced test result. I think that also applies to each and every form of mental questioning: "When did the conflict arise?" or "How many drops does the patient need?" are examples of impermissible questions, because in so doing, testers switch on their mental apparatus, which all too easily blocks the testing process.

Testing yields the best results when one has a relaxed, playful attitude in which the test result, at the moment of testing, is a matter of total indifference. For myself, testing is something that I enjoy without any sense of concentration or effort. EEG specialists talk about a relaxed, alert and happy Alpha state, and are familiar with the disruptive phenomenon of "Alpha block" as soon as strong stress upsets inner equilibrium. Good testing thus to a certain extent resembles meditation, in which one gives oneself over to a relaxing activity. The longer one performs testing, the better one seems to get at it, so that testing ability seems to be trainable.

12.4 Testers should be more energetically healthy than their patients

Testers with a good, conflict-free energy system test markedly better. Therefore, testers should be in an energetically better condition than their patients. Ultimately, testers do not test patients directly, but rather indirectly via their own energy field (cf. **Fig. 3.1**). The requirement for a harmonic energy field of the tester's would seem to be self-evident, but it often is not! At the Psychosomatic Energetics seminars, one can find therapists in droves who have poor energy values provoked by geopathies, emotional conflicts and the like – so it is no wonder that such therapists can only produce false test results.

> • **Note**
> Surprisingly, a small study of dowsers, conducted by myself and certified engineer Günter Engelhard, resulted in the exact opposite: the dowsers with the worst REBA test values got the best results. They might possibly be more sensitive to the negative geo-radiation, whereas energetically healthy persons balance out the geo-radiation and thereby can test out worse. [12]

Just as psychoanalysis requires self-analysis for analysts and – to mention a more banal example – surgeons, before operating, are required to wash their hands, precisely so should testers have a "clean", harmonious and open energy system and have experienced on themselves the methods of Psychosomatic Energetics. Beginners can make do with the Brunler-Bovis ampoule in their pants pocket, as well as possibly the Geovita ampoule, but these are not good options over the long term, since the entire test result is somewhat falsified thereby. We therefore absolutely require self-therapy during PSE training, which, by the way, is also very useful to the therapist as self-experience.

12.5 Testing children

For children less than 6-8 years old, the requirement that all other persons including the mother leave the room during testing can often not be enforced, so the mother must remain in the room. The formerly-promoted surrogate testing using the mother (who, with the Brunler-Bovis ampoule in the Yin region – and thereby energetically neutralized – holds the child by the arm while the mother is tested) I no longer recommend, since it is too uncertain. Instead of testing a surrogate, I prefer to test the child itself using the arm-length test. My youngest patient was 14 months old and only recently capable of sitting up, and the entire test, lasting about five minutes, was very relaxed and completely problem-free; the mother, sitting 6 feet away, could be seen by the child the entire time.

With children, kinesiological testing using the arm-length reflex test is literally child's play, in which one, without applying any muscle tension whatsoever, very lightly brings their arms together (**cf. Fig. 12.1**). Since children are energetically open, they still exhibit very strong and well-defined test reactions.

Because of their short attention span, one should limit oneself to as few test results as possible, such as

- Determining the Vital and Emotional values with the REBA Test Device in steps of 20%, then
- clarifying whether geopathy is present,
- which Chakra is disturbed,
- which conflict is present,
- whether Vital and Emotional REBA test values are normalized by the found Chavita and Emvita and finally
- what the size of the found conflict is; here the Causal value is enough to determine therapy duration.
- Sometimes one will also need one acute agent or another.

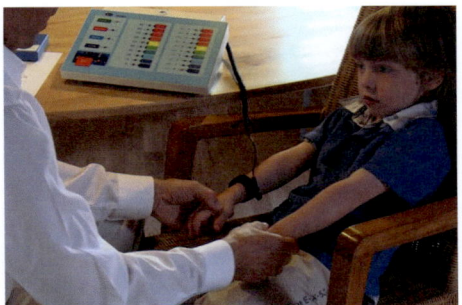

Fig. 12.1 – Testing a child with the kinesiological arm-length test and the REBA® Test Device. (With the kind permission of www.cmd-crossmedia.com.)

This quick testing lasts five minutes at the most, seldom longer, and demands of the tester a lot of practice and a great deal of sensitivity and tact. Therefore, one should only test small children after having acquired a fair bit of work experience. If one is relaxed and perfectly natural, then even these small patients will be quite free and easy and exhibit the necessary trust, because "it doesn't hurt at all and is fun". Sometimes, they will want to "help you" with the device and push a button or two, but that can usually be prevented, and offered as a reward at the end of the session. Children are fundamentally very rewarding patients from the viewpoint of PSE, because their energy systems are still very open and the therapy effects are thus very well-defined. In studies with children, the success rate with PSE was over 90%, while the rate for older persons went down to 70%. Rewarding indications include all forms of juvenile anxiety, behavioral disorders, ADHD, nocturnal bedwetting, unclear stomachache with no somatic equivalent and similar symptoms.

12.6 Testing animals

More and more pet owners are looking for gently effective and holistic forms of therapy, and because PSE is a kind of nonverbal psychotherapy, it is ideal particularly for animals with behavioral disorders. When it comes to household pets, the psychoenergetic disorders of the owner often have an amplifying effect, so it is advisable in many cases to treat animal and master together. Like mothers and their children, they often share a common conflict. Unlike humans, animals respond very quickly and visibly to the method, while we humans occasionally defensively put up unconscious resistance to conflict dissolution; energetically as well, we are, through our character type, more hardened and inflexible than animals are.

Overall experience to date indicates that conflicts, once eliminated, are gone forever. The results achieved are thus usually permanent – unless, of course, new external problems surface. I've learned through personal reports from veterinarians that they have had very good experiences especially when it comes to competitive-sport animals. For instance, an Olympic gold medal in dressage was won with the aid of PSE, which probably would not have been possible without the PSE (oral communication from the trainer). The dissolution of conflicts elevates an animal's overall energy state and thereby its performance.

Those who have an empathic relationship with animals very quickly sense that they have a rich emotional life. Empirical naturopathy has long known that animals can be treated through emotionally-acting energy agents such as Bach Flowers, homeopathic high potentiations or direct energy transfer (Reiki, Therapeutic Touch). Often, however, the results obtained are not far-reaching nor lasting enough. Some therapists – particularly veterinarians – have specialized in the PSE treatment of animals, who respond as well as or even better than children do to this method. Since the REBA Test Device has an effective radiation range of about 4-5 feet, there is no need to attach the electrodes to the animals (**cf. Fig. 12.2**). Unlike humans, animals only have a Vital and Emotional body, but otherwise testing is much like that for humans.

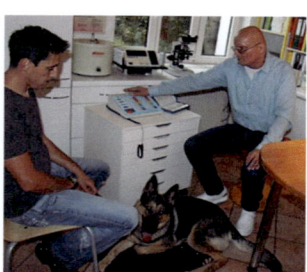

Fig. 12.2 – *PSE testing of animals, demonstrated by the Austrian veterinarian Rudolf Hauck. (Photo: Michaela Muschitz)*

If no REBA Test Device is available, you work with the

Basic Test Kit, placing ampoules in sequence near the resting animal, using your arm-length or a tensor as indicator.

For large animals like horses, put ampoules in a small bag around the animal's neck with a strap. Surprisingly, geographic stress is sometimes found in dogs, although this is a case of fleeing from radiation. The master's orders take precedence over the animal's instinctive behavior. For large hoofed animals, the stall sometimes makes avoidance impossible, so that geopathies can also be seen here, even though horses, cows, sheep etc. avoid geo-radiation.

13 Psychosomatic Energetics in Everyday Practice

The following describes real-world cases from daily practice which demonstrate the possibilities and limits of the method. The cases cover various areas of specialization that illustrate the current therapeutic spectrum of Psychosomatic Energetics, although they by no means provide a comprehensive overview: PSE is young yet and the areas of application are thus still in flux. The yearly Expert's Meeting of "Certified Energy Therapists" (the professional designation for therapists trained in PSE) provides new looks at new operational areas and demonstrates synergies with other methods which can provide support for PSE. The following compilation also contains some naturopathic recipes and proven therapeutic strategies which can usefully be applied (in part independently of PSE).

13.1 Anxiety, AIDS, addiction

There is a widespread assumption that discourse is essential when treating the mind, however that is not necessary with PSE. Children, the mentally handicapped or very old persons frequently can hardly talk about their emotional problems, and often lack the intellectual capacity to be adequately addressed at this therapeutic level. There are also many normal adults who are incapable of talking about their emotional problems, because these topics are either repressed or denied. Mild to moderately severe emotional elements in particular are one of the domains of PSE, starting with behavioral disorders on up to depressive states and anxiety diseases.

Specialists estimate that every 5th to 10th person suffers from **anxiety disease** at some point in life. This can be a situational short-term test anxiety, but also a social phobia or claustrophobia. What is often found in daily practice is a vague fear accompanied by excessive worries and apprehensions lasting for months. In PSE, a response to Anxiovita can provide indications of this and steer the therapy in the right direction, as shown in the following case.

Part 3 Clinical practice

- **Case study**

Ms. K has been suffering for over 10 years from chronic fatigue, which the University clinic has classified as "chronic fatigue syndrome". Numerous therapeutic attempts have thus far proven unsuccessful. During testing, the ampoules Anxiovita and the conflict "Restless, hectic" respond. My suspicion of a generalized anxiety ailment, which often masquerades as stubborn exhaustion, is soon confirmed. Upon inquiry, the patient reports being worried about all manner of things. After four months of PSE therapy, the symptoms have permanently disappeared, the patient once again feels fully fit, seems generally more carefree and, in her own words, no longer broods nearly as much as she used to.

Restless and inattentive children are a big problem in the modern world – one which has always existed, to be sure, but is on the rise due to a modern lifestyle with too little child-appropriate activity, very high pressure to get good grades in school and the "psychiatrization" of what is actually normal behavioral variation [3]. In today's constant sensory assaults, children can no longer find the necessary inner calm needed to collect themselves, and are overwhelmed by media messages from smart phones, PCs and television. They often get poor grades in school, which then triggers a visit to the doctor. If, as an alternative position, one looks for causes, one often finds the obvious: domestic electrosmog in the form of computers and television sets in children's bedrooms. If children suffer in addition from energy blocks due to geo-radiation and from emotional conflicts, it frequently leads to behavioral disorders and a sharp drop in performance at school, as the following case makes clear.

- **Case study**

10-year-old Michael suffers from disruptive behavior disorders such as fidgetiness and inability to concentrate, and therefore gets poor grades in school. The school psychologist mentions hyperkinetic syndrome and recommends transferring him back to private school from public school. Testing reveals geo-radiation stress and a conflict with the theme "Tense". The size of the conflict suggests a Central Conflict. The father confirms in conversation that Michael, as a Sanguinic, exhibits the typical character traits of the Hysteric personality type. Such people tend to want to be the center of attention, are very competitive and above all take everything to its maximum. In so doing, they overexert themselves much more than is normally healthy with respect to strength and energy reserves. For this reason, the parents must set particularly strict limits for Michael, since by his very nature he tends to overstep the bounds. The parent should reduce activities such as watching TV and playing computer games to a minimum, so as to avoid inflaming Michael's already overstimulated nervous system even more, which has more than enough to do dealing with the conflict theme. In addition, immediate relocation of his bedside to a neutral spot is strongly recommended, for which an experienced dowser is recommended. The conflict is treated for a number of months. A year later, I learn from a neighbor of theirs who brings her child in for therapy that Michael is doing very well and that things couldn't be better.

ADHD (attention-deficit/hyperactivity disorder) is almost always due to large conflicts and often geopathy as well, plus not infrequently electrosmog. The children affected usually have Vital and Emotional values less than 40%, which makes them fidgety and sometimes turns them into problem children. Sometimes, intestinal flora dysbiosis, chronic tonsillar foci and the like get added to the mix. In my opinion, the often-accused food-coloring and chemical hypersensitivities are consequences and not the actual causes, since healthy children easily tolerate brightly colored sweets.

Experience in everyday clinical practice suggests that the self-healing powers of the Psyche are much greater than is generally assumed. It is often claimed that emotional disorders can only be cured through psychological intervention, i.e. psychotherapy or behavioral therapy. However, in the majority of cases, this is not exclusively so – or at least only for very pronounced disorders for which, due to severe deficits in personality development, psychotherapy and behavioral therapy has become necessary. On the other hand, for many emotional disturbances, energy treatment is often enough, e.g. to markedly improve an **addiction situation** or even heal it. Obviously, self-control and discipline are just as necessary as a positive social environment, since all of this will not work by itself, but rather only supports the individual's own efforts.

> • **Case study**
> 50-year-old Mr. S Is long-term unemployed and has been an alcoholic since he was a teenager. On top of that, he is a heavy smoker. I examine him in the context of a pilot project to study the possibilities of Psychosomatic Energetics in dealing with addiction. The energy test reveals strikingly low Vital and Emotional values of 20%. The high Causal value of 80% shows him to be above-averagely sensitive – a fairly common finding among addicts. There is also a Central Conflict with the theme

> "Rage". In the post-test discussion, the caregiver confirms that Mr. S would never exhibit aggression, a typical personality trait of the Depressive character type to which he evidently belongs.
>
> Mr. S is prescribed the appropriate homeopathic compound remedies for four months in all. A few months later, the caregiver relates the following to me: "After a number of odd jobs, an employer has offered him a permanent position. Mr. S stopped drinking fairly soon after the PSE therapy. He now says that he can drink a beer at a party, but it never turns into too many anymore. He's smoking much less. After four years of misery and woe, he not only has a permanent job, but in the fall is to be hired in his original occupation (computer science). He's had a compact car for a few weeks, loves life and the people around him, and a new relationship might be in the works. He calls me regularly and shares with me his success and progress stories."

This case reveals the central role that personal well-being plays in maintaining a self-determined and healthy lifestyle. It was only when the man psychoenergetically returned to his middle – after his Central Conflict had been eliminated – that he was able to overcome his self-destructive addiction. Thus, the definition of the World Health Organization (WHO) is understandable, which considers well-being and self-determination to be important features of true good health. When talking about well-being, it is important (especially when it comes to addiction) to distinguish genuine from false well-being: heroin addicts may feel good after having taken their fix, but this is an artificially s(t)imulated sense of well-being. True well-being has no need for drugs, and only without them can it be the mark of quality of a self-determined lifestyle.

In the case of chronic fatigue syndrome (CFS), we are very often dealing with depressive exhaustion states which should accordingly be treated as depression (Chapter 13.2). These cases often involve unrecognized severe geopathy along with very large active conflicts. To make matters worse, there are often intestinal fungal infections as well, which alone often lead to crippling fatigue and a constant feeling of befuddlement. One sometimes also finds other focal diseases such as dental foci. The allegedly responsible Coxsackie, mononucleosis and herpes virus titers are, in my assessment, simply the consequence of a weakened immune system, and not the actual cause. Even Borrelia, besides a neurotic iatrogenically-created disease development, is often more a hodgepodge of disorders which, in the view of PSE, can be otherwise explained.

In the newer terminology, psychovegetative symptoms are designated as "**somatoform complaints**", previously referred to as vegetative dysregulation or neurasthenia. At the beginning of the previous century, these complaints were considered to be a pastime of bored aristocrats having nothing better to do with their time. Even now, modern medicine's linguistic innovation still betrays a hint of a certain disdain, although PSE makes it perfectly clear that psychovegetative symptoms cause real and excruciating pain. It's just the patient's bad luck that, in the realm of the invisible where the blocks are located, conventional medicine cannot cope and has no solutions to offer.

For acute exhaustion, vitamin B complex and mineral injections (Zentramin) have sometimes proven useful. Phosetamin as an oral medication and Horvi Psy 4 comp 1 drops are often useful as a first aid.

13.2 Emotional ailments – Central Conflict dissolution

The first case illustrates the classical effect of a dissolution of the Central Conflict; healing it has mostly a strongly catalytic effect in the form of a clear, positive personality transformation.

> **• Case study**
> A 40-year-old personal assistant complains about **mobbing** at work. She says that her boss is always on her case, that according to him she can't do anything right. Because of this, for years she has had trouble sleeping, is constantly exhausted and has been to a number of different clinics. Her fear of long-term unemployment means that she can't quit, since women of her age have trouble finding work. The PSE test reveals very depressed Vital and Emotional values of 20% each, as well as a large Central Conflict with the theme "Helpless, at the mercy of" in the first Chakra. The typical core symptoms (likes to be alone, strategically oriented, rationalistic, does not like chitchat, takes her time to warm up to others) show her to be a typical Melancholic. It becomes clear to me that a good personal assistant would need to have many Melancholic character traits. The fact that, Mobbing aside, she feels very good in her job likewise supports the correctness of the diagnosis.
> I see her again nine months later (therapy for the Central Conflict alone took seven months). She seems completely transformed and explains, to my surprise, that she

> is still working at the same place and still has the same boss. She invites me to guess what it was that changed. My guess is that she has given notice, but she surprises me by saying that she simply changed her mental attitude. She laughs inside at her boss now, something she'd not been able to do before. Her work makes her happy again, and the further motivation is that her mobbing boss is retiring soon. His successor is a very nice person and she's already looking forward to working with him.

Although I am not familiar with the character type of the mobbing boss, he might well be a Sanguinic. Sanguinics by nature have low self-esteem that is in constant need of external validation. Melancholics don't know this and tend to overlook it because that's not the way they are. On the contrary, because they are unshakably self-assured and for the most part not very empathetic, they, in the eyes of Sanguinics, commit one inexcusable error after the other without (as presumably in the case of the personal assistant above) at all being aware of doing so.

Added to which which is the fact that Sanguinics are by nature competitive. Masterful job performance, such as the personal assistant's, puts pressure on them, making them feel forced into a competitive situation which really only exists in their imagination. They thereby feel under constant challenge and often degraded, especially if the colleague does not signal submission. The Melancholic does not catch any of this and is then surprised at the harsh reaction as in the case above, where the mobbing probably represents a kind of psychological self-therapy to the boss, i.e. by somehow managing to win the imaginary contest with his assistant. One can see from what has been said that both protagonists have taken their characterological worldview as a standard, thereby overlooking that the other person has a completely different one.

Basically, PSE therapy by no means leads inevitably to divorce, quitting and separation, as can be seen in the case of the mobbed personal assistant described above. Instead, her improved self-esteem leads to greater personal integrity, as the personal assistant is better able to set out limits and clearly maintain her autonomy. Because she now feels well and stable inside, her boss's attacks largely bounce harmlessly off her. Improved self-demarcation after Central Conflict treatment is particularly striking in the case of the Choleric, for whom it represents the central emotional problem, as the following example illustrates.

> **• Case study**
> At age 48, this independent masseuse contracts **fibromyalgia**, whose intensity

rises constantly. She is in agonizing pain day and night, and can no longer work, so at age 60 she takes early retirement. She hasn't had a pain-free day for about 13 years. Despite all attempts with various rheumatism clinics, naturopaths and naturopathic physicians, she receives not the slightest alleviation. Emotionally, the patient seems extraordinarily gentle and compliant, friendly and warm – in sharp contrast to her symptoms.

In the energy test 50% Vital, 10% Emotional (!), 90% Mental and 40% Causal. An enormous Central Conflict (#9, "rage, exploding") is found in the upper abdomen with the values 90% Vital, 90% Emotional, 20% Mental and 80% Causal. Placing the test ampoules for Rage (Emvita 9) and for Chavita 3 yields normal readings in the remedy test of 100/100/100/80, which gives good hope for a positive therapy outcome later on. At the follow-up check two months later, she says that it's like a miracle. After just three days, all symptoms had completely disappeared. She didn't think it was possible, but despite unfavorable autumn weather, the rheumatism is now as good as gone. I now test personal values of 100% Vital, 100% Emotional, 90% Mental and 80% Causal. Since the Central Conflict continues to test out large, it is treated for an additional four months. Curious afterwards, I ask her if there'd been any changes after she took the "Rage drops". She reported on vivid dreams with fierce interpersonal confrontations and discussions which she first plays through and anticipates noncommittally in the subconscious. She can now say No in real life and not just in dreams, and is starting to learn to stand up for herself. She realizes that she had put up with too much in the past. It had always been her misguided inclination to try to please everybody.

Eliminating the Central Conflict often leads to emotional maturation (and sometimes genuine developmental) leaps, along with downright spectacular growth steps and positive personality changes. However, the changes are often unnoticeable and hardly perceptible even to those affected, so that, interestingly, the difference is only noticed by others such as family members or friends who had not seen the patient for a long time. Therapists need to know this so as not to be needlessly disappointed. Evidently, the ability to perform an accurate self-assessment is much less pronounced than we think.

13.3 Psychiatric ailments

In cases of **moderate to mild depression**, one can – as is customary in naturopathic practices – initially prescribe high doses of St. John's wort, 300 mg 2-3 times daily (warning: sunlight). One should not forget about intestinal flora as an important site of neurotransmitter formation! For seasonal winter depression, one sometimes needs light in the form of high Alpine visits, sunlamps or light radiation (in psychiatric outpatient departments etc.), as well as vitamin D 2000-4000 IU daily. There are more than a few depression cases brought on by geo-radiation. My Austrian colleague Otto Bergsmann was able to show that geopathy provokes a lab-verifiable highly significant serotonin deficiency – a deficiency now recognized to be an important factor in the onset of depression. Mild to moderate depression cases are very common in clinical practice. PSE is likewise quite effective and often enough by itself, as the following two case studies show, which my colleague Dr. Birgitt Holschuh-Lorang has treated and documented.

> • **Case study**
> Monika, 59. The patient has suffered from depression for years, and has therefore taken early retirement. She complains of anxiety, sleep disorders, feels weak and has little drive despite taking Mirtazepin and Maprotilin. The first examination with the REBA Test Device reveals vitality reduced to 30% and an equally reduced reading for emotional resilience. The patient has no trouble identifying with these values as far as her state of health is concerned. Over 4 therapy sessions in all, 4 unconscious conflicts block energy uptake, whose themes are "Experiencing life as a struggle", "Retreat and hurt feelings", "Rage" and finally "Disrupted self-esteem". Therapy is very simple and consists of taking the corresponding Chavita and Emvita remedies associated with each conflict theme, mornings and evenings 12 drops each. At the end of treatment, the values for vital energy and emotional resilience have climbed to 90%, and this is clearly reflected in the patient's state of health. She feels much more active and stable, the fears have disappeared, she sleeps well, her drive is noticeably improved, she can perceive her goals and implement them. The antidepressants are no longer needed.

> • **Case study**
> Ingo, 23, has complained for several months of strong inner unrest; he feels very tense. Because of his parents' separation and his grandmother's death, he is in

> a depressive mood. He doesn't feel up to the demands of his studies. Despite psychotherapy and initially taking Fluoxetine, then Ciprolex, he is not doing any better. The results of the first testing session reflect this clearly reduced state of health: a Vital reading of only 20% and an Emotional value of a mere 25% are measured. Six therapy sessions are needed to resolve the conflict themes "Flight from reality", "Retreat and hurt feelings", "Feeling closed in", "Frustration" and "Perseverance" with the corresponding homeopathic compound remedies Chavita and Emvita. Thanks to the energy increase as a consequence of the treatment, with an improvement of the Vital reading to 100% and the Emotional to 95%, he experiences a noticeable improvement in his sense of well-being, saying that he's doing great, that he's feeling more and more able to deal with the demands of his studies and he got a good grade on the final exam. He feels well-balanced, is no longer restless, has plenty of drive. The thoracic pressure is gone, he no longer needs Cipralex.

In terms of life expectancy, **severe depression** is a more serious disease than cancer. One of the main reasons for this is suicide – but also chronic sleep deprivation with obesity, an expression of elevated levels of stress hormones as well as other internal consequences of stress. The self-destructive phenomenon of suicide allows a clear study of the secret dynamics of highly active conflicts – a dynamism which has a self-destructive effect on the conflict host. Before the act itself, many suicides exhibit a peculiar aggressiveness and/or high spirits, whereas earlier they had been depressed and withdrawn. To the uninitiated, this looks like improvement, and is therefore often wrongly interpreted as such by unsuspecting relatives. In my estimation, however, the high spirits and not only to be viewed as an emotional sign of incipient self-aggression, as traditional psychiatry assumes, but rather, from the viewpoint of the conflict, a sign of conflict activation, which in a certain sense "takes the wheel" and drives the patient into suicide. The rage, frustration etc. of the conflict thus directs itself in a self-destructive manner against the patient himself – which, as has been already mentioned, does not matter in the least to the conflict, because it is single-mindedly interested only in the constant staging of its conflict contents. One should speak openly with suicide patients about their secret desires and intervene appropriately.

In cases of severe depression, there is no avoiding allopathic adjuvant medication in the initial phase, e.g. the modern serotonin antagonists (Paroxetin is very good). In uncertain cases with risk of suicide, one should try to establish co-therapy with a psychiatrist – for forensic reasons alone. The Emotional values are usually under 10%, sometimes even 0%! I'd also like here to point out a valuable differential-diagnostic possibility, available only to energy testers. If serotonin antagonists absolutely do not respond in the test, then this empirically indicates emotional (neurotic) depression. If, on the other hand, serotonin antagonists exhibit a positive test reaction, then this points to a serious neurotransmitter deficiency. When it comes to conspicuous clinical depression, I occasionally do not shy away from prescribing an allopathic antidepressant during the initial phase of treatment, and I have often had very good results with this. Not infrequently, one will also note that an allopathic antidepressant which has been taken for a long time loses its effectiveness (tests energetically neutral); it should then be swapped out for another more effective medication.

In therapy-resistant depression cases (an emotionally very excruciating disease against which the usual antidepressants have failed), I have for decades enjoyed excellent results with Trancylpromin – but it must be applied correctly (a diet low in tyramine, no hard cheese, red wine etc.). Noticeable improvement often sets in after just 4-5 days, but if nothing is happening after three weeks, then the patient is a non-responder. For manic-depressive patients, PSE therapeutic results are usually poor due to the patient's erratic emotional state, who thus does not take the remedy regularly, so an attendant is needed to supervise administration of the PSE remedies.

Experience has shown that **psychoses** are tricky cases, which is why specialist co-therapy is a good idea. Psychotics usually have very low Mental values of less than 20% and frequently oversized conflicts which have to be eliminated in a laborious protracted process. Added to which, the personality disorders can sometimes also persist long after the psychosis has abated (residues). In the case of juveniles for whom timely treatment has begun right after onset of the disease (conflict dissolution with PSE and parallel treatment, properly performed, with antipsychotics such as Clozapin, Risperidon etc.), there are often no remaining personality deformations and very good healing courses. Especially in the initial phase, patients often exhibit substantial additional worsening during treatment of the usually active Central Conflict (often Chakra 1 or 7 themes!), which can be taken to be conflict resistance. However, using the "bottle method", one can usually maneuver successfully around these dangerous reefs.

13.4 Venous and arterial circulatory disorders

Psychosomatic Energetics is effective not only for emotional ailments, but physical ones as well. Those who from the very start consider alternative medicine to be no more than a placebo will of course find this assertion implausible, but I'd like to put forward a patient as an example, one who suffered for decades from stubborn varicose ulcers (**Ulcera cruris**). These circular sores in the ankle region, often up to an inch or two in diameter, usually appear as consequence of deep venous thrombosis due to congenital connective-tissue insufficiency. If it persists for years, the disease is usually considered to be therapy resistant, i.e. it does not disappear on its own and it often resists all attempts at treatment. Usually, the only recourse is consistent mechanical compression therapy or an operation. For the patient I'd like to present, however, that was ineffective, which is why she finally came in for PSE therapy.

> **• Case study**
> Ms. J, a 47-year-old patient, is slender and athletic, and she takes great care with her diet. She is happily married and has two children. Her biggest problem is the lower-leg sores located above both ankles with about half-inch-deep wound craters (cf. Fig. 13.1). Because the sores often have an unpleasant smell, she's disgusted with herself. She has tried everything, but nothing has helped permanently. Her mother and grandmother had also had it, so it is probably hereditary. Psychosomatic Energetics testing found reduced Vital and Emotional values of around 60%. The pelvis responded as disturbed segment with the conflict "Helpless"(Emotional remedy 3). When asked about it, it occurred to her that she often did feel helpless and at the mercy of her dominating parents and other people – and she is likewise helplessly at the mercy of her *Ulcera cruris*. After taking Emvita 3 and Chavita 1 for a number of months, the leg sores heal up completely for the first time in over a decade, with no need for any additional therapeutic measures. Her situation has now been stable for several years. A brief relapse was dealt with by eliminating an additional conflict.

Other cases of lower-leg sores were treated by various therapists with comparable success, so it is unlikely to have been due to pure chance. However, to be on the safe side, I'd like to add that there are also some cases in which PSE therapy brought no improvement for leg sores. Nevertheless, the successful treatments do demonstrate that PSE can have a clear effect on blood flow and the tissue healing. Yogis come to mind, who meditate in the snow for hours; they can consciously change their subtle energy and thereby increase blood circulation so much that they do not get frostbite. This applies as well to arterial circulatory disorders, and many patients report, after successful PSE therapy, to have warm hands and feet for the first time in their lives.

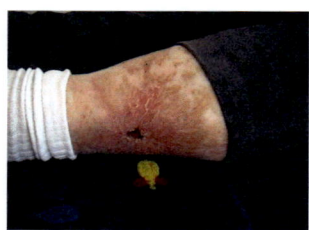

Fig. 13.1 – Ulcus cruris *healing up.*

The following case is quite impressive.

> • **Case study**
> Male patient, middle-aged businessman, heavy smoker, somewhat overweight, has advanced **Claudicatio intermittens** (OAD St.II). He was only able to walk about 150 feet or so without pain, and the distance was getting ever shorter. The internist treating him was considering leg amputation would be necessary if he did not quit smoking – which, however, he did not do, and sought alternative-medicine aid. PSE revealed a large conflict in the pelvic region with the theme "In control". After its elimination four months later, the patient can for the first time take longer walks again with no pain, but he continues to smoke. The next round involved a conflict in the third Chakra with the theme "Frustration" being active. After it has been eliminated four months later, the patient gives up smoking on his own, and the pain-free walking distance has increased even more.

By the way, I have seen good results in comparable cases with ozone-autologous-blood infusions.

13.5 Cardiovascular diseases

Cardiovascular diseases top the mortality statistics in the Western world. The known causes to date are based on unhealthy lifestyle and genetics. One should know that more than 99% of human cholesterol is produced in the liver, and that lack of an exogenous supply does fairly little therapeutically; in addition, both eggs and butter are an important source of lecithin. LDL should be below 100 mg/dL (www.ldl-unter-hundert.de), but coenzyme Q10 should be administered to protect muscle tissue when taking high doses of statins [53]. Patients should be advised to eat a Mediterranean diet with lots of fish, olive oil, garlic, fresh vegetables, fresh white bread and salads, as well as red wine in moderation. The resveratrol found in red wine is produced primarily in oak barrels for dark reds such as Cabernet or Shiraz.

Sunlight, for instance, can make possible a brief vacation in the South during the winter, or the administration of vitamin D (2000-4000 IU daily), can have protective effect. Much can be changed regarding the emotional causes of an unhealthy lifestyle by eliminating the conflicts. For instance, many smokers and overweight persons often have, as has been said previously, large and unconscious frustration-generating conflicts. In general, I don't think much of artificial vitamin and food supplement intake, apart from genuine deficiencies of e.g. folic acid, iodine (as iodide 200 μg per day) or vitamin D. By the way, all the large meta-studies of artificial vitamin supplementation have so far had negative results.

> • Note
> A folic acid deficiency, quite common, is usually caused by bad intestinal flora. Too little folic acid lets the homocysteine level go down, which in turn is an important cause of arteriosclerosis. The elevated presence of superannuated erythrocytes in darkfield microscopy, i.e. erythrocytes with a whitish shimmering aged membrane is, in my experience, predominantly due to folic acid deficiency. The primary cause is usually found in bad intestinal flora (occasionally also caused by poor diet with very little fresh foods). The folic acid deficiency inhibits the formation of new erythrocytes, which is why darkfield microscopy shows the aforementioned "old folks home" in the form of superannuated erythrocytes. These old erythrocytes transport oxygen less effectively. Patients often feel tired, wheeze after strong physical exertion (stress-induced shortness of breath with no cardiac or bronchial cause), often have chronic ailments such as cancer (where, according

> to Otto Warburg, oxygen deficiency is known to play a role) and calcify more quickly – occasioned by the oxygen deficiency in the intima vessels of the arterial vascular walls. Treatment is easy, since regenerating the intestinal milieu often also improves the folic acid deficiency; in addition, one can prescribe folic acid tablets.

For **hypertension** patients, good results can be achieved in some cases through conflict dissolution and administering Simvita, although that is hardly ever enough. One should test out the appropriate hypertension remedy for tolerance; ACE inhibitors and calcium antagonists often test out very well energetically. This is due to the relationship of the ACE inhibitors with snake venoms, which likewise have a roborant and immune-system stimulating effect. Since in my practice I have available all the modern options for monitoring blood pressure, from the 24-hour blood-pressure recording to the stress EKG; since I also work with specialists on problem patients, I feel confident, after decades of activity in this area, to give a comprehensive opinion at this point.

My summary, after more than 20 years of my own intensive follow-up checks, is simply this: objectively verifiable and long-lasting blood-pressure reduction is only possible with mainstream medications.

There is an often-voiced objection (which actually does not hold true) to the effect that hypertension medications allegedly have so many side effects, because the benefit in the form of lower blood pressure outweighs them all by far. The lay public should know that the litigation mania of American lawyers has meanwhile led, worldwide, to elaborate formulations in the package insert designed to forestall any possible lawsuit by simply issuing warnings concerning almost anything that could possibly happen. Unfortunately, the lay public is thereby no longer able to assess what is actually relevant and is, regrettably, needlessly frightened.

Some anti-hypertensive medications have turned out to be particularly gentle and useful, which is why I preferentially prescribe them. This includes a mixture of a mild diuretic chemical substance together with an Indian plant *Rauwolfia serpentina* (sold under the trade names Briserin, Triniton etc.). For mild to moderate hypertension, these mixtures have over the decades proven to be very effective and low in side effects. From the 1960s to the 80s, they were Germany's top-selling anti-hypertensives. Nowadays, unfortunately, these preparations are considered to be outdated by specialists, probably simply because the pharmaceutical industry no longer researches nor promotes them – which, however, in no way reduces their outstanding efficacy.

The aforementioned agent is 50% plant origin and thus extremely inexpensive; it has been put to the test in millions of cases over the decades. In my clinical practice, it has always proven to be very reliable and effective, with a gentle action, i.e. it only lowers blood pressure when actually necessary, so there is no danger of over-therapy.

The second group of substances that have proven to be biologically well-tolerated and useful are the so-called ACE inhibitors. Originally developed from snake venom and closely related to it, the angiotensin inhibitors have retained the immune-system-elevating, overall-energetically-stimulating, "fit-making" and biologically-stimulating characteristics of the original snake venom. We now know these valuable biological characteristics from specially prepared detoxified preparations such as the Horvi Snake Venoms which many naturopaths and naturopathic physicians apply successfully, particularly in chronic disease cases. Besides the aforementioned advantages which make them valuable biologically over a broad spectrum, ACE inhibitors also have blood-pressure-lowering properties.

Basically, from a biological standpoint, all chemical anti-hypertensives are better than their reputation. Most patients tolerate them excellently and can take them without reservation for years, although some monitoring in the first months, as well as later on, is not a bad idea. As with all blood-pressure agents, a prescription will be necessary, i.e. they cannot be purchased without further ado at pharmacies by laypersons, which makes sense considering the advisability of qualified monitoring. Moreover, experience has shown that blood-pressure agents can sometimes be reduced or even terminated if they have been taken for a long enough time. However, one should not raise patients' hopes (with these to be sure rather infrequent cases from clinical practice) that they might not necessarily have to take the medicine forever.

I have had good long-term results with existing coronary heart disease cases, with clearly improved resilience using heparin injections (5000-7500 IU as an off-the-shelf injection subcutaneous in the abdomen twice weekly for a total of 3-4 months). After the injection – which willing patients can administer themselves after simple instruction – patients should engage in moderate exercise, which promotes capillary formation in the coronary arteries. In cases of cardiac arrhythmia, one should always search for head foci (teeth, nasal sinuses, with the Organ Test Kit). In cases of long-standing atrial fibrillation with TIA and risk of apoplexy, I recommend Marcumarisation and have seen good results with it, both prophylactically and with respect to overall energetic state. Cases of cardiac insufficiency respond well to *Scilla maritima*, hawthorn, mineral supplements (Tromcardin,

Trophicard), Strophantin (Strodival) – the appropriate combination can easily be tested out with the remedy test.

13.6 Allergies

Allergic diseases such as hay fever, **asthma** and neurodermitis take on an ever-growing medicinal significance in our modern society. About a fifth of adults have allergies, as do a third of the children, and the rising figure of sick children means it's not hard to see that the number of allergy sufferers is constantly increasing. Environmentally conscious critics place the responsibility for this on the rising number of environmental toxins. And in fact, one can show in Japan that the number of allergies is higher on city streets with high traffic density than in rural areas. The answer in this case was found to be soot particles clinging to pollen, thereby intensifying the allergic reactions.

Further confirmation for the environmental theory of allergy would seem to be the fact that allergies are virtually unknown in primitive societies. Ecologically oriented people make environmental toxins exclusively responsible for allergies, which is certainly partly true. But the main cause of the rising number of allergies is due not only to environmental toxins, but to the lack of *dreck* (dirt mud filth) in our modern world, which the immune systems of primitive societies still have to cope with. For example, Amazon Indians basically all have intestines full of parasites which keep the immune system so busy that it has no time left over for the production of such silly things as allergies. One Japanese researcher's curiosity led him to infect himself with tapeworms, at which point he promptly lost his allergies.

Nowadays, experts recommend that mothers of allergy-at-risk babies – i.e. one or even both parents are allergy sufferers – continue breast-feeding as long as possible, just as they do in primitive societies. Breast-feeding supplies the developing infant's immune system with protective anti-allergic substances from the mother. In addition, they recommend a lot of contact with dirt and not so much hygiene as soon as the child begins crawling around. Best of all would be growing up on a farm, particularly for children at risk of allergy. Of course, best of all would be to prevent allergies from the very beginning, by starting with the baby and its mother. One easy possibility along this line would be inoculations of the newborn child with eubiotics (e.g. Mutaflor suspension daily on the tongue for a few weeks) as well as early elimination of psychoenergetic blocks. In this manner, outbreak of allergy can be prevented in many cases.

Research in **psychoneuroimmunology** has shown that the mind and the immune system are intimately interlinked. Numerous studies confirm that long-term emotionally depressing and disheartening situations weaken the immune system. Logically enough, cancer patients with a positive attitude have a higher life expectancy, which is what therapies such as the well-known Simonton method are based on. Moreover, immunological reactions can be trained and conditioned, so that patients can learn to view the future more optimistically. So, within certain limits, immune function can be trained to take a desired course; with some restrictions, this of course also applies to allergies.

In acute allergies such as **neurodermitis** attacks, one can see the close relationship to intestinal flora in the fact that Colibiogen injections for acute allergically triggered symptoms often effect very rapid relief – often even more so than high-dosage cortisone. Kanne Brottrunk (bread drink), by normalizing intestinal flora, has a rapid inflammation-relieving effect, and can also be rubbed into the skin externally, for example applied after a shower with a damp sponge. In cases of bronchial asthma, one sometimes finds a subliminal sinus inflammation as focus, as well as, for many allergies, dysbiosis (Organ test ampoule "Colon"responds). Not infrequently, PSE conflict treatment is followed by clear improvement of an allergy. In addition, I recommend specific desensitization in the form of hypodermic or oral medication such as is generally customary in mainstream medicine. Combined with naturopathic procedures, I have often achieved my best results this way.

A very useful therapy with children is homeopathic potentiation of autologous blood (generally), autologous urine (asthma) or mother's milk (for milk crust). Add a few drops to a 30 mL medicine glass with 30% alcohol (available inexpensively at most drugstores; first remove the stopper, add the drops of blood then replace the stopper), then vigorously rap the glass 100 times on a hardcover book; this results in a C1-Korsakoff potentiation. Add a few drops from this C1 glass to another 30 mL glass with alcohol and rap as above (C2); continue for 6 glasses until a C6 potentiation has been reached. Now the child is given six drops daily of the C6 for three weeks in his milk bottle, then likewise the C5 as well, and so forth down to C1.

For active **hay fever**, I have seen the best results from Colibiogen injections. One ampoule injected intramuscular per week will keep the symptoms under control.

There are also good compound preparations from certain firms, such as DHU hay fever agent/Luffa, comp (Omida). For house-dust allergy, the homeopathic physician Wiesenauer recommends Sabadilla D6 globuli 3x5 globuli for 3 weeks, 1 week rest, then repeat. Pollinosis S capsules from Ronneburg have proven themselves in my practice for oral desensitization, preferably pre-seasonal. Snake venoms (Horvitrigon pure toxin forte 2x10 drops daily OP Horvi) prophylactically, presumably as suppressor cells are thereby activated and immune-moderating portions promoted. By the way, in many of its preparations, Sanum therapy is based on similar effects, in that the immune system is in a sense diverted away from the allergy.

I'd also like to mention foci and intestinal flora disorders which, as important hidden causes, can both provoke and prolong allergies. For neurodermitis patients in particular, nothing is going to work without first cleansing the disturbed intestine (often fungi and anaerobes!), just as asthmatics often have sinusitis as a focus. One of my most remarkable cases came at the beginning of my professional career, when I diagnosed a tonsillar focus in a young woman with severe neurodermitis. Even though her tonsils looked normal and she had no tonsil-related symptoms, I was able to persuade my ENT colleague to remove the seemingly healthy tonsils because of the severity of the clinical picture. The patient reported that, during the tonsillectomy, the pus squirted up to the ceiling – and the very next day her neurodermitis was gone!

Regarding neurodermitis, here is yet another typical case study.

• **Case study**
Jonas is a lively eight-year-old boy who has suffered since infancy from pronounced neurodermitis. Despite his above-average body size, Jonas is visibly undernourished because, says his mother, he apparently suffers from dietary intolerance to milk and wheat (according to kinesiological testing done by a previously consulted therapist). Because of the presumed food allergy, he has needed a special diet for years which, to all appearances, has led to his obvious undernourishment. Like starving third-world children, Jonas's individual rib bones are clearly visible, and he has an unhealthy pale facial tone.
The REBA Test Device finds a very low Emotional reading of 30% which matches his sub-depressive condition. Underlying Jonas's condition is an enormous psychoenergetic conflict with the theme "Wrong thinking" in the seventh Chakra. The cause of the conflict can be found in intrauterine stress situations. In addition, Jonas has disturbed intestinal flora, as the test ampoule "Colon" (Organ test kit)

indicates. First, a considerable fungal infection (candidiasis) needs to be treated with nystatin and Amphotericin lozenges (4 weeks). Besides the typically bright red tongue of the fungal-infection patient, with mucus-whitish rear third of the tongue (colonic reflex area), Jonas has a sore anus and a craving for sweets – all of which indicates fungal infestation of the intestines, which is confirmed by a stool test (fungal breeding ground). Later, the intestinal flora are built up with eubiotics (Mutaflor and/or Colibiogen, plus bifidus bacteria and Hylak drops) and the intestinal milieu is acidified with Kanne Brottrunk (bread drink, available at health food shops, two shot glasses daily mixed with apple juice).

Additionally, after showering, Kanne Brottrunk (bread drink) is rubbed into the skin. I also prescribe gamma linoleic acid as capsules and as salve. After this, Jonas's neurodermitis is completely healed except for small residues on the hands and the inside of the elbows, which quickly disappear after applications of St. John's wort oil and Cardiospermum salve. Thankfully, Jonas can once again eat anything, including the alleged dietary allergens; he gains weight noticeably, and has a fresh healthy facial skin tone. In addition, his school work improves, so that, according to his mother, he is no longer so fidgety and distracted.

In my experience, the great majority of supposed **food allergy** sufferers consists of people with severe intestinal flora dysbiosis, whereby the intestinal mucous membrane has been rendered extremely hypersensitive, like the feel of a shirt on sunburned skin which one can hardly stand to wear. Once the intestinal flora are improved and the agitated immune system (which is often also irritated by foci and geopathy, as well as psychoenergetic conflicts), the alleged dietary intolerance often disappears as well! By the way, very similar processes also lead to apparent heavy-metal stress (amalgam), where an already severely disturbed metabolism completely decompensates if a heavy metal is added to the mix. It is therefore urgent to normalize a disturbed metabolism, which means that heavy metals can then much more easily be dealt with (and excreted more from the now healthy organism, as urine tests confirm).

13.7 Hormonal disorders

Infertility is very often triggered by severe geopathy, less often by electrosmog. Besides geopathy, childless couples often have large conflicts the pelvic or head region. The sixth Chakra blocks the hormonal system, while the seventh Chakra blocks the pelvis via the high/low coupling. For infertile males, I prescribe Unizinc and Testiculus Spl. or Damiana (Cefagil). Good for women are Pascofemin or Gynaecoheel for stimulating the hormonal system. The thyroid gland and its fertility-stimulating effect should not be neglected here, say with Jodid 200 µg 1×1 over 6 months and/or iodine-containing seafood such as seaweed, saltwater fish etc.

Another hormonal organ which often triggers remote effects is the **thyroid gland**, first as a metabolic motor, but also from an energetic standpoint (Chakra 5). Many people feel much better at the seashore simply because their craving for iodine is satisfied. Even today, iodine deficiency is for many people, especially teenagers, an important dieases factor easily remedied by a few months of iodine therapy (Jodid 200 1×1 daily, or as a "wild dosage" as seaweed, Sushi etc.) and frequent dining on saltwater fish. When it comes to hyperthyroidism, I have heard very little good about Lycopus preparations and, in cases of manifest non-regressible diseases, I basically tend to recommend radioiodine therapy even for young persons, rather than having them constantly take outright toxic thyreostatics. Radioiodine therapy is much gentler than any operation, and of course the risk of hypoparathyroidism is also not present.

Hashimoto thyroiditis can sometimes be brought well into line with intensive PSE therapy [43].

13.8 Adjuvant therapy in malignancy cases

Worry and grief and emotionally harmful events are often associated with a later outbreak of cancer (psycho-oncology). However, studies on the influence of traumas on subsequent emergence of cancer (Bergelt, Johansen) have yielded no or very weak correlation. A pioneering study by the Stanford psychiatrist David Spiegel in 1989 showed that group therapy increased life expectancy among breast cancer patients by a significant 18 months. More recent studies such as one by Pamela Goodwin in Toronto arrived at contrary results with respect to survival time. At any rate, the quality of life of patients who took part in group therapy was considerably better, and this is what the well-known Simonton method is based on.

Around the turn of the century, famous surgeons such as Wagner-Jauregg noticed that cancer sometimes disappeared in patients with newly-acquired infectious diseases such as tuberculosis or malaria. This led to the development of an immune therapy which tries to simulate the condition, either by artificially inducing fever (hyperthermia) or administering weak pathogens (Sanum therapy, Pyrogenium etc.). A holistic view of carcinosis has thereby received the crucial encouragement that even advanced cancers considered completely untreatable spontaneously disappear in some – admittedly extremely rare – cases (to be sure, the probability is estimated to be just 1 case in 80,000!). The idea that something like this is at all possible fascinates many. From a scientific standpoint, it would seem to be worthwhile looking into the causes of these spontaneous cures, and making them available to a larger circle of patient.

> Anita Moorjani [99] describes an impressive near-death experience followed by complete healing of an advanced malignancy. Similarly impressive is the book *A Glance into Eternity* [2] by the neurosurgeon Eben Alexander describing his near-death experience, after which he also was cured of incurably septic meningitis.

In malignancy cases, one almost always finds severe geopathy, unless a patient has moved before the test and thereby was unknowingly liberated from a "cancer bed" in which the patient had previously been "stewing" for years. As has been said, cancer patients often have an active Central Conflict located precisely at the site of the primary tumor or the strongest metastasis. It seems extremely likely that the Central Conflict has a direct influence on carcinogenesis; however, since virtually every person has a Central Conflict acting as a subliminal energy block, I don't wish to place an equals sign between cancer and Central Conflict. The actual reason for my restraint is the danger of unwitting imputation of guilt, which can unnecessarily unnerve and cripple a patient. Dissolution of the Central Conflict improves the overall state of health, leads to more optimism and *joie de vivre* and to a better overall immunological situation.

Naturopathic immune therapy usually involves mistletoe injection. Mistletoe was first recommended by the founder of Anthroposophy, Rudolf Steiner. According to the doctrine of signatures, mistletoe acts as a plant parasite in cancer cases. The lectins in mistletoe have a weak immune effect as well as a certain mood-elevating influence. Because mistletoe thrives in the presence of geo-radiation, it seems likely that it energetically compensates geopathy. I myself seldom use mistletoe for carcinomas because I am so convinced of the top-priority necessity of geo-radiation cleansing – and besides, there are more effective naturopathic agents.

Sanum medications have proven themselves in immune therapy, for example Utilin S (strengthening "agent", OP Sanum) as injection of two ampoules per week (or else as capsules or suppositories). Snake venoms (Horvi) are often quite effective, for instance in the form of Horvi X 44 2×10 drops, or Horvitrigon pure toxin forte 2×10 drops sublingual. Plant pigments (beetroot etc.) can be useful [122]. Selenium 100 µg and zinc (for instance Unizink) as well as AE-Mulsin forte (5 drops daily) are very effective for immune stimulation and as roborant. Bromelain is very good for prevention of metastasis and nonspecific enzyme therapy (or eat pineapple more often). Thymus and NeyTumorin (Vit-Organ) as injections or infusions have also proven themselves. It is also worthwhile to strengthen the intestinal flora (Kanne Brottrunk (bread drink), dysbiosis agents). I have also seen good results from stimulating the citric-acid cycle, i.e. with Ubichinon from Heel.

13.9 Neurological diseases

Neurological systemic diseases such as **multiple sclerosis** often give the impression that, during the initial examination, the patient has every bad thing that one's most vivid imagination could dream up – e.g. active Central Conflict plus geopathy plus dental focus plus severe intestinal dysbiosis with submucosal fungi and/or overgrowth. Later on, the poor abused nervous system can recover after administration of B complex (yeast), lecithin (Buerlecithin and eggs), saltwater fish (polyunsaturated fatty acids) and cellular therapy (VitOrgan etc.). If the process is too far advanced, then one will have to be satisfied with a standstill. In general, allopathic agents such as interferon and the like block the naturopathic regeneration process very little, which is why I advise continuing with the usual medication.

In **dementia** cases, PSE will sometimes detect geopathy or conflicts, whereby the symptoms will improve markedly after the causes have been eliminated. Yet another frequent problem is **migraine**, of which the following is a typical case.

> **• Case study**
> Ms. J has suffered for years from weekly-recurring and at times extremely severe migraine, as well as occasional exhaustion, cold hands and feet, and dry scaly skin. Her mother and grandmother had the same symptoms for their entire lives, so she's convinced that it's congenital. Testing with Psychosomatic Energetics reveals very low energy readings (Vital and Emotional 20% each) as well as a large complex with the theme "Helpless". In addition, I discover a very disruptive geopathy (Geovita, placed in the Yin region, normalized the Vital and Emotional values to 100% each). The severe geo-radiation stress is later confirmed by an experienced dowser. The bed is shifted to a neutral location and the conflict is eliminated after a few months with homeopathic compound remedies (Chavita 1 and Emvita 3). At a follow-up check six months later, she is doing noticeably better. Another conflict is found in the sixth Chakra with the theme "Restless". When this one is eliminated after a few more months, all symptoms have disappeared. For the first time, she has normal skin and warm hands and feet. In addition, although the migraine persists, it recurs much less frequently.

Chronic pain states are a well-known nuisance in practical medicine. Most of these patients take a lot of allopathic medications, which makes treatment more difficult, and they have often already undergone a medical and naturopathic Odyssey. One often finds many large conflicts, often including the conflict "Uneasiness" in the sixth Chakra, as well as conflicts dealing with tension and restlessness. Many of these patients have depressive emotional states and very low Emotional values. Not infrequently, severe geopathy is involved (often with a maximum zone in the head region), which is nearly always overlooked by those who had treated him before, but which sometimes represents the actual key to the elimination of therapy resistance. For trigeminal neuralgia, I recommend a Janetta-style operation, but in addition, I have had good results using PSE as an adjuvant method.

13.10 Rheumatological diseases

When it comes to **chronic inflammatory diseases**, PSE is only of significance as a complement to mainstream medicine. Many naturopathic procedures have been disappointing here, and there are actually few which effectively help. I learned from the rheumatologist and PSE therapist Dr. Martin Scharm that rheumatoid arthritis patients often have a fifth-Chakra block and that PSE can be useful as an adjuvant to mainstream medicine, but I myself have little experience in this area.

For acute **rheumatoid diseases** such as acute lumbar sciatica, cervical syndrome etc., osteopathy and neural therapy are indispensable.

Acute pain states can often be quickly be checked by hourly administration of 5 drops of Paravita or Simvita (one needs to first test out what responds, and sometimes Neurovita tests positively as well). The painful segment is often identical with the active conflict, in which case the high/low coupling of the conflicts should be kept in mind, i.e. sixth Chakra conflicts tend toward lumbar sciatica, third Chakra conflicts to cervical spine and shoulder symptoms. PSE is often successful – and that very quickly – with the often-blocked sacroiliac joints or Atlas blocks. Applying the suitable Emvita and Chavita test ampoules often immediately brings the Atlas back into normal position! In addition, leg-length difference almost always disappears, as long as it is not due to structural leg lengths, which is very rarely the case. In addition, leg-length differences can be corrected by the Thorn method: infiltrate the sacroiliac joint neural-therapeutically, say, with Xylocaine 2% (very often also reacts painfully).

If not too advanced, PSE is often successful in cases of **arthrosis and soft-tissue rheumatic diseases** including fibromyalgia, but also arthritic and functional spinal column misalignments. When it comes to rheumatic diseases, particularly arthrosis and soft-tissue rheumatic forms, overall deacidification and detoxification have top priority. Because of the large quantities of acids which accumulate in rheumatism patients, an external supply of alkaline substances is usually just a stopgap. Good general deacidification is done by injecting homeopathic lactic acid (in the form of Sanuvis, Lacto-purum and the like). Also important is cleansing the intestinal flora, by which the organism's largest source of acid is switched off; in the intestines, enormous amounts of toxins accumulate in the form of bacterial toxins and metabolic waste byproducts. Additional acid sources include, as I've said, focalization and geopathy.

Locally, a great deal can be achieved with hyperthermia (ABC plaster, cantharides plaster), cupping and the Baunscheidt method (possibly with St. John's wort/Jukunda) in order to stimulate detoxification processes. Also very helpful are injection cures with local mistletoe wheals – such as Viscum Mali 2% from Wala, which, mixed twice weekly with procaine/Xylocaine, is whealed with a #20 needle in the painful region. With a #10 series, there have been, empirically, permanent results in over 60% of cases, and that even for moderately severe done arthrosis and coxarthrosis. Occasionally, this can lead to local reddening, which can be taken as a good response. Also very effective are intra-cutaneous choline wheals (PGM). I have often had excellent results with ear acupuncture (for example with permanent needles) for otherwise therapy-resistant cases. In many cases, manual techniques are indispensable, such as the Thorn method and chirotherapeutic manipulation. At the end of treatment, it has proven to be a good idea to give the patient some specific behavior guidelines – such as not to lift heavy weights by bending over, but rather by starting from a kneeling position and lifting up with a straight spinal column. For building up cartilage, one can recommend sulfate-rich baths (Klopfer sulfur bath).

I would like to present a typical case in order to illustrate the full range of therapeutic possibilities.

> • **Case study**
> Ms. A has suffered for years from **lower back pain** which radiates into the legs. According to the orthopedist, it's a case of "pseudo-radicular sciatic neuralgia with sacroiliac joint blockage". During her third pregnancy, her lower back pain was often intolerable. She struggles bravely with no painkillers through pregnancy and the nursing period. After the delivery, she is tormented by stubborn shoulder-neck tension from carrying the two small children. Testing with the REBA Test Device reveals reduced Vital readings of 30%. She says she is often tired, which she attributes to lack of sleep because of nursing. As conflict, the Emotional remedy #5 with the theme "Hectic, nervous" responds. She confirms that she is internally often very uneasy, even though those around her are mostly unaware of it. The patient takes Emvita 5 and Chavita 2 for a month – and then, because she once again feels very good, she at some point forgets to continue taking the remedies. After another month, the old complaints gradually return. After resuming Emvita 5 and Chavita 2, she's immediately pain-free again: evidently, the conflict was not quite healed, so she had to continue taking the remedies.

13.11 Emotionally/physically conditioned ailments

For the majority of diseases, physical and mental causes are inseparable. Here is a case from daily practice which may be considered to be average with respect to diagnosis, therapeutic recommendation and course of therapy.

Part 3 Clinical practice

> • **Case study**
> A 50-year-old office worker has been feeling severely exhausted for quite a while, even after a weekend, which he often spends in bed due to exhaustion. He has trouble staying asleep and often feels totally whacked out in the morning. In addition, he suffers from constantly recurring lower back pain. Although he enjoys his work and is happily married, daily life is becoming increasingly unbearable. In the morning, he often would much prefer not to get up at all, even though constant lying around in bed does nothing for him either. His family doctor has examined him thoroughly and already referred him to a number of specialists, which led to an initial consideration of a sleep disorder, but despite many examinations nothing was found which could reasonably explain his symptoms. He rejects a recommendation of psychotherapy because, in his opinion, his exhaustion is not due to any mental condition.
>
> At the initial examination, I test some very poor energy values. With Geovita, I find a very strong geo-radiation stress. The dowser who was called in confirms my hypothesis and recommends moving the bed to an unstressed location, which leads to the sleeping problems as well as the lower back pain largely disappearing within a few weeks. In addition, the organ ampoules test out a "biliary drainage disorder" as well as dysbiosis, both of which are treated for a few months with bitter substances and eubiotics. Yet another conflict is found in the pelvic region with the theme "Helpless". At the follow-up check six months later, the patient is energetic once again and feels considerably better, his life feels worth living once more.

In the case described above, an unfortunate cycle of mutually-reinforcing disturbances arose. Experience has shown that geopathies often lead to exhaustion states and sleep disorders. Poor sleep disrupts the autonomic nervous system, whereby intestinal peristalsis becomes subliminally stressed, leading to an increase in digestive and putrefactive bacteria. In addition, nocturnal tension causes the fine biliary tracts to cramp up, which leads to headaches and exhaustion. The patient feels helplessly at the mercy of the entire disease process and its constant pain, which leads psychoenergetically to the activation of a conflict with the name "Helpless" located in the pelvis, which in turn disrupts pelvic energy and further aggravates the lower back pain. Ultimately, the entire thing turns into a self-maintaining cycle that can only be stopped by treating all the important individual disruptions.

13.12 Spiritual crises

The term "spiritual crisis" describes a state of psychic emergency that can appear during the exercise of certain spiritual practices – usually after mystical experiences and unusual states of consciousness. One often observes these disruptions in young persons whose personalities are not yet very developed, who have Causal values of 80% and above. As an expression of so-called transpersonal states of consciousness, spiritual crises can overlap with psychiatric diseases. Here is how the Czech psychiatrist Stanislav Grof (considered to be a pioneer in transpersonal psychology) puts it:

> "It is extremely important to adopt an even-handed approach and to be able to distinguish between spiritual crises and authentic psychoses. While, on the one hand, traditional approaches tend to pathologize mystical states, there is the contrary risk of glorifying pathological states – or, even worse, of overlooking an organic problem." [55]

I'd like to describe a typical instance of a spiritual crisis.

- **Case study**
Claudio S, 41 years old, has an unusually high Causal value of 100%, which is characteristic of very high sensitivity and unusually great spiritual permeability. Claudio works as a therapist in the healthcare system, and is very interested in esoteric procedures and naturopathic methods. He is already well acquainted with various different spiritual practices, and he says that he reacts very strongly even to the faintest stimuli. Two years ago, as self-therapy he tried out an esoteric light-wave therapeutic device which, according to the manufacturer, was supposed to be completely harmless. After a very brief exposure of certain energy centers, Claudio experiences a total collapse and an outbreak of schizophrenia which renders him unable to work. Since then, he has been in constant therapy with a psychiatrist and is taking antipsychotic medications.
When I test him using Psychosomatic Energetics two years after the outbreak of his disease, Claudio has a Mental value of only 10%. Values that low are typical of psychoses. One after the other, very large conflicts are found during separate PSE consultations spaced several months apart; thematically, they deal with "Wrong thinking, restlessness and tension". The conflicts are eliminated with homeopathic

> Emvita compound agents, while at the same time he takes low-dosage allopathic medications for his disease. After more than a year of PSE therapy, Claudio is able to work again to a limited extent, and after that his situation stabilizes more and more.

Like a highly sensitive instrument, spiritually advanced persons respond particularly intensely and enduringly to psychoenergetic influences. Spiritually active persons are well advised to know their Causal value in advance, and if it is high, to be especially cautious. Furthermore, large conflicts seem to be activated by particular practices, so that a thrust of external energy not only stimulates the people in question, but also brings to light their inner psychic blocks. They should thus first have their conflicts treated before exposing themselves to strongly transformative spiritual processes. This agrees with the recommendation of many spiritual systems to cleanse oneself mentally and physically before getting involved in them.

13.13   Limits to PSE

Every effective medical and psychological method has certain limits which, if exceeded, renders them ineffective. I would briefly like to present some of these limits, which are determined partly by clinical picture and partly by patient behavior or therapist error. One can spare oneself much disappointment and misapplication by being aware in advance of the limits of the method **and** by proceeding realistically. Basically, very advanced somatic clinical pictures calling for repair or substitution are unsuitable for PSE treatment. Psychic processing of unconscious conflict themes calls for a certain minimum of intelligence: with the mentally handicapped, it has been my experience that the same conflict themes tend to reappear after a while, presumably because they were psychically not rightly processed.

False dogmas: PSE therapy motivates many people to make positive changes in their lives. This is difficult if they are convinced that they're incapable of change, say because unconscious dogmas, ideological principles, social considerations or similar reasons supposedly hinder their doing so. Those who, due to their ailment, enjoy social benefits therefrom (keyword: pension neurosis) or derive some other emotional advantage (keyword: subconscious revenge) often feel little inclination to seriously work on changing their situation. When it comes to [members of] overly strict families and authoritarian groups or societies, PSE therapy is often ineffective, since every psychological improvement in the form of self-confidence, initiative and individualism is nipped in the bud straightaway because it shakes the foundations of authoritarian systems.

Lack of discipline and low tolerance for frustration: patients who have no patience and expect healing to be quick and easy are not suitable for PSE treatment.

Rigid personality structures: above-averagely neurotic persons with a long history of illness are a difficult problem in clinical practice. The same goes for those with psychiatrically defined personality defects, i.e. so-called borderline disorders, or mentally impaired persons. Experience has shown that they can only be helped a little bit, and in fact only by way of alleviation, if that. In difficult cases, PSE therapy should be supplemented and accompanied by techniques such as psychotherapy and behavioral therapy, by hypnosis and by any allopathic remedies and other conventional methods that might be necessary.

False indication: is present whenever a particular disease can be causally and rationally treated in another manner, for instance fractures, malaria and the like. A false indication is also present if conventional therapy would make sense except for the fact that it is not feasible due to a lack of medical progress. Therapists should be aware of this problem and inform patients of the hopelessness of the situation. Understandably, desperate people in terminal stages of severe diseases will grasp at straws. With such patients, therapists often lack the courage to decline the therapy, but they should nevertheless make it clear how low the expectation of a positive result is in their case. Usually, patients will still want to be treated, as the following case illustrates.

> **• Case study**
> Mr. M has suffered for years from Duchenne's muscular dystrophy (a congenital muscular paralysis). He is no longer able to walk and has recently begun to use a wheelchair. His older brother has already died of the disease. Testing with Psychosomatic Energetics reveals very low Vital values of less than 10%. In the space of a year, a number of large conflicts are eliminated, and in addition other naturopathic agents are tested out and administered. Unfortunately, results are very limited, and after a brief improvement lasting a few weeks, the disease resumes its course, apparently totally immune to influence. After the end of PSE treatment, I learn

> from his family that the patient is on artificial respiration, is no longer able to be transported, and therapy had to be discontinued.

Duchenne muscular dystrophy is currently considered incurable, yet there is the possibility that stem-cell therapy or some other specifically-acting therapy will someday change the situation. As a matter of principle, I consider such ailments as unsuitable for treatment by PSE alone, presumably because specific disease processes are involved such that simply stimulating the self-healing powers alone cannot cure them. This also applies to other severe diseases such as malignancy, for which I first and fundamentally recommend conventional therapy, and view adjuvant alternative-medicine treatment as a supplement.

Failure of therapy: PSE results are negative in an estimated 10% of cases (25% for older persons). I consider a PSE course of therapy to be unsuccessful when there is no clear improvement after dissolution of 4 to 5 conflicts. It usually takes one and a half to two years to get to this point. After that, the chances of improvement are empirically limited (but not totally hopeless); I nevertheless recommend discontinuing therapy in such cases. It is currently not clear why these failures crop up at all, nor do we know how we might reduce the failure rate. Still, there are patients every now and then who, even after long-term PSE therapy, suddenly react with a positive breakthrough, so that persistence is sometimes rewarded.

13.14 Successful practice management

Therapists wanting to successfully apply such a complex and demanding method as PSE should take some tried-and-tested advice to heart. Whenever possible, PSE should be combined with other diagnostic and therapeutic techniques in order to increase diagnostic reliability, to better persuade patients and to improve the success rate. As mentioned previously, darkfield microscopy is a good diagnostic adjuvant to PSE. Foot reflexology therapy achieves good agreement with the Organ Test Kit. Equally valuable is segment electrography (AMSAT, earlier known as Impulse Dermogram) which, like the Chakras, enables segmental main-emphasis diagnostics.

I have been practicing thermoregulation diagnostics for many years, and moreover have a degree in it and researched it a lot, but I gave it up because ultimately its therapeutic gaps were too big. The same goes for Iridodiagnosis, which (for me at least) provides fairly unreliable indications, compared to such precise techniques as the Organ Test Kit. (Perhaps it takes more experience than I have in order to use it.) Other energetic diagnostic methods such as psychokinesiology have a strong mental orientation, which drastically increases the error rate and makes the method interference-prone. Bioresonance procedures and Mora techniques are successfully used by some PSE therapists, but I have no personal experience along these lines. The high homeopathic potentiations used by PSE make it impossible to resonate medication information with computerized and other technological methods, for which reason we strongly advise against the use of such. Radionics devices have turned out to be completely unreliable diagnostically compared to PSE.

The best and most valuable investigative methods continue to be an anamnesis and a thorough physical examination. One often learns that, with respect to some recently discharged hospital patients, significant findings were simply overlooked, yet very important. In the patient's interest, one should insist that these cases be mainstream-medicine pre-examined and appropriately treated according to the rules of mainstream medicine, before beginning a course of complementary-medicine procedures. This is also a good idea for legal reasons and, if a patient absolutely refuses to do so, the refusal should be documented by a notarized written statement.

Due to multi-morbidity, most patients have ailments such as generative spinal-column symptoms, which are treated, if needs be, with an injection series of mistletoe wheals. PSE is then, as it were, the central thread of long-term therapy lasting for months, which is supplemented by other forms of therapy. I have already mentioned other useful procedures for making PSE more attractive and for keeping patients in line with faster-acting therapeutic effects; these include: EMDR, Energy Psychology (Tapping), Bach Flowers (these can be tested out like Emotional remedies; usually only one will respond), phytotherapeutics such as St. John's wort, colon hydrotherapy, neural therapy, chirotherapy, Dorn method, classical homeopathy, TCM and ear acupuncture, Spenglersan therapy and many more.

As co-therapist, one absolutely needs a good dowser (addresses available in the specialist section of www.rubimed.com and in Chapter 19: **Useful addresses**), one who can also measure electrosmog, who does not do shielding, prices moderately (roughly that of a good workman) and can reliably identify maximum morbific zones without having been informed of their location in advance. A good dowser should also have enough power of persuasion to motivate patients to move their bed to a neutral location. Other important co-therapists include a biological dentist who can reliably detect and treat foci, as well as broad-minded physicians of various areas of specialization (ENT, gynecology, urology, surgery).

Information is provided during training regarding billing options in clinical practice. These days, a good media presence (printed matter, Internet website, speeches at naturopathic associations etc.) is essential. Important key figures such as pharmacists, masseurs, barbers, teachers etc. can be won over as valuable multipliers for a PSE practice if one correctly explains to them the advantages and unique selling points of PSE. Even though we have no statistical proof and no long-term history over many decades, we do have strong indications emerging from clinical experience that psychoenergetic harmonization with PSE pays off for patients in the long run.

13.15 The testing process

Correct application of the testing sequence has been recorded and is available on a training DVD which every PSE trainee receives at no cost during the Basic Seminar.

Make absolutely sure beforehand:

- No geopathy at the testing site, no electrosmog (place cell phone at a distance, turn off Wi-Fi and Bluetooth etc.)
- Patients should not have any medications in their pockets nor be wearing any energetically disruptive amulets etc.
- Relaxed atmosphere, no disruptive factors, no inner expectations
- Testing site should be very familiar to the tester (better results)
- No spectators if at all possible (have them wait outside), or if so (small children), then the mother should be no closer than 4-5 feet from the testing site.

General advice:
Testing can be done either with the patient lying down (better for beginners, more objective) or sitting (more democratic, harder because patient observes and "co-operates"). Which test is chosen has no significance for the end result; the arm-length test is the simplest and very reliable.

13.15.1 A testing sequence

1. What are the patient's energy values? (> Fig. 13.2)
Next, testing the following test ampoules takes place with the device reset to 0%.
   Note: if the tester wants to subliminally stress the patient, which sometimes makes testing easier (for beginners), select a test stimulus of 10-20% in the Vital or Emotional value (depending on which of the two levels has the poorer readings, e.g. for Vital 30% and Emotional 50%, choose 20% Vital value to continue testing with).

2. Is there any geo-radiation stress? (> Fig. 13.3)
Note: segment determination with the Geovita ampule should only be performed as an exception; recommending a dowser for a house call is better.
   If electrosmog is suspected, test Phosphorus D 21 (seldom, frequency mostly below 5%).

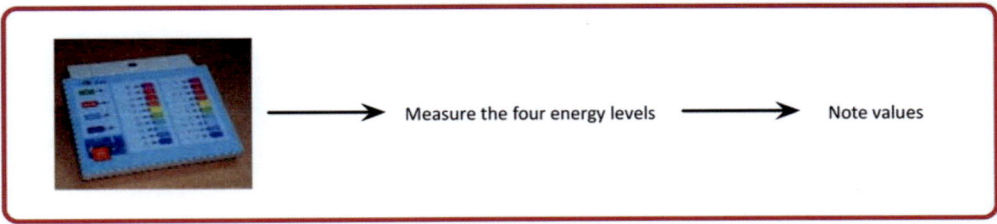

Fig. 13.2

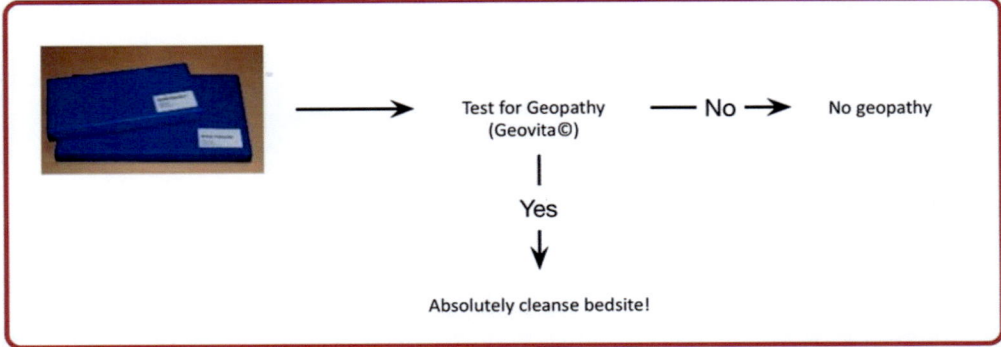

Fig. 13.3

3. Which Chakra is testable? (> Fig. 13.4)

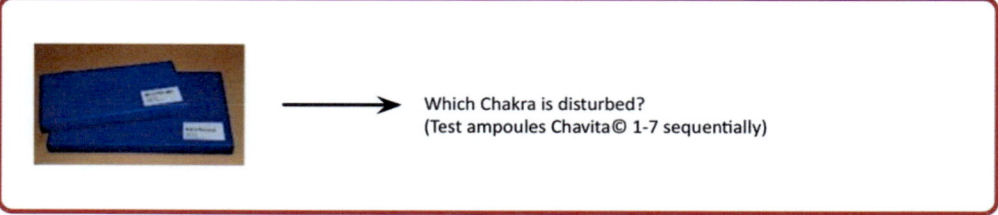

Fig. 13.4

4. Which conflict is active? (> Fig. 13.5)

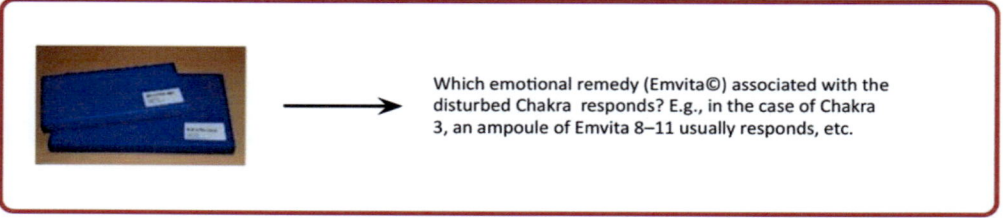

Fig. 13.5

5. How large is the conflict? How long must it be treated? (> Fig. 13.6)

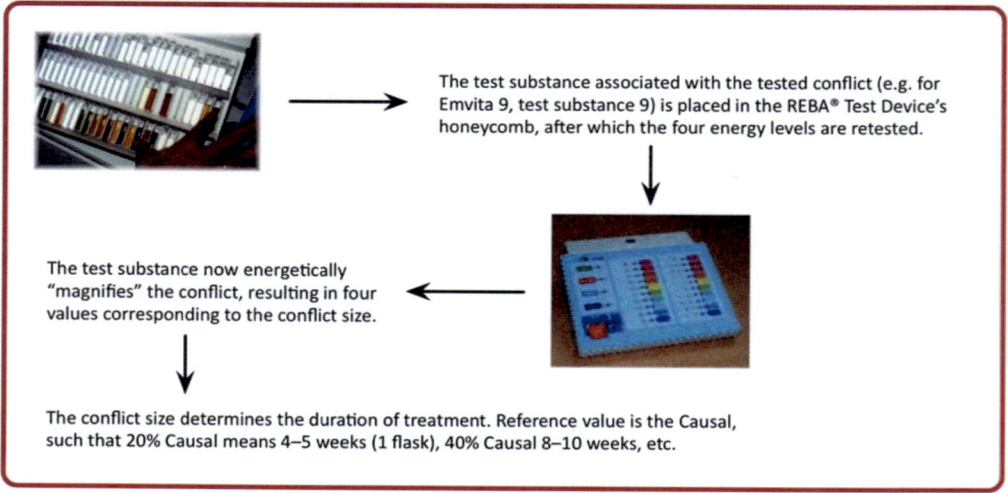

Fig. 13.6

6. Which of the four acute agents respond? (> Fig. 13.7)

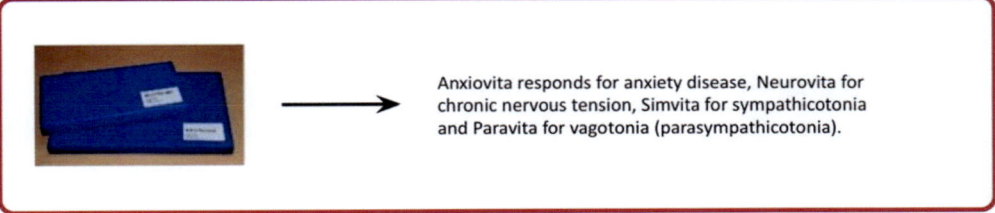

Anxiovita responds for anxiety disease, Neurovita for chronic nervous tension, Simvita for sympathicotonia and Paravita for vagotonia (parasympathicotonia).

Fig. 13.7

7. Remedy test (intermediate check) (> Fig. 13.8)

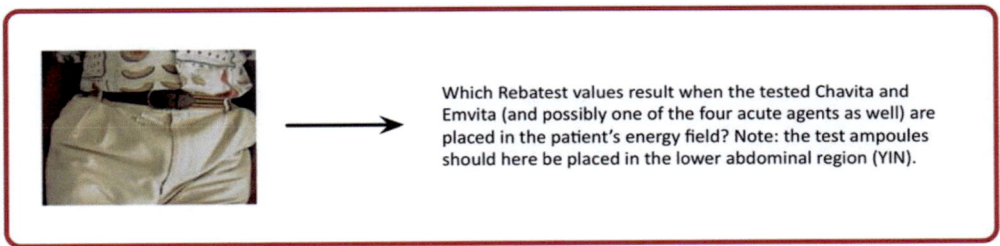

Which Rebatest values result when the tested Chavita and Emvita (and possibly one of the four acute agents as well) are placed in the patient's energy field? Note: the test ampoules should here be placed in the lower abdominal region (YIN).

Fig. 13.8

8. What is the metabolic situation? (> Fig. 13.9)

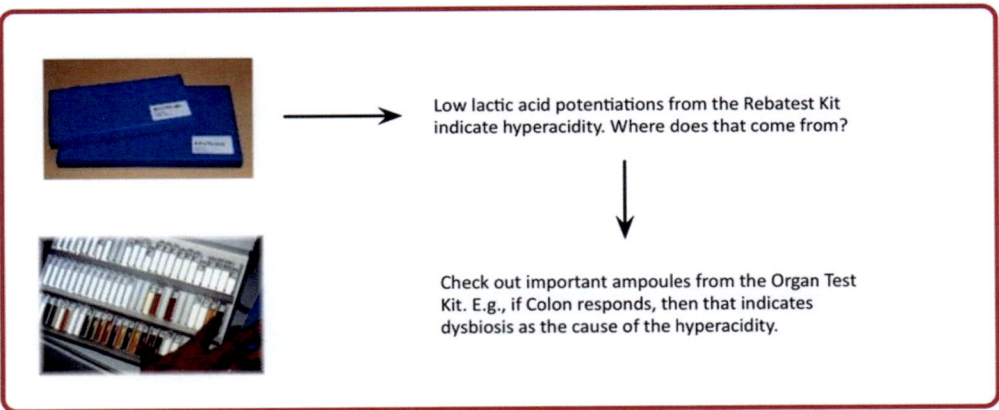

Low lactic acid potentiations from the Rebatest Kit indicate hyperacidity. Where does that come from?

Check out important ampoules from the Organ Test Kit. E.g., if Colon responds, then that indicates dysbiosis as the cause of the hyperacidity.

Fig. 13.9

9. Concluding remedy test (> Fig. 13.10)

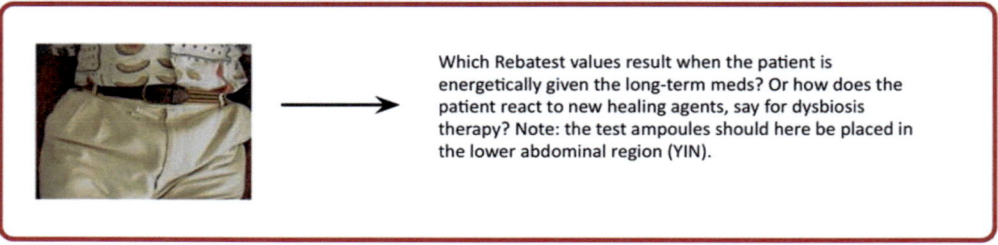

Fig. 13.10

10. Discussing test results
Discussing the test results, as described thoroughly in this book. Setting up the next appointment, depending on conflict treatment duration (for every 20% Causal: 1 flask of Emvita/Chavita = 5 weeks; example conflict with 80/80/10/80 = next appointment 20 weeks later).

General advice:

- Follow-up test normally only after complete dissolution of the tested conflict (often after 2 months, very often 4-5 months are needed).
- For intermediate tests, please **do not** test for new conflicts, but rather only, 1: use the test substances to measure the size of the conflict currently being treated, and, 2: check the effectiveness of the therapy (Emvita and Chavita should markedly improve low test values).
- If 1 above does not apply (conflict values unchanged) but 2 does (agents work as before), it is possible either that the patient has not taken the medication or they have been rendered ineffective due to improper storage or the like. If so, then reissue the prescription. If neither 1 nor 2 apply, then there has probably been a – thankfully rare – misdiagnosis, and in this case a new conflict search can be initiated.
- Other consultations during ongoing PSE therapy are permissible (for psychotherapy and/or application of some other coterminous therapy), but they can never be the grounds for any modification of the current course of PSE therapy. (**For acute crises, an additional acute agent might also be needed!**)

Part 4
PSE Therapist training – Studies – Case studies – PSE's accomplishments

14 Training

14.1 Studying the basic works

A complete understanding of this book is predicated upon already having read other books. These include, first of all, the fundamental works on Psychosomatic Energetics whose titles are **New Life through Energy Healing** [7] and **Healing through Energy Medicine** [8]. Both of these extensive books thoroughly describe the history of energy medicine, the Chakras, the individual conflicts and the character types. These books also impart important depth-psychology knowledge and insights, e.g. the levels of the unconscious and the phenomenon of spiritual maturation. These books are written to be understandable to a lay audience, and are aimed both at therapists as well as patients, and can thus be recommended to interested patients wanting to deepen their knowledge of the system. This textbook and the aforementioned foundational works form a unity, which is why I recommend reading the fundamental works in parallel, while one is working through the textbook, since then the most important building blocks, of which the method is composed, are added in as needed.

For those who are pressed for time, I recommend reading at least the chapters dealing with conflict origins, conflict contents, the Central Conflict and character types in the fundamental works so as to understand the background topics of this textbook. Those who have already read these books, and are now working with the method, are in need of practical and clearly illustrative cases from daily practice so as to extend their knowledge; this goal can be met with the four Psychosomatic Energetics readers, which contain practice-relevant articles from various areas of specialization. Volume 4 has an index to facilitate lookup. The readers are ideal both for deepening and extending knowledge. Therapists wanting even more extensive information can get it by attending the Psychosomatic Energetics seminars; the Intensive Seminar in particular presents the method in its full scope, and also includes an examination for "Certified Energy Therapist".

Further recommended books on PSE can be found at www.igpse.ch.

14.2 Training program in detail

A standardized training and testing plan has been developed and proven itself over many years. Training includes instruction with a set daily program, PowerPoint presentations and seminar scripts, practical work with the method, standardized testing using the REBA Test Device, and recapitulation of the background knowledge which is set down in the recognized specialist literature for PSE. The training plan is under the control of the chief instructors, who are guided by the specialist literature.

Every healing method relies upon the talent and conscientiousness of the therapists which make use of it. Therefore, there are uniform and intelligible standards for Psychosomatic Energetics training. The medical councils of a number of German states recognize the training seminars in the context of their training regulations; corresponding efforts on the part of the professional associations are also being undertaken in other regions as well for nonmedical practitioners.

Training takes place in-service over a number of steps:

1. A 1½ day basic seminar is obligatory (and a prerequisite to obtaining a REBA Test Device). The Lower Saxony medical council, e.g. recognizes the basic seminar with continuing education points.
2. Highly recommended are one or more days of practice under the direction of a training leader for practical experience and deepening the theoretical knowledge of the basic seminar and of practical testing ability.
3. Obligatory is a 1½ day advanced seminar to extend the theoretical knowledge. Some German medical councils recognize the advanced seminar with continuing education points.
4. Highly recommended are one or more practice days (under the leadership of a senior trainer) for practical experience and deepening the theoretical knowledge of the advanced seminar and practical testing ability with more complex types of problems.
5. For admission to the intensive seminar, 5 documented cases supervised by a recognized training leader are obligatory.
6. Obligatory is a 4-day intensive seminar. The Baden-Württemberg medical council, e.g. recognizes the intensive seminar with continuing education points.
7. At the end of the intensive seminar, there is an obligatory written as well as a practical examination.

8. Also obligatory is proof of having undergone PSE self-therapy. This therapy can take place with any certified PSE therapist, even before training.

Self-therapy – independently of any small or large disturbances to overall well-being – makes clear to trainees the workings of unconscious conflicts and the strengthening of their own vitality more impressively than any theoretical intensive schooling: they feel for themselves what the vitality released by the melting away of conflicts can do for them on their Vital and/or Emotional level.

The courses are booked during the course of a year, or also at longer intervals, in order to accumulate enough practical knowledge between the individual training steps and, if possible, specifically to deepen them on practice days with other users at the same level of training. At the beginning, every participant receives a training pass and certify their training by means of certificates and stamps issued by the training leaders and by iGPSE.

Only persons with permission to practice medicine with humans or animals (doctors, nonmedical practitioners, naturopathically oriented psychotherapists, naturopaths, veterinarians, animal nonmedical practitioners etc.), who are permitted to be active in their profession or are about to begin doing so. Those with any other form of qualification must show whether they are permitted to practice medicine, make diagnoses and perform therapy. In special cases, with a person's valid petition – e.g. for research purposes – the Board of Directors may issue a special authorization for training – which, however, does not take the place of official permission to heal. After the four-day intensive seminar, training closes with a written and practical examination. In the practical and written examination, participants demonstrate that they know the course contents regarding Psychosomatic Energetics and that they know how to put them to practical use (including certain standards of quality: good testing ability, sufficient concentration, mastery of the technique in various areas of application etc.). Those who pass the examination are graduates and receive from the IGPSE Board of Directors a certificate as "Certified Energy Therapist" which is valid for 5 years and is renewed when users certify their regular continued training recognized by the IGPSE (International Society for Psychosomatic Energetics).

The International Society for Psychosomatic Energetics encourages their certified therapists to continue their education and training. In the first place, the research and study which they support thereby is constantly generating new knowledge and insights; secondly, the exchanges and conversations of PSE users at specialist functions serves to generate new experiences. For the participants, it has to do regularly with medical specialists having years of experience who have dedicated themselves to various different areas of expertise and who are therefore in an excellent position to accurately evaluate the spheres of activity of their specializations and of PSE. Advanced and continuing education is considered to be necessary, practical and useful by the International Society for Psychosomatic Energetics.

For trainees there are – depending on successful conclusion of the basic or advanced seminar – reasonable-cost options for practical training in small groups on the so-called practice days. Upon request, there can even be single-day individualized training in one's own practice. For certified energy therapists there is, as a rule, the yearly multi-day Expert's Meeting with diversified workshops, demonstrations and lectures. In addition, there has been, for more than a decade at the yearly meeting known as the Medical Week in Baden-Baden (Germany), a lecture day for Psychosomatic Energetics at which speakers report on new experiences and what they have learned in their daily practice (accessible only to doctors).

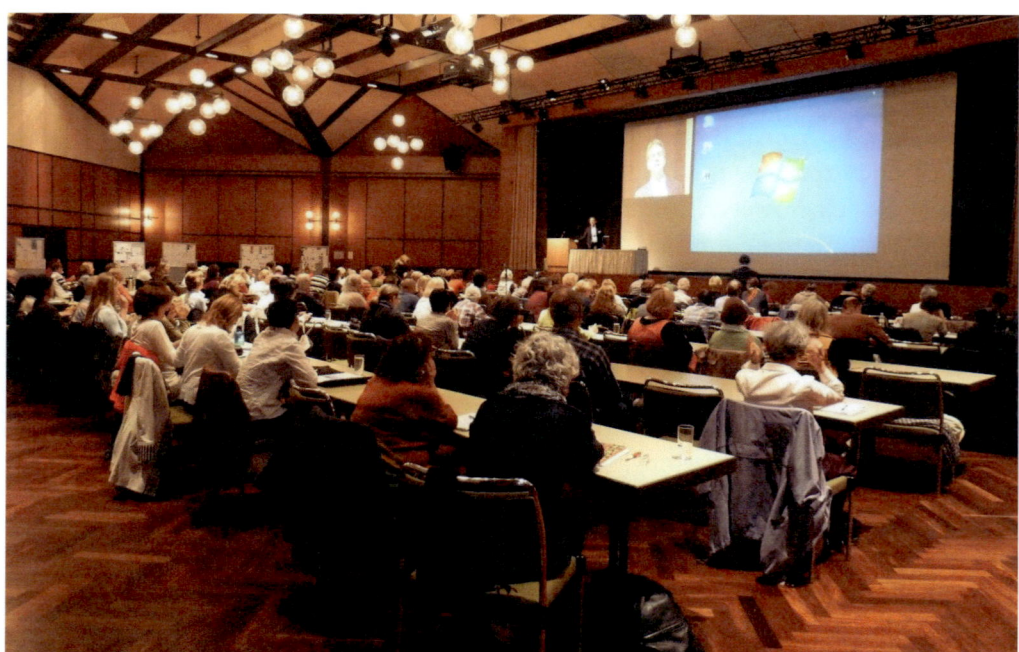

Fig. 14.1 *– Expert's meeting 2013 in the Inselhalle in Lindau on Lake Constance.*

In order to renew their IGPSE certificate, PSE experts must be able to show participation in a specific **advanced or continuing** education session during the five-year validity period of their certificate. The minimum obligation is a one-time visit to the yearly Expert's Meeting, which only certified energy therapists are allowed to attend (**cf. Fig. 14.1**). This is for continuing education, where new findings are presented, present knowledge is deepened and reports are given concerning synergy with other areas of the sciences and the humanities. The level at the Expert's Meeting is high, but the expenses are kept as modest as possible so as to allow as many experts as possible to have an optimum continuing education experience, as well as to promote networking among certified energy therapists.

15 Studies

There are currently more than a dozen clinical studies with more than 2000 patients dealing with Psychosomatic Energetics (PSE). Additionally, some theoretical work has been done in the area of applied mathematics. This work is presented below in chronological order based on publication date.

15.1 Clinical study at a general practice in Bregenz (Austria)

In a clinical study [10] performed in the years 2000-2003 at their general-medicine co-practice by the general practitioners Dr. Reimar Banis and Dr. Ulrike Banis, more than 300 randomly chosen patients took part, who had come in for treatment at least twice and who had been treated using PSE for at least 8 months. Table 15.1 below details the therapeutic results for 336 patients who had come in at least twice for PSE testing over the course of a three year span. Every patient was assigned to just one group corresponding to each patient's primary symptomatology (even if other diagnoses might be present) – i.e., there were no multiple assignments possible.

Therapy result	Count (n)	Excellent	Good	Moderate	Poor	Dropout	Result (good / excellent)
All clients	336	55	215	54	10	2	270 (80.4%)
1 Psychosomatics/psychiatry	194	31	122	34	6	2	153
1.1 Psychoses	10	5	3	2	—	—	8 (80%)
1.2 Depression	48	7	31	8	2	—	38 (79.2%)
1.3 Sleep disorders	26	2	19	4	—	—	21 (80.7%)
1.4 Neuroses	19	5	8	4	2	—	13 (78.9%)
1.5 Anxiety disease	23	5	8	4	2	—	13 (82.6%)
1.6 Exhaustion	68	6	47	13	1	1	53 (77.9%)
2 Neurology	56	9	35	8	3	1	44 (78.7%)
2.1 Neurological (e.g. paresis)	11	1	9	—	—	1	10 (90.9%)
2.2 Migraine	6	—	5	1	—	—	5 (83.3%)
2.3 Chronic pain	39	8	21	7	3	—	29 (74.4%)

Therapy result	Count (n)	Excellent	Good	Moderate	Poor	Dropout	Result (good / excellent)
3 Internal medicine	41	9	25	7	—	—	34 (82.9%)
3.1 Cardiological	9	3	5	1	—	—	8 (88.8%)
3.2 Infection susceptibility	14	3	8	3	—	—	11 (78.6%)
3.3 Gastrointestinal	18	3	12	3	—	—	15 (83.3%)
4 Adjuvant tumor therapy	18	1	16	1	—	—	17 (94.4%)
5 Children (ADHD et al.)	12	2	9	1	—	—	11 (91.7%)
6 Skin	12	2	6	3	1	—	8 (66.7%)
7 Gynecology	3	—	3	—	—	—	3 (100%)

Tab. 15.1 – Clinical study in a general practice. Results after elimination of at least two conflicts, evaluation of PSE therapy results vis-à-vis school grades or dropout then followed (n = 336).

Assessment of the therapeutic results was done by the participating doctors and was supported by the patients' statements (very good, good, moderate, poor, therapy discontinued). Various disease groups were created so as to facilitate comparisons. The majority of patients (circa 57%) had psychosomatic/psychiatric complaints.

On average, after two consultations at intervals of about 4-5 months – i.e. after approximately 8-10 months of therapy – Psychosomatic Energetics yielded good to very good results in 80.4% of the patients. Additional therapy was not applied in the majority of cases; when it was, it was usually short-term routine medications such as those prescribed by the family doctor for everyday indispositions. As a rule, chronically ill patients maintained their routine allopathic medications, only reducing them after consulting with the physicians co-treating them once there had been some improvement (but only in exceptional cases).

The individual assessment of the study shows that particularly good results were seen for the diagnostic groups that were usually considered to be particularly problematic, such as cases of chronic anxiety (mostly generalized anxiety), neurological cases (in particular paresis and neuralgia), juvenile disorders such as ADHD, migraine headaches and cases involving adjuvant tumor therapy. Below-average success rates were achieved in cases of skin disease, chronic pain, neurosis and chronic fatigue, evidently because other components also had to be treated in order to improve the success rate (or the PSE therapy duration in the study was too short).

15.2 Mathematical modeling

The goal of the lecture ([9], Vol. 2) is to formulate some thoughts regarding future PSE research. A simplified mathematical model of the dynamics of PSE course of treatment is presented by Dr. Mark Friedman of the Mathematical Sciences Department, University of Alabama, Huntsville (USA). Earlier, Dr. Friedman had published a similar work on acupuncture. The description of PSE in the work comes from Dr. Reimar Banis, general practitioner in Switzerland.

15.3 Clinical study at a general practice in Saarlouis (Germany)

Another clinical study [63] comprised 224 cases which were treated with PSE in a German general-practice clinic in the years 2003-2005. The precondition for a sufficiently long therapeutic timespan was at least 3 patient visits. As a rule, after the initial examination, the checkup took place 3-4 months later, so the resulting minimum treatment time was 6-8 months. Of course, patients were also included who had been treated for a longer time. The mean treatment time was 14.8 months, i.e. clearly longer than in the first clinical study.

As in the first clinical study, "grades" (very good, good, satisfactory, sufficient, deficient: Table 15.2) were assigned based on patient testimony in the assessment of therapeutic results. The best therapeutic results were achieved with children and teenagers. Therapeutic success (inclusion criterion: "very good" to "satisfactory") with PSE in this group was 97.5%; in the 19-40 year group it was still 88.2%; for the 41-60 group 82%, and in the 60+ group 68%.

Summing up, in comparing the two clinical studies, what stands out is the somewhat differing therapeutic results of 80.4% versus 85%. It seems to me that this is due, first, to the differing evaluation of the terms "satisfactory" or "moderate" in assessing the therapeutic results: a moderate result tends to be somewhat poorer than a satisfactory one. Thereby, in this study by Dr. Holschuh-Lorang, there probably tended to be (at the level of fewer percentages) more subjects assessed as having been successfully treated. Besides which, the total duration of therapy in the second study was, at nearly 15 months, almost twice as long as in the first one (8 months). After all, experience tells us that a longer therapy time will result in a higher success rate.

Group	Very good	Good	Satisfactory	Sufficient	Deficient	Result (%)
Neurological/psychiatric	19	16	7	4	11	74
Vegetative	10	20	12	4	3	85
Internal medicine	18	14	6	2	2	90
Dermatological	3	10			1	93
Oncological	6	4	0	0	1	91
Immunological	7	10	3		1	90
Other	10	11	4	2	2	86
Total (n = 224)	73	85	32	13	21	85

Tab. 15.2 – PSE therapy results in a general practice after elimination of 3 conflicts (evaluated vis-à-vis school grades; n = 224).

Both clinical studies clearly show that, for the common general-practice clinical pictures, good to satisfactory results can be achieved with PSE in four out of five cases – provided that at least two (better yet three) large conflicts are eliminated. Empirically, this takes about 8-15 months. Compared to other psychotherapeutic and naturopathic techniques, this therapy time span would seem to be acceptable, keeping in mind that these are, as a rule, lasting therapeutic results. It should also be particularly emphasized that, empirically, PSE patient clientele consists of the chronically ill who have undergone numerous frustrating prior therapeutic attempts, and thus whose possibility of being cured can usually be rated as somewhat unfavorable. With a high proportion of such difficult cases, the results obtained are effectively doubled. Dr. Holschuh-Lorang writes as follows in her summary:

> "The fact that this method is not merely a matter of temporary improvement of symptoms in the patients treated, but rather of stable healing success, is shown by the (by now long-standing) follow-up checks of many patients who, at intervals of six months to a year, come in for their "energy check" and exhibit amazingly good energy values after having received sufficient basic treatment."

15.4 PSE as a complementary diagnostic and therapeutic procedure in a neurological practice

In a small clinical study 2005-2008 at a neurological/psychiatric practice [34], Dr. Thomas Coenen treated a total of 31 patients with somatoform disorders and anxiety disease with PSE. After 14.5 months average treatment time, 23 patients in all saw the treatment to its conclusion. After conclusion of treatment for the 23 patients, the average summation of their Reba test readings (adding together the Vital, Emotional, Mental and Causal percentages) improved from 135 to 185, their subjective estimate of their state of health went from 3.7 to an average of 2.4 (measured in German school grades, where 1 = very good, 2 = good, 3 = satisfactory, 4 = sufficient, 5 = deficient, 6 = insufficient). 16 of 23 patients (thus 70%) designated the therapeutic results as good to very good, 2 patients reported no improvement of the original complaints.

15.5 Adjuvant homeopathy (drops) for juvenile behavioral disorders (Jupident study)

Ten foster-home children ages 9-14 were treated for 12 months (2004-2005) four times by the internist Dr. Wolf Hemsing with the methods of Psychosomatic Energetics. They were administered the appropriate emergency drops found for each case, as well as the Chakra and Emvita remedies. The children came from psychosocially problematic situations and predominantly had learning and performance disorders, plus displaying some behavioral problems. Examination with Psychosomatic Energetics [61] revealed that they all had low energy values. The assessment of their caregivers reported a noticeable (and to some extent considerable) improvement in learning, performance and behavioral criteria.

15.6 The Butterfly Project (Schmetterlings-Projekt) with Austrian grade-school students

A clinical study with the project name "Butterflies" [107] was initiated in Austria by the retired school principal and kinesiologist Gerlinde Paukert. She looked into whether preventive treatment with PSE might favorably influence school performance and overall behavior of the children. Her thinking on this was that an improved energy system and dissolution of conflicts would have to be a good proactive measure, such that children would learn better and with more enjoyment. She had chosen a first grade in elementary school (student participant age 6-7 years), a first grade in high school (age 10-11 years) and a beginning college class (age 19-20 years). With the agreement of the school management supported patronized sponsored, the teachers and the parents, all the students were tested with the REBA Test Device and then provided with the drops at no charge (sponsored by Rubimed AG). Although participation was completely voluntary, all the students took part. Since the project was sponsored by the International Society For Psychosomatic Energetics (IGPSE) and carried out by Ms. Paukert at no charge, there were no resulting expenses for students and parents. Ms. Paukert wrote:

> "The energy situation has improved for all children and teenagers, having risen between 7% and 25%. The effects are noticeable both on the physical as well as the mental and emotional levels. Concentration, overall health and mood are clearly higher, the classroom atmosphere is better, and the interchange in class means feeling better in school. The second test year exhibited a more harmonious classroom and a leveling out at a markedly higher energy level. The time and materials (drops) cost is also an absolutely noteworthy aspect (by way of comparison, an hour of work was priced at about $45). The entire project was carried out at no cost to the parents.
> If you look at the cost reduction in a single school year (minus 28%), this result – quite apart from the personal value – is quite interesting from an economic standpoint. Underlying all of these facts and figures are the fates of children: large and small, at times dramatic, stories."

Ms. Paukert's commendable pioneering work clearly shows that the earlier energetic treatment is begun, the lower the resulting costs are (Table 15.3). Her study also shows that even lower costs ensue if, for example, an additional second year (Table 15.4) of PSE treatment is done. The thing is, PSE treatment is, as a rule, self-limiting, so that less and less time and effort is needed to maintain a person in a psychoenergetically normal state once the conflicts have been eliminated.

Type of school	Time per student (min.)	Number of flasks	Cost
Elementary school	145	2.9	$150
Junior high school	145	4.0 + 38%	$165 + 13%
High school	155	7.3 + 152%	$210 + 43%
Elementary school	145	2.9	$150
Junior high school	145	4.0 + 38%	$165 + 13%

Tab. 15.3 – *Estimated costs for one semester in the first year.*

Type of school	Time per student (min.)	Number of flasks	Cost
Elementary school	90 – 38%	2.4 – 17%	$95 – 28%
Junior high school	114 – 22%	3.5 – 12.5%	$145 – 12%

Tab. 15.4 – *Estimated costs for the second year of care.*

Summing up, it can be said, with Ms. Paukert, that it would be desirable to examine every first-year student for geopathic stress and psychoenergetic conflicts, well before any possible difficulties at school arise. In this economical, painless and effective manner, a great deal of good can be done and high social costs avoided. At the end of her multi-year study, she writes:

> *"in closing, I would just like to express my personal conviction that high energy values serve to harmonize personality, resulting in more resilience, willingness to work, motivation, joy – and success is then just around the corner. Social competence also changes for the better and there is suddenly a new "class atmosphere" in school. Classmates are more friendly and less aggressive amongst themselves, cooperation takes priority over competitiveness."*

15.7 Butterfly Project (Schmetterlings-Projekt)

In the years 2005-2008, 14 preschool children were examined and treated with PSE three times by general practitioner Dr. Birgitt Holschuh-Lorang [64]. After six months of treatment, the energy values of all the children were clearly improved. A prophylactic energy check made it possible for the children, after treatment of their unconscious emotional conflicts, to have a better energetic charge, thus making them better able to cope with daily stresses. The treatment results are substantiated by the kindergarten teacher's positive commentary.

15.8 Burnout syndrome and exhaustion states – results of a clinical investigation (2007-2009)

From July 2007 to 2009, 304 inpatients at a private clinic for psychosomatics in southern Germany were additionally treated with PSE by general practitioner Dr. Ulrike Güdel Banis [14]. The large number of successfully treated patients, who have found a way out of their burnout condition, shows that the PSE (Psychosomatic Energetics) method is an important component on the path to recovery.

15.9 My "Butterfly Project" (Schmetterlings-Projekt) in a Children's Village in Vorarlberg (Austria) – positive experiences with PSE

In 2008 and 2009, a total of nine children displaying behavioral problems, who lived in the Children's Village in Bregenz (Austria), were tested with the aid of PSE by general practitioner Dr. Ulrike Güdel Banis [15]. All and all, the girls profited considerably more than did the boys: the average increase for the girls was more than 30%, for the boys about 14%. The treatment results are corroborated by the caregiver's positive commentary.

15.10 Chronic pain: tissue's cry for energy flow – clinical practice experience with PSE since 1998

In a clinical study of 102 patients (24 male, 78 female), general practitioner Dr. Ulrike Güdel Banis has performed at least three PSE test series since 1998 in 1.5 years [16]. Treatment outcome and main area of symptoms in the time span from 1998 until publication in 2009 were evaluated. Most frequent among the chronically ill patients were emotional problems (65% of cases), exhaustion (50%) and pain syndrome (31%). The therapy outcome was 39% very good and 39% good (overall 78%); the outcome was 18% satisfactory and 4% poor (overall 22%).

15.11 How stable are healing successes? Long-term study results of applying Psychosomatic Energetics

The study undertaken by general practitioner Dr. Birgitt Holschuh-Lorang [65] comprised 153 patients who, in the time span of 2001 to 2009 were treated with PSE for at least 3 years in my clinical practice. Question: was the symptomatology in fact lastingly eliminated? 72% of the cases were evaluated as very good, 12% as satisfactory; only 16% of cases received an evaluation of sufficient or deficient. The emotional equilibrium of most of the patients was significantly improved.

15.12 Multicentric clinical study of Psychosomatic Energetics

A multicentric clinical study [11] running over 4 years, carried out by myself as head of the study, comprised 11 participating clinical practices and 1002 patients. The study summarizes the treatment results that a large number of therapists have experienced with Psychosomatic Energetics. The average therapy time ran to 15 months over 4 sessions in all. Very good, good and satisfactory therapeutic results were achieved in 86.5% of cases. Considering that, in a PSE practice, predominantly problem patients are treated, the achieved therapeutic outcome looks even more impressive. One sees particularly good therapeutic outcomes with children and teenagers, as well as with patients with psychosomatically-determined clinical pictures.

16 What PSE is capable of

In this concluding chapter, I'd like to address the issue of what can be achieved with Psychosomatic Energetics (PSE). Were talking here about a general overview, since so many specific areas have already been thoroughly covered.

Frequent questions include:

- how diagnostic accuracy can be evaluated with respect to overall well-being and general patient assessment;
- whether PSE is congruent with clinical findings;
- how the therapy outcomes are;
- how the long-term results look;
- for which clinical pictures PSE is particularly successful;
- what therapists think of the method;
- finally, whether (and if so, when) PSE has unique characteristics vis-à-vis other forms of therapy.

Diagnostic accuracy. Ultimately, every psychodiagnostic method should be measured by its ability to describe patients' overall emotional situation, well-being, behavior and the main thread of their biography fully and accurately. Based on clinical practice experience to date, this is true of PSE. Patients generally confirm that which PSE has previously ascertained out. This applies, first, to the testing of patients' energy values (Vital, Emotional, Mental, Causal), but also to the theme complex of the respective conflict, its unconscious tendencies and, above all, the associated character type when dealing with the Central Conflict.

Congruence with clinical findings. From a medical standpoint, it is very helpful and important that the PSE diagnosis virtually always agree with clinical findings. Casually put, PSE therapists do not live in some kind of "special universe" but rather absolutely arrive at clinically sound and objectively valid findings. Thus, in depression cases, the PSE Emotional values are significantly reduced and improve in synchrony with the clinical course of healing, which can be monitored thereby. In cases involving psychosis, the PSE Mental value is significantly reduced and improves as the schizophrenia symptomatology subsides, so that, here as well, the course of healing can be monitored. In short, the PSE findings agree with the clinic. Added to which, with the aid of the PSE remedy test, allopathic medications with optimum efficacy can be selected – an option with great future potential which has so far seen little use.

It should be emphasized here that PSE diagnosis has a far greater scope than standard mainstream-medicine diagnostics. The broader diagnostic horizon vis-à-vis conventional medicine can help make presumably subjective health disorders objectively testable. Because of this, many patients can again feel that they're being taken seriously, whereas prior mainstream-medicine attempts were unable to objectivize anything, which led to their initially being dismissed as hypochondriacs. Since mainstream medicine knows nothing about energetics, it knows nearly nothing about an extremely important pathogenic cause, which would seem to be crucial for many ailments, as well as for the origin and persistence of chronic diseases.

16.1 The effects of energy deficiency

Decades of experience with hundreds of patients has shown that a long-lasting subtle-energy deficiency can often mean that one can no longer adequately cope with daily life. Among children and teenagers, this leads to concentration disorders, disinterest in school and poor perseverance; they exhibit a lack of educability, various behavioral disorders (sometimes accompanied by increased aggressiveness) and, in introverted children, general withdrawal tendencies as well. One gets the feeling that they are driven by unknown forces into self-destructive behavior and cobnsequent failure at school.

Many adults with energy deficiency complain of a lack of resilience, tiredness and elevated irritability. Vegetatively-tinged complaints such as tension, sleep disorders and generally feeling unwell are additional typical symptoms. If one allows everyday life to have its effect on such people and then tries to evaluate it, one gets the distinct impression that they no longer actively shape their lives, but rather have literally become victims of circumstance. If, as therapist, one inquires as to when the problem began, it often turns out to be several years in the past, so that the accompanying lack of energy has presumably also been present for a number of years.

In the case of energy-deficient persons, PSE will test out low energy values of, e.g. Vital and Emotional 20% each (instead of the normal reading of 90-100%). If later on, in the context of a medical examination, the causes of the energy deficiency are identified and eliminated, then the described symptoms usually disappear as well. One may therefore conclude from this that long-term energy deficiency can lead to mental and physical illness, and also to failure at school or at work. One may also more generally conclude that subtle energy in general can be considered to be vital for mental and physical well-being, and that it sees to it that one can cope well with other persons in the everyday social give-and-take.

If one then prescribes the appropriate Emotional remedy and it is taken for some months, this will lead to a gradual melting away and dissolution of the conflict in question. In this process, patients often undergo a slow but constant psychophysical self-healing process (often without any other therapeutic influence) which enables persons to again become self-confident, socially competent, mentally balanced and emotionally resilient – in short, thereby leads them back to their psychic center.

16.2   Therapeutic results

Children still have a largely open energy system and, in the experience of PSE, respond especially well to energy therapy, as the following case illustrates.

> **• Case study**
> A five-year-old boy comes in with his single-parent father, behind whom he hides the entire time, not saying a single word to me. The boy is strikingly pale, extremely thin, and the father says that, unlike his siblings, he is very prone to infection. Also striking is his extreme shyness whenever he is not with his three siblings and encounters other children. The reason for bringing him in is the question as to whether or not he is ready for school, whether he can cope. The anamnesis reveals that, right after he was born, he was operated on for a severe heart disorder. The Vital and Emotional readings I test out are very low, and I find a large conflict with the theme "Panic" (**cf. Fig. 16.1**).
> Five months after beginning PSE therapy, his energy values are once again normal. For the first time, the boy looks tanned, strong and healthy. The father says that he no longer sits around the house all day by himself, but rather has become much more open and plays out on the street with other children. To my surprise, he now speaks to me directly and assertively while I'm talking with his father: "So, how long is this going to go on?" He says this in a very self-assured manner,

> giving me the evil eye and with arms akimbo. His father reports that he goes up to other children and he defends himself in confrontations, which he had been unable to do before. He no longer has any infections and, happily, enrolling him in school will now be possible.

In the next case of a boy with behavioral disorders, the foreground problem this time was not introversion but rather extreme extraversion.

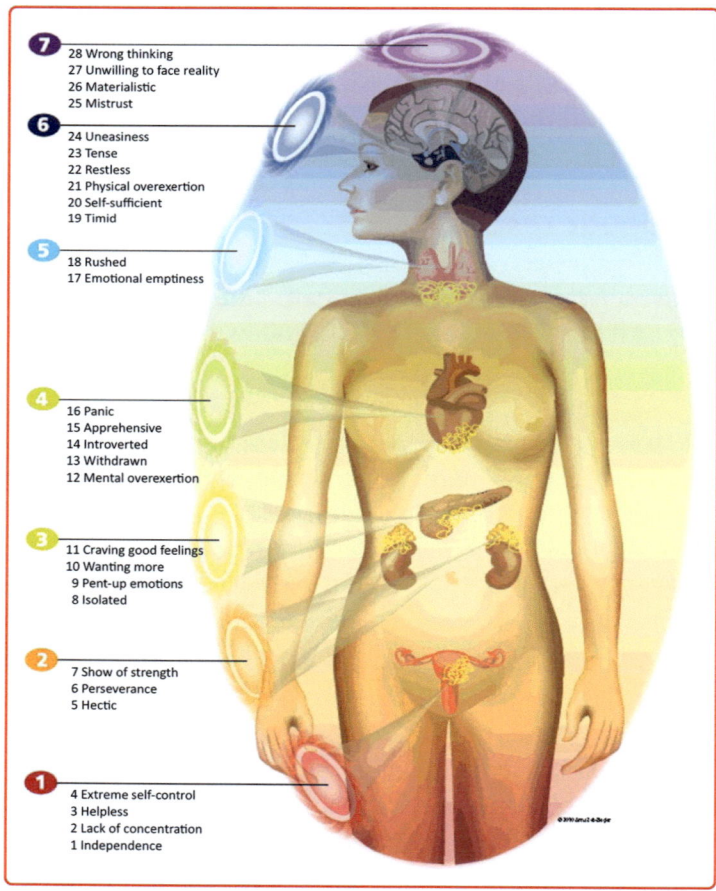

Fig. 16.1 – *The 28 conflict themes of PSE, which can be related to specific bodily segments. (Modified from a drawing by Anna Zeis-Ziegler, Sinntal Jossa)*

> **• Case study**
> A 10-year-old boy comes in with his parents, who say he has highly variable grades in school, sometimes the best in class but at other times very low grades. He is at times extremely restless, running around the classroom during class time and annoying his fellow students. The parents have been told that he'll have to be sent to a special school if this behavior continues. Testing reveals very diminished Vital and Emotional values. The energy block found is a large conflict with the theme "Restlessness" (cf. **Fig. 16.1**). After four months of conflict therapy, the boy is markedly calmer and can now concentrate. He is now friendly with his classmates and pedagogically accessible once more. To the parents' relief, he will be able to remain in the regular school.

These two cases of juvenile behavioral disorder make it clear that both introversion (here in the form of extreme shyness) as well as its opposite, extroversion (with provocative behavior), can have energetic causes. These juvenile behavioral disorders can be eliminated by PSE, and behavioral patterns renormalized. One can see comparable results for PSE therapy with adults, in which behavior as well as emotions are likewise redirected from abnormal back to normal. Besides an emotionally equilibrating effect in anxiety and depression cases, PSE also has an overall vegetative harmonizing effect. Vegetative dysfunctions are therefore among the primary indications for PSE therapy. All chronic ailments having a functional aspect – i.e. triggered and maintained by an entire mix of causes, such as pain states, various forms of digestive ailments, but also etiologically unclear diseases – are generally a domain of PSE.

In adults, conflict treatment often also positively affects social competence and thereby the overall job situation. In this context, I would like to present the following example.

> **• Case study**
> A blue-collar worker, single, comes in for PSE treatment because, since his childhood, he always stuttered whenever he got excited. Although he no longer thinks that it might be curable (since he has tried so many times already), he nevertheless now wants to try an alternative therapy option. His colleagues at work make fun of him because of his stuttering, and he's so shy on dates that no lasting relationship ever comes of them. In the test, he has a large conflict in the Neck Chakra with the theme "Rushed". He confirms that, and exhibits all

> the typical characteristics of a Phlegmatic/compulsive character type – a person who tries to control his subconscious fears through pedantry and inner tension. After the conflict has been eliminated, his stuttering mostly disappears, and the small remnant doesn't bother him, for the first time in his life. He even shows up at a homeowner's meeting and, for the first time, publicly and energetically speaks his mind – an impressive experience for a person who heretofore always stayed in the background.

Clinical practice work with PSE shows that a subtle-energy deficiency leads to reduced resilience, willingness to work, ability to concentrate, as well as to self-destructive behavior in the form of addiction or social withdrawal; in this process, unconscious emotional conflicts are considered to be causal. If the conflicts are identified and eliminated, this often leads to clear positive changes in the subjective experience of those who undergo the treatment; they go on to become more self-confident, act with more autonomy and can once again take their fate into their own hands.

The previously cited studies (Chapter 15) illustrate especially well which kinds of **clinical pictures** PSE is particularly successful with. In particular, children and teenagers respond very well to PSE. Causally unclear and chronic psycho-vegetative ailments, as well as the typical everyday psychiatric diagnoses of general medicine (such as generalized anxiety, burnout syndrome and mild to moderate depression) are all in the domain of PSE therapy. The **long-term results** of PSE are empirically very good, this being well illustrated in the aforementioned long-term clinical study of the general practitioner Dr. Birgitt Holschuh-Lorang (Chapter 15.10). In the meantime, many cases have had follow-up checks for more than 10 years, and they show continuing good results.

16.3   Therapists' experiences

Time and again, medical colleagues and nonmedical practitioners, as well as naturopaths, report on their astonishing results with PSE. The following statements come from an intensive seminar in Weggis (Switzerland) in October 2003; they were made by participating therapists in response to my query regarding impressive experiences with PSE.

- **Case studies**
- Dr. H. H.: I would just like to add how happy I am, and tell you about a patient who, since the middle of last year, has been completely stuck in a depression that was virtually unresponsive to antidepressants: after just one week of medication with Chavita 2 and Emvita 6, he noticed such a clear improvement that, as he told me, he was able to smile again for the first time in 3 to 4 years. I still can't quite believe it yet, but there were clear improvements – and even breakthroughs – in the other patients as well who received the benefits of this medication. I am very happy to have become acquainted with your method and, since then, I enjoy my work much more.
- P. D.: A hyperactive youngster was able, within six weeks, to once again concentrate on school work. The atmosphere improved at home as well. Unfortunately, the problems with his mother only got worse, but now she is also in treatment and her relationship with her son is gradually improving.
- E. B. O.: Girl, 4½ years old, was always tired, already on the couch half an hour after getting up. Her only active time was after 5 PM. Pediatrician found nothing, lab results negative. Patient readings 40/50/95/80. Therapy: Emvita 10 (40/50/65/40) 2X 4 drops. Just a week after beginning therapy, she became somewhat more active, showed somewhat more interest in playing, although never more than 30 minutes, then she went back to the couch. As treatment continued, she got more and more active, more curious, after 7 January 2003, no more noon-hour nap, now a small beaming bundle of energy.
- A.F.D.:
  - Case 1: Girl, special class, only speaks at home, always smiling, irresolute, no opinion of her own – after PSE treatment good posture, self-confident, braver, says what she thinks and now wants to go to the normal school.
  - Case 2: A bed-wetter was dry after four weeks.
  - Case 3: Woman with migraine and PMS considerably better after one month.
- G.: A patient just happens to mention, after the first follow-up check, that he had quit smoking with no problem whatsoever; he had been a heavy smoker.
- L.: The first couple I tested had wanted a child for a long time. Geopathy tested out for both of them. About 1½ months later, she was pregnant.
- Dr. J. G.: Many good results with patients who had already undergone multiple psychotherapies (outpatient and inpatient) with no satisfactory result – all in all, significantly quicker treatment.

- Dr. F.E.B./L.J.B.:
  - Case 1: Therapy-resistant sight defects for years. Various ophthalmologists find nothing and depression – after therapy symptom-free.
  - Case 2: Ten years of pain on Galea and Trichotillomania on up to baldness and wig. After therapy symptom-free, normalization without wig.
  - Case 3: Sexual abuse theme with depression for high government official, after therapy symptom-free, radiant woman 1¼ years later, is writing a book.
- Dr. E. R. P.: Eight-year-old boy, for 1 year 2 tablets Ritalin, because child cannot concentrate, not particularly restless, parents description: stubborn and hard to control, "dreamer". Tested Chakra 1, Emotional remedy 2, conflict Causal value 80, after 6 months discontinued, child can concentrate well, is now attending secondary school (treated 3 years ago, no new problems since then).
- J. J. H.: Four-year-old boy came in with neurodermitis since infancy. During these years was treated only homeopathically. Treated with REBA, after 2 months no more skin problems, situation now stable for six months. Had bad bed location with geopathy and Ch 2-E7, precisely there the skin was at its worst. Bed was relocated and from then on situation improved.
- E.R:
  - Case 1: Female alcoholic just wants "Energy Check" without talking about her dependency, signs up on her own for an Antabuse cure.
  - Case 2: Hard-boiled authoritarian school principal is suddenly ready to discuss things.
  - Case 3: Woman mobbed at the workplace becomes self-confident, can defend herself and looks forward every day to work.
  - Case 4: Tinnitus improves in a short span of time.

16.4 Special qualities of Psychosomatic Energetics – an overview

Many of the diagnostic and therapeutic characteristics of PSE are unique and cannot be obtained to this extent by any other natural method. Compared to other methods, these are distinctly unique features of PSE. The outstanding advantages and special qualities of the method include:

1. A kind of **"X-Ray snapshot" of the subtle-energy system** can be taken with it. The usual subtle-energy test procedures are unable to test the energy system to the extent that PSE can – and above all not quantitatively and with the same degree of discrimination between various subtle-energy levels.
2. PSE offers **reliable quantitative test values** for the four energy levels in percent. The four energy levels contain differing qualities and psychophysical functions, such that it makes sense to test them individually.
3. **The healthy and unhealthy can be clearly discriminated with PSE.** As is known, many naturopathic diagnostic techniques tend to pigeonhole almost everyone as sick, which is not the case with PSE – i.e., the method reflects reality.
4. The test values obtained **usually agree with the patient's subjective feeling as well as clinical diagnoses**. Hence, one finds low Emotional values in depression cases or low Mental values for psychoses. With clinical improvement, the test values also improve, thereby enabling progress monitoring.
5. Thanks to the standardized REBA Test Device and standardized test procedure, the **results obtained from different testers are roughly comparable** and hardly vary even over longer timespans.
6. Further outstanding advantages to PSE include ascertaining the **disrupted energy center, of the acute emotional conflict**, as well as determination of its size. One thereby learns how much energy the conflict has robbed the patient of, how conscious the conflict is and likewise for how long, empirically, it needs to be treated.
7. Precise **determination of conflict size** also enables progress monitoring (not possible for other comparable techniques to this degree of precision) where, for example, even during the several months of treatment, one can clearly determine whether patients are regularly taking their medications – or whether the medications are having any therapeutic effect at all.
8. In addition, PSE is able to reliably establish **character type**. Normally, personality determination calls for intensive and lengthy depth-psychological investigations, yet PSE can do it quickly. PSE makes use of the same four character types of ancient times (Melancholic, Choleric, Phlegmatic and Sanguinic). Since specific characters have specific talents, preferences and dislikes, knowing the character type enables one to derive appropriate life-counseling guidance. Knowing character type can also enable one to develop more understanding for one's fellow humans – who, after all, sometimes "march to the beat of a different drummer".

9. PSE can reliably **detect geopathic stress and electrosmog**, as independent investigations by experienced dowsers on site have shown time after time. So-called "geo-radiation" is empirically an important cofactor, either as a direct or a co-cause. Due to habituation and a lack of sensitivity or knowledge etc., many victims at some point no longer notice geo-radiation stress. The same is true to a lesser degree for electrosmog, which, as we know, is physically less harmful, yet nevertheless can be subjectively very disturbing. PSE can clearly identify those affected and check the result of cleansing, whereby one can either take prophylactic measures against illness or eliminate impediments to healing.
10. Using special PSE organ test ampoules, **functional stresses** such as disturbed intestinal flora, biliary drainage and pancreatic functional disorders can be identified. For many people with long-term ill health (fatigue, vertigo etc.), eczema, chronic pain, as well as digestive disorders of unclear etiology (with nausea, irritable colon symptomatology etc.), experience has shown that they play a key role, yet are unpardonably ignored by conventional medicine, because it is ignorant of such hidden and hitherto hard-to-objectivize disease causes (using conventional means).
11. In addition, PSE can recognize and correctly treat **chronic focal stresses** such as paranasal sinusitis.
12. With the aid of the test procedure known as **"filtering"**, the interrelationships of various different ampoules among each other can be detected and thereby reveal **causalities between various harmful factors**. Moreover, with the aid of the REBA Test Device, one can also test out the energetic strength of a specific stress, which plays an important role in establishing the urgency of therapy, as well as in arriving at a prognosis.
13. Finally, the REBA Test Device can reliably **predict the therapeutic efficacy of numerous medications**. Analogously, the harmfulness of specific substances can be ascertained, i.e. to sidestep side effects. It is important to mention that, in this process, effective and individually well-tolerated orthodox-medicine medications test out just as strongly as homeopathic medications do – i.e., when it comes to effective therapy, there is ultimately no essential difference between them. PSE can thus confirm the thesis that any good therapy is ultimately based on the same mechanisms, which makes it clear that orthodox medicine and complementary medicine belong together, although, to be sure, they simply address different regions of the organism.

In short, the method offers many enormous advantages which no other alternative-medicine method can match to a like degree. PSE is thus unique and, quite logically, has come to be considered indispensable in many complementary-medical practices. Some specific important questions and issues can only be answered and solved with PSE. Moreover, PSE is one of the few modern complementary-medicine techniques which adheres to standardized teaching content, is subject to external quality management, includes a high-quality internationally standardized training program whose final intensive seminar closes with a written and oral examination.

PSE is understood to be a supplementary method for mainstream medicine and comes into play either when, in chronic illness cases, one wishes to accomplish a bit more, or if mainstream-medicine or standard psychological/psychiatric therapies are not effective enough. PSE is based on ancient energetic thinking found not only in shamanism, but also in Asian forms of therapy such as traditional Chinese medicine (TCM) or spiritual life-traditions such as Indian Yoga.

These traditions (of which nowadays mainstream medicine and psychology are not cognizant) maintain that subtle harmony and enough energy – i.e. sufficient quantity and quality of life energy (Ch'i or Prana) – are an important precondition for health and healing, but also for *joie de vivre* and overall well-being. Psychosomatic Energetics agrees with this 100% and treats its patients accordingly – often with profound and lasting success.

Part 5
Appendices

17 List of the 28 Conflict Themes

The following list of the 28 PSE conflicts is a compact listing of the key symptoms for each conflict theme (synonymous with the "emotional remedies" sold under the name Emvita), as well as the composition of the respective homeopathic compound agent. Like many highly effective homeopathic complexes, they contain mineral, animal and vegetable ingredients. In this process, the organ acts as a resonance aid with respect to the affected segments (e.g. Ovar/Testis for the pelvic Chakra). Unlike ordinary homeopathics, the highest PSE potentiations respond to the conflict only and are fully absorbed by it energetically, which is why it does not result in any homeopathic medication pictures.

17.1 Conflict Theme 1

Independence, puberty conflicts, not being good enough on one's own, feelings of inferiority.

Composition:
1. Kalium carbonicum C 800
2. Calcium carbonicum LM 16
3. Lachesis LM 18
4. Naja D 21
5. Pulsatilla D 21
6. Ovar/Testis D 21

17.2 Conflict Theme 2

Lack of concentration, distracted, lost in thought, wistful, not grounded.

Composition:
1. Calcium phosphoricum C 800
2. Veratrum album LM 16

3. Cuprum metallicum LM 18
4. Vipera berus D 21
5. Ovar/Testis D 21

17.3   Conflict Theme 3

Loss of control, weak-willed, helpless as a baby, bedwetting, defecating in bed, incontinence.

Composition:
1. Apis C 800
2. Hepar sulfuricum LM 16
3. Conium LM 18
4. Bovista D 21
5. Ovar/Testis D 21

17.4   Conflict Theme 4

Extreme self-control, sadomasochistic, destructively aggressive, emotions not permitted by suppressing emotions, perversions, psychopathic (extreme form), apathetic, indifferent, alexythemia.

Composition:
1. Platinum C 800
2. Petroleum LM 16
3. Stramonium LM 18
4. Apis D 21
5. Ovar/Testis D 21

17.5   Conflict Theme 5

Hectic and hyperkinetic symptoms, excitable, nervous.

Composition:
1. Bufo C 800
2. Pulsatilla LM 16
3. Cuprum metallicum LM 18
4. Zincum metallicum D 21
5. Phosphorus D 21
6. Glandula suprarenalis D 21

17.6   Conflict Theme 6

"Stiff upper lip", wanting have self-control despite feeling helpless, somatized fears.

Composition:
1. Phosphorus C 800
2. Secale cornutum LM 16
3. Arsenicum album LM 18
4. Lachesis D 21
5. Glandula suprarenalis D 21

17.7   Conflict Theme 7

Show of strength, arrogant, defiant, snappish, secretly inferior, exceeds one's limits.

Composition:
1. Lachesis C 800
2. Lycopodium LM 16
3. Anacardium LM 18
4. Phosphorus D 21
5. Glandula suprarenalis D 21

17.8 Conflict Theme 8

Isolated, uninterested, dull, hiding something unhappy, lazy.

Composition:
1. Ammonium carbonicum C 800
2. Graphites LM 16
3. Chininum arsenicosum LM 18
4. Opium D 21
5. Calcium carbonicum D 21
6. Pancreas D 21

17.9 Conflict Theme 9

Exploding, all bottled up inside, destructive rage, wanting to deliberately behave badly, irascible, attacks of raving madness.

Composition:
1. Lycopodium C 800
2. Tarantula LM 16
3. Sulfur LM 18
4. Hepar sulfuris D 21
5. Pancreas D 21

17.10 Conflict Theme 10

Greedy, insatiable, never satisfied, demanding, power-mad, dictatorial, inconsiderate, compulsive, aggressive, always wanting more.

Composition:
1. Hepar sulfuricum C 800
2. Lachesis LM 16
3. Aurum triphyllum LM 18

4. Petroleum D 21
5. Agnus castus D 21
6. Pancreas D 21

17.11 Conflict Theme 11

Inner dissatisfaction, craving good feelings, addictions, anorexia, bulimia.

Composition:
1. Ferrum metallicum C 800
2. Ignatia LM 18
3. Secale cornutum D 21
4. Cuprum metallicum D 21
5. Pancreas D 21

17.12 Conflict Theme 12

Too tense mentally, constant effort to collect one's thoughts, mental laziness, dyslexia.

Composition:
1. Apis C 800
2. Naja C 800
3. Ignatia LM 16
4. Barium carbonicum LM 18
5. Graphites D 21
6. Opium D 21
7. Glandula Thymus D 21

17.13 Conflict Theme 13

"Gutshot", deeply injured and withdrawn, disinterested, self-centered, autistically self-involved, bad regression, withdrawn.

Composition:
1. Bothrops C 800
2. Calcium carbonicum LM 16
3. Graphites LM 18
4. Anacardium D 21
5. Glandula Thymus D 21

17.14 Conflict Theme 14

Tight and tense, fear of going crazy, unable to breathe deeply and freely, compulsions, closed in.

Composition:
1. Stramonium C 800
2. Moschus LM 16
3. Sulfur LM 18
4. Hyposcyamus D 21
5. Plumbum D 21
6. Calcium carbonicum D 21
7. Glandula Thymus D 21

17.15 Conflict Theme 15

Sinister-terrible, left alone, very frightened, phobias.

Composition:
1. Apis C 800
2. Zincum metallicum LM 16
3. Lachesis LM 18
4. Phosphor D 21
5. Glandula Thymus D 21

17.16 Conflict Theme 16

Heartbreak, feeling of being inundated by a huge horrible wave, panic attacks, mortal terror.

Composition:
1. Aconitum C 800
2. Opium LM 16
3. Ambra LM 18
4. Secale cornutum D 21
5. Zincum metallicum D 21
6. Glandula Thymus D 21

17.17 Conflict Theme 17

Drained of thought and emotion, Devil-may-care attitude, indifferent, emotionless, loveless, frozen emotions.

Composition:
1. Chininum arsenicosum C 800
2. Graphites LM 18
3. Pulsatilla D 21
4. Barium carbonicum D 21
5. Glandula Thyreoidea D 21

17.18 Conflict Theme 18

Hasty-impulsive, superior, thoughts faster than actions, stuttering, feeling like a victim of circumstance, deep feeling of leading the wrong life.

Composition:
1. Agaricus muscarius C 800
2. Cuprum metallicum LM 18

3. Jodum D 21
4. Bufo D 21
5. Glandula Thyreoidea D 21

17.19 Conflict Theme 19

Unwilling to see things clearly, dispirited, diplomatic, timid, indecisive.

Composition:
1. Magnesium carbonicum C 800
2. Zincum metallicum LM 18
3. Calcium carbonicum D 21
4. Hypophysis D 21

17.20 Conflict Theme 20

Snooty, conceited, self-involved, proud, vain, narcissistic, self-satisfied, modest, submissive, false pride.

Composition:
1. Belladonna C 800
2. Ignatia LM 16
3. Apis LM 18
4. Magnesium carbonicum D 21
5. Phosphorus D 21
6. Pulsatilla D 21
7. Cantharis D 21
8. Hypophysis D 21

17.21 Conflict Theme 21

Restless-tense, nail-biting, physically overtaxed, sympathicotonically overdriven, irritated, unable to relax, restless movements.

Composition:
1. Lachesis C 800
2. Chamomilla LM 18
3. Magnesium carbonicum D 21
4. Arsenicum album D 21
5. Hypophysis D 21

17.22 Conflict Theme 22

Restlessness, mentally overdriven, prolonged worries, no relaxation, mental nervousness.

Composition:
1. Chamomilla C 800
2. Jodum LM 16
3. Anacardium LM 18
4. Crotalus D 21
5. Phosphorus D 21
6. Ambra D 21
7. Hypophysis D 21

17.23 Conflict Theme 23

Tense, cramped, helpless, impulsive, thoughts faster than actions, quirks.

Composition:
1. Cuprum metallicum C 800
2. Rhus toxicodendron LM 18

3. Agaricus muscarius D 21
4. Hypophysis D 21

17.24 Conflict Theme 24

Constant uneasiness, persistent pain, Dysesthesia, bodily dysesthesia, depression, hopelessness.

Composition:
1. Crotalus C 800
2. Phosphorus LM 16
3. Chamomilla LM 18
4. Ignatia D 21
5. Hypophysis D 21

17.25 Conflict Theme 25

Distrust, withdrawn, determination, unwilling to give an inch.

Composition:
1. Conium C 800
2. Magnesium carbonicum LM 16
3. Apomorphinum hydrochlor. LM 18
4. Plumbum D 21
5. Lycopodium D 21
6. Cerebellum D 21

17.26 Conflict Theme 26

Wanting everything for oneself, dog-eat-dog mentality, avarice, stinginess, hypochondria, obsession with poverty, possessive, putting having over being, egotism, life as a permanent struggle for survival.

Composition:
1. Arsenicum album C 800
2. Lycopodium LM 16
3. Plumbum LM 18
4. Millefolium D 21
5. Cerebellum D 21

17.27 Conflict Theme 27

Visual, acoustic, olfactory illusions, incapable of clear sensory perception, drugs, hallucinations, unwilling to see reality.

Composition:
1. Helleborus C 800
2. Mandragora LM 16
3. Anacardium LM 18
4. Anhalonium (Peyotl) D 21
5. Cerebellum D 21

17.28 Conflict Theme 28

Overvalued, excessive mental illusions, psychosis, wrong thinking, false dogmas and rigid doctrinal beliefs.

Composition:
1. Mandragora C 800
2. Helleborus LM 18
3. Hyoscyamus D 21
4. Cerebellum D 21

18   Character Type Questionnaire

Introduction
For each statement, try to answer as spontaneously as possible, and without too much delay, whether or not you agree with it. Even if a statement is just mostly applicable, or for the most part or in most cases, you should answer Yes.

Statement List
- Being lonely is for me one of the greatest punishments I can imagine. (c)
- I am prepared to take risks and love variety. (s)
- Each day is a new beginning for me, and I tend to quickly forget the small concerns of the previous day. (s)
- I generally appraise a situation quickly and know what needs to be done. (m)
- Precision and perfection are very important to me. (p)
- I tend to make careless mistakes and prefer to ignore details, because I often race ahead with my thoughts, and I concentrate on The Big Picture when it comes to problem solving. (m)
- I am a bit too aloof and distrustful. (m)
- I can only feel good if others feel good as well. (c)
- In the interest of keeping the peace, I often act against my own will, then secretly get angry at myself for doing so. (c)
- I prefer clear and orderly procedures in my daily routine. (p)
- People sometimes accuse me of being too chaotic, but I can get along well even with such disorderliness. (s)
- My desk and other personal articles are always tidy, with no superfluous paraphernalia. (p)
- Way down deep, I am very emotional, and I have the feeling that life is withholding something from me. (c)
- I have trouble saying no because I'm afraid of hurting other people's feelings. (c)
- Festive parties and "Wine, Women and Song" are very important to me. (s)
- I tend to see a higher meaning behind everything, and I am inclined to profound musings. (m)
- I don't mind being alone even for longer periods of time, and I often even seek out solitude. (m)

- Self-control and accuracy are very important in life. (p)
- I have trouble initiating contact with others in a roomful of strangers. (m)
- I tend to feel personally responsible for everything and to take over things that are of general group interest. (c)
- I am not a group person, and I sometimes have the uneasy feeling that my independence is jeopardized in a crowd. (m)
- I much prefer my accustomed routine. (p)
- I am a very reliable person. (p)
- I find it very easy to charm other people into doing what I want. (s)
- I empathize well with others, and I suffer with them. (c)
- I like to be the center of attention at any social gathering. (s)
- Most things in life should be well planned out in advance and happen at a moderate pace. (p)
- I tend to procrastinate for a long time before finding the best solution. (p)
- I am quick to become enthusiastic, and just as quick to regret my rash impulsiveness. (s)
- I feel very good when I am praised. Praise is very important to me. (c)
- I constantly have new ideas and plans that keep me on the go. (s)
- I always try to abide by the rules. (p)
- I try very hard to avoid confrontation, even if I'm right. Later on, that annoys me. (c)
- I try to extract maximum profit from every situation. This includes, for example "celebrating parties as they come". (s)
- When setting up a new technical device, I read the instruction manual carefully. (p)
- I hate small talk – trite chitchat about everyday life is a waste of time and a bother. (m)
- It's not what one talks about, but simply the fact that one is talking and how one is talking that's so important to me. (c)
- I think that, above all, life should be fun and enjoyable! (s)
- I'd rather work alone than in a group, and I prefer to read non-fiction books when I want or need to learn something interesting. (m)

Evaluation

The classifications should not be known to the subject before the evaluation. Their meanings:

s – Sanguine/hysterical type (H. Jung's Lively type)

m – Melancholy/schizoid type (H. Jung's Independent type)
c – Choleric/depressive type (H. Jung's Thoughtful type)
p – Phlegmatic/obsessive-compulsive type (H. Jung's Controlled type)

Count up all the Yes answers for each letter. Usually, each of the four character types will have one or more Yes answers, but the greatest number will be in the character type that the subject incorporates. As a rule, the subject's character type will have 2–3 Yes answers more than in the others. The remaining answers give an idea of how well-balanced the person is, since the more traits that are in common with the other character types – as can be determined from the distribution of the answers – the more mentally "rounded" the subject is considered to be.

Examples:
- s 10 ; m 3 ; c 4 ; p 2 = Clearly Sanguine type of the disharmonic variety, some obsessive-compulsive component (often chaotic hedonist).
- s 7 ; m 4 ; c 4 ; p 4 = Sanguine type of the harmonic variety, with balanced character traits, often a mature person (identifiable by high causal readings).
- s 8 ; m 6 ; c 2; p 3 = Unclear situation (difference between "s" and "m" is only 2 answers!). Should be cleared up with the Character Type Test Kit.

Clinical tests:
For example, the TCI (Temperament and Character Inventory) personality structure test of the Viennese Test System (Schuhfried, Vienna) tests for four character traits that can be paired with the four "Riemann Types" as follows: Curiosity (Hysteric), Damage avoidance (Hysteric), Reward-dependent (Depressive) and Persistence (Obsessive-compulsive). Such tests are of interest to clinical psychologists. There are many other clinical tests besides this one, similarly structured and potentially very helpful for research purposes, but to my mind usually not very practical in daily clinical practice.

19 Useful Addresses

19.1 Information about Psychosomatic Energetics products

Rubimed AG
Grossmatt 3, 6052 Hergiswil, SWITZERLAND
Tel: 041 630 0888 (Switzerland country code: 0041)
Website: www.rubimed.com (with list of therapists)
North America: www.terra-medica.com (USA)
and www.biomedicine.com (Canada)

19.2 Psychosomatic Energetics seminars

Basic seminar, Advanced seminar, Practice days, Expert's seminar and Intensive seminar with examination for "Certified Energy Therapist".
Further information available at:
Internationale Gesellschaft für Psychosomatische Energetik (IGPSE)
[International Society for Psychosomatic Energetics]
Seminar organization:
Ms. Caroline Buck
Dörflistrasse 4, CH-6056 Kägiswil, SWITZERLAND
Telephones for application, registration or information:
Switzerland +41 44 586 04 86
Germany +49 6 837 2133 81
Or at: seminar@igpse.ch

19.3 List of qualified dowsers

Austria:
Verband für Geobiologie [Geobiological Association]
Koppstrasse 89–93/3/2, 1160 Vienna, AUSTRIA
Tel: 01 408 18 83
Germany:
Forschungskreis für Geobiologie [Geobiological Research Group]
Adlerweg 1, 69 429 Waldbrunn-Waldkatzenbach, GERMANY
Tel: 0 62 74–91 2100
Switzerland:
Inquire at Rubimed AG, Tel.: 0 41 630 08 88
Or at: www.rubimed.com: (listed by area of specialization)

19.4 Foci, milieu diseases

Luffa-Schwamm (Loofah sponge]:
Stadt-Apotheke Leutenberg, Hauptstrasse 35, 07 338 Leutenberg, GERMANY
Tel: 03 67 34 222 19
Website: www.luffa.de

19.5 Biological dentists

Bundesverband der naturheilkundlich tätigen Zahnärzte Deutschlands e. V.
[Federal Association of German Naturopathic Dentists]
Von-Groote-Str. 30, 50 986 Cologne, GERMANY,
Tel/Fax 02 21 - 376 10 12
Website: www.bnz.de
Internationale Gesellschaft für Ganzheitliche Zahnmedizin e.V. (GZM)
[International Society for Holistic Dentistry]
Seckenheimer Hauptstrasse 111, 68 239 Mannheim, GERMANY,
Tel: 06 21 47 64 00, Fax: 47 3949,
Website: www.gzm.org

Schweizerische Gesellschaft für Ganzheitliche Dentistry (SGZM)
[Swiss Society for Holistic Medicine]
Postfach 969, 3 011 Bern 7, SWITZERLAND
Tel: 031 311 9757,
Website: www.sgzm.ch

19.6 Yearly PSE lecture event (since 1998) at the Medizinische Woche [Medical Week] Baden-Baden

www.medwoche.de

20 Bibliography

[1] Adler E. Allgemeinerkrankungen durch Störfelder [Systemic Illnesses Due to Disturbance Fields]. Heidelberg: Verlag für Medizin Dr. Ewald Fischer; 1973

[2] Alexander E. Blick in die Ewigkeit [A Glance into Eternity]. Munich: Ansata; 2013

[3] Allen F. Normal: Gegen die Inflation psychiatrischer Diagnosen [Normal: Countering the Inflation of Psychiatric Diagnoses]. Cologne: DuMont; 2013

[4] Aschner B. Lehrbuch der Konstitutionstherapie [Manual of Constitutional Therapy]. Stuttgart: Hippokrates; 2000

[5] Bachler K. Der gute Platz [The Right Place]. 11th Ed. St. Pölten: Residenz; 2007

[6] Bachler K. Erfahrungen einer Rutengängerin [A Dowser's Experiences]. 18th Ed. St. Pölten: Landesverlag; 2003

[7] Banis R, Holschuh-Lorang B. Repetitorium – Medikamente der Psychosomatischen Energetik [Review Manual – The Medications of Psychosomatic Energetics]. Hergiswil (CH): Rubimed AG; 2013

[8] Banis R, Hrsg. Lesebuch der Psychosomatischen Energetik [Psychosomatic Energetics Reader]. Vols. 1-4. Hochheim: CO'med; 2004–2008

[9] Banis R. "Multizentrische Praxisstudie zur Psychosomatischen Energetik" [Multicentric Clinical Study of Psychosomatic Energetics]. Schweiz Z Ganzheitsmed [Swiss Journal of Holistic Medicine] 2010; 22(5): 269–272

[10] Banis R. Durch Energieheilung zu neuem Leben [New Life Through Energy Healing], 4th Ed. Petersberg: Via Nova; 2012 (English, Italian, Russian editions)

[11] Banis R. Heilung durch Energiemedizin [Healing through Energy Medicine]. Petersberg: Via Nova; 2012 (English, Italian editions)

[12] Banis R., Banis U. "Psychosomatische Energetik – Ergebnisse einer Praxisstudie" [Psychosomatic Energetics – Results of a Clinical Study]. Schweiz Z Ganzheits-med [Swiss Journal of Holistic Medicine] 2004; 16(3): 173-178

[13] Banis R., Engelhard G. Forschung zur energetischen Standardisierung von Rutengängern. Wetter – Boden – Mensch [Research into the Energetic Standardization of Dowsers. Weather / Ground / Man] 2007; 2

[14] Banis U. "Chronischer Schmerz" [Chronic Pain]. Lecture at the Medical Week. Baden-Baden; 2009

[15] Banis U. "Schmetterlingsprojekt in Voralberger Kinderdorf" [Butterfly Project

in a Vorarlberg (Austria) Children's Village]. CO'med, Zeitschrift für Komplementär-medizin [Swiss Journal of Complementary Medicine] 2009; 8

[16] Banis U. "Schmetterlingsprojekt" [Butterfly Project]. Lecture at the Expert's Meeting in the Roggenburg Cloister, Allgäu (Germany); October 2010

[17] Banis-Güdel U. Wie wirkt Psychosomatische Energetik? [How Does Psychosomatic Energetics Work?] Kirchzarten: VAK: 2010

[18] Bergsmann 0. Risikofaktor Standort- Rutengänger-zone und Mensch [Risk Factor Location: The Dowser Zone and Man]. Wien: Facultas; 1990

[19] Beuchelt H. Konstitutions- und Reaktionstypen [Constitutional and Reaction Types]. Heidelberg: Haug; 1971

[20] Bischoff SC, Ed. Probiotika, Präbiotika und Synbiotika [Probiotics, Prebiotics and Symbiotics]. Stuttgart: Thieme; 2009

[21] Blofeld j. Rad des Lebens [The Wheel of Life]. Zurich: Rascher; 1961

[22] Bohm W. Die Wurzeln der Kraft (Chakras – die Kraft der Lotusblumen) [The Roots of Power (Chakras – The Power of the Lotus Blossom)]. Munich: O.W. Barth; 1966

[23] Boorstein S. Transpersonale Psychotherapie [Transpersonal Psychotherapy]. Munich: Scherz; 1988

[24] Borck C. Anatomien medizinischen Wissens [Anatomies of Medical Knowledge]. Frankfurt/Main: Fischer; 1996

[25] Bösch J. Spirituelles Heilen und Schulmedizin [Spiritual Healing and Orthodox Medicine]. Bern: Lokwort; 2002

[26] Boyesen G, Boyesen ML. Biodynamik des Lebens – Grundlagen der biodynamischen Psychologie [Biodynamics of Life – Fundamentals of Biodynamic Psychology]. Essen: Synthesis; 1987

[27] Boyesen G. Über den Körper die Seele heilen[Healing the Soul via the Body]. Munich: Kösel; 1988

[28] Boyesen G. Von der Lust am Heilen [The Joy of Healing]. Munich: Kösel; 1995

[29] Breidert M, Hofbauer K. "Placebo: Mißverständnisse und Vorurteile" [Placebo: Misunderstandings and Prejudices]. Deutsches Ärzteblatt Int [German Medical Journal Int] 2009; 106 (46): 751-755

[30] Brugh JW. Weg der Erfüllung – Selbstheilung durch Transformation [The Path to Fulfillment – Self-Healing through Transformation]. Interlaken: Ansata; 1985

[31] Calaprice A, Ed. Einstein sagt [Einstein Says]. Munich, Zürich: Piper; 1996

[32] Candi: Radiästhetische Studien [Radiesthetic Studies] 3rd Ed. St. Gallen: RGS, 1982
[33] Choa KS. Grundlagen des Pranaheilens [Fundamentals of Prana Healing]. Freiburg: Bauer; 1996
[34] Coenen T. "PSE als komplementäres Diagnose- und Therapieverfahren in der nervenärztlichen Praxis" [PSE as Complementary Diagnostic and Therapeutic Procedure in Neurological Practice]. In: Banis R, Ed. Lesebuch der Psychosomatischen Energetik [Psychosomatic Energetics Reader]. Vol. 4. Hochheim: CO'med; 2008
[35] Dalai Lama. Logik der Liebe [The Logic of Love], Munich: Goldmann, 1989
[36] Daskalos SA. Die esoterische Praxis [The Esoteric Practice]. Duisburg: Edel; 1994
[37] Dethlefsen T. Krankheit als Weg [Disease as Pathway]. Gütersloh: C. Ber-telsmann; 1983
[38] Diamond J. Der Körper lügt nicht [The Body Doesn't Lie]. Kirchzarten: VAK; 1983
[39] Diamond J. Die heilende Kraft der Emotionen [The Healing Power of Emotions]. Kirchzarten: VAK; 1994
[40] Dossey L. Heilungsfelder – wenn die Seele den Körper heilt [Healing Fields – When the Mind Heals the Body]. Amerang: Crotona; 2012
[41] Dürckheim K. Hara – Die Erdmitte des Menschen [Hara – Man's Earth Center]. Weilheim: O.W. Barth; 1967
[42] Elbers F. Zur Rolle des Vertrauens in internationalen Geschäftsbeziehungen [The Role of Trust in International Business Relationships]. Munich: Grin; 2009
[43] Els B. "Psychosomatische Energetik und Hashimoto-Erkrankung" [Psychosomatic Energetics and Hashimoto's Disease]. Report-Naturheilkunde [Naturopathy Report] 2010; 6:28
[44] Emoto M. Messages from Water. Tokyo: Hado Kyoi-kusha; 1999
[45] Evans-Wentz WY. Das Tibetanische Totenbuch (oder die Nachtod-Erfahrungen auf der Bardo-Stufe) [The Tibetan Book of the Dead, or, the After-Death Experiences on the Bardo Plane]. Olten & Freiburg: Walter; 1971
[46] Fromm E. Die Kunst des Liebens [The Art of Loving] (1956). 60th Ed. Frankfurt: Ullstein; 2003
[47] Gedeon W. Von der biologischen Medizin zur Ganzheitsmedizin [From Biological Medicine to Holistic Medicine]. Heidelberg: Haug; 1991

[48] Gerber R. Vibrational Medicine for the 21st Century. New York: Eagle Book/ Harper & Collins; 2000
[49] Gershom Y. Kehren die Opfer des Holocaust wieder? [Will the Holocaust Victims Come back?] Dornach: Verlag am Goetheanum; 1997
[50] Gopi Krishna. Kundalini. Weilheim. O.W. Barth; 1968
[51] Govinda Lama A. Die psychologische Haltung der frühbuddhistischen Philosophie [The Psychological Attitude of Early Buddhist Philosophy]. Wiesbaden: R. Löwit; 1961
[52] Graf K. Störfeld Zahn [Disturbance Field: Tooth]. Munich: Urban & Fischer in Elsevier; 2010
[53] Gröber U. Arzneimittel und Mikronährstoffe [Medications and Micronutrients] Stuttgart: Wiss. Verlagsgesellschaft; 2007
[54] Grof S. Das Abenteuer der Selbstentdeckung – Heilung durch veränderte Bewusstseinszustände [The Adventure of Self-Discovery – healing through Altered States of Consciousness]. Munich: Kösel; 1987
[55] Grof S. Geburt, Tod und Transzendenz [Birth, Death and Transcendence]. Reinbek: Rowohlt; 1991
[56] Guggenbichler N. Menschen im Stress [People in Stress]. Bad Homburg: VAS; 2012
[57] Harner M. Der Weg des Schamanen [The Way of the Shaman]. Munich: Hugendubel; 1990
[58] Hartmann E. "Yin Yang – Über Konstitutionen und Reaktionstypen" [Yin/ Yang – Constitutions and Reaction Types]. Waldbrunn: Forschungskreis f. Geobiologie [Geobiology Research Group]; 1986
[59] Hartmann E. Krankheit als Standortproblem [Disease as a Location Problem]. Heidelberg: Haug; 1986
[60] Hellinger B. Ordnungen der Liebe [Love's Hidden Symmetry]. Heidelberg: Auer; 1997
[61] Hemsing W. "Adjuvante Homöopathie mit Tropfen bei verhaltensgestörten Jugendlichen (Jupident Studie)" [Adjuvant Homeopathy with drops for teens with behavioral disorders (Juopident Study)]. In: Banis R, Ed. Lesebuch der Psychosomatischen Energetik [Psychosomatic Energetics Reader]. Vol. 3. Hochheim: CO'med; 2007

[62] Hoffmann S. Neurosenlehre, psychotherapeutische und psychosomatische Medizin [Neurosis Theory, Psychotherapeutic and Psychosomatic Medicine]. Stuttgart: Schattauer; 1999

[63] Holschuh-Lorang B. "Psychosomatische Energetik in der Allgemeinmedizin. Ergebnisse einer Praxisstudie" [Psychosomatic Energetics in General Medicine. Results of a Clinical Study]. Schweiz Z Ganzheitsmed [Swiss Journal of Holistic Medicine] 2006; 18(7-8): 368-371

[64] Holschuh-Lorang B. "Schmetterlingsprojekt" [Butterfly Project]. In: Banis R. Ed. Lesebuch der Psychosomatischen Energetik [Psychosomatic Energetics Reader]. Vol. 4. Hochheim: CO'med; 2008

[65] Holschuh-Lorang B. "Wie stabil sind Heilerfolge?" [How Stable are Healing Results?] Lecture at PSE Expert's Meeting. Constance; June 2009

[66] Hröbjartsson A, Götzsche PC. "Is the placebo powerless? An analysis of clinical trials comparing placebo with no treatment". N Engl J Med 2001; 344(21): 1594-1602

[67] Hröbjartsson A, Götzsche PC. "Is the placebo powerless? Update of a systematic review with 52 new randomized trials comparing placebo with no treatment". J Intern Med 2004; 256: 91-100

[68] Huxley A. Die ewige Philosophie [The Perennial Philosophy], Munich: Piper, 1987

[69] Huxley A. Pforten der Wahrnehmung [The Doors of Perception]. Munich: Piper; 1970

[70] Issels J. Mehr Heilungen von Krebs [More Cancer Cures]. Bad Homburg: Helfer; 1980

[71] Jäger W. Suche nach dem Sinn des Lebens [Searching for the Meaning of Life]. Petersberg: Via Nova; 1997

[72] Johari H. Das große Chakra-Buch [The Big Chakra Book]. Freiburg: Bauer; 1987

[73] Jones C. Die letzte Reise – Eine Kulturgeschichte des Todes [The Final Journey – A Cultural History of Death]. Munich/Zurich: Piper; 1999

[74] Jung CG. Der Mensch und seine Symbole [Man and his Symbols]. Freiburg: Walter; 1982

[75] Jung CG. Die Psychologie des Kundalini-Yoga [The Psychology of Kundalini Yoga]. Freiburg: Walter; 1998

[76] Jung CG. Über psychische Energetik und das Wesen der Träume [Psychic Energetics and the Nature of Dreams]. Zurich: Rascher; 1948
[77] Jung H. Persönlichkeitstypologie [Personality Typology]. Munich/Vienna: Oldenbourg; 2000
[78] Kafkalides A. The Knowledge of the Womb. Heidelberg: Mattes; 1995
[79] Kanne W. Krebs ist vermeidbar! [Cancer is Preventable!] Thannhausen: Deni Druck; 2002
[80] Klußmann R. Psychosomatische Medizin [Psychosomatic Medicine]. Heidelberg: Springer; 1998
[81] König K. Mit dem eigenen Charakter umgehen [Getting Along with Yourself]. Düsseldorf/Zurich: Walter; 2001
[82] Kübler-Ross E. Über den Tod und das Leben danach [On Death and Life Thereafter]. Güllesheim: Silberschnur; 1991
[83] Leadbeater CW. Der sichtbare und der unsichtbare Mensch [Man Visible and Invisible: Examples of Different Types of Men as Seen by Trained Clairvoyance]. Freiburg: Bauer; 1986
[84] Leadbeater CW. Die Chakras [The Chakras]. Freiburg: Bauer; 1986
[85] Lechner J. Armlängenreflex-Test und systemische Kinesiologie [Arm-Length Reflex Test and Systemic Kinesiology]. Kirchzarten: VAK; 2002
[86] Lechner J. Störfelder im Trigeminusbereich und Systemerkrankungen [Disturbance Fields in Trigeminal Region and Systemic Ailments]. Bad Kötzting: Verlag für ganzheitliche Medizin; 1999
[87] Leuner C. Lehrbuch der Katathym-imaginativen Psychotherapie [Manual of Katathym-Imaginative Psychotherapy]. Göttingen: Huber; 1994
[88] Lowen A. Der Verrat am Körper [The Betrayal of the Body]. Reinbek: Rowohlt; 1983
[89] Malin L. Die schönen Kräfte – eine Arbeit über Heilen in verschiedenen Dimensionen [The Beautiful Powers – A Work about Healing in Various Dimensions]. Frankfurt: Zweitausendeins; 1986
[90] Mann AT. Das Wissen über Reinkarnation [Knowledge about Reincarnation]. Frankfurt: Zweitausendeins; 1995
[91] Markides K. Der Magus von Strovolos (Daskalos) [The Magus of Strovolos (Daskalos)]. Munich: Knaur; 1988

[92] McDougall J. Theater des Körpers – ein psychoanalytischer Ansatz für die psychosomatische Erkrankung [Theaters of the Body: A Psychoanalytic Approach to Psychosomatic Illness]. Stuttgart: Internationale Psychoanalyse; 1991
[93] Meinhold W. Das menschliche Bewusstsein [Human Consciousness]. Düsseldorf/Zurich: Walter; 1998
[94] Meinhold W. Der Wieder-Verkörperungsweg eines Menschen durch die Jahrtausende – Reinkarnationserfahrung in Hypnose [A Man's Re-Incorporation Path through the Millennia – Reincarnation Experiences under Hypnosis]. Freiburg: Aurum; 1989
[95] Meinhold W. Krebs – eine mystifizierte Krankheit [Cancer – A Mythologized Disease]. Düsseldorf/Zürich: Walter; 1996
[96] Mertens W. Einführung in die psychoanalytische Therapie [Introduction to Psychoanalytic Therapy]. Vol. 3. Stuttgart: Kohlhammer; 1990
[97] Mewes C. Charaktertypen – wer passt zu wem? [Character Types – Who is Compatible with Whom?] Illertissen: Media Maria; 2011
[98] Milgram S. Das Milgram-Experiment. Zur Gehorsamsbereitschaft gegenüber Autorität [The Milgram Experiment – Willing Submission to Authority]. 14th Ed. Reinbek: Rowohlt; 1997
[99] Moorjani A. Heilung im Licht. München: Arkana; 2012
[100] Motoyama H. Chakra, Nadi of Yoga and Meridians, Points of Acupuncture. Tokyo: Institute of Religious Psychology; 1972
[101] Motoyama H. Chakras – Bridge to Higher Consciousness. Wheaton/Illinois: Quest Books; 1995
[102] Motoyama H. Diagnostic Methods in Western & Eastern Medicine – a Correlation between Ki Energy and Environmental Conditions. Tokyo: Human Science Press; 1999
[103] Motoyama H. Measurements of Ki Energy Diagnoses & Treatment – Treatment Principles of Oriental Medicine from an Electrophysiological Point of View. Tokyo: Human Science Press; 1997
[104] Murphy M. Der Quantenmensch – ein Blick in die Entfaltung des menschlichen Potentials im 21. Jahrhundert [Quantum Man – A Look into the Development of Human Potential in the 21st Century]. Munich: Integral/Scherz; 1998
[105] Nietzsche F. Menschliches, Allzumenschliches. Ein Buch für freie Geister. [Human, all too Human. A Book for Free Spirits].1878 & 1880

[106] Panikkar R. Gott, Mensch und Welt [God, Man and World]. Petersberg: Via Nova; 1999
[107] Paukert G. "Projekt Schmetterling – Förderung von Schulkindern" [Putterfly Project – Fostering Schoolchildren]. Lecture at the Medical Week, Baden-Baden 2005
[108] Pierrakos J. Core Energetik – Zentrum deiner Lebensenergie [Core Energetics – The Center of Your Life Energy]. Essen: Synthesis; 1987
[109] Popper KF. Logik der Forschung [The Logic of Research]. 11th Ed. Tübingen: Mohr Siebeck; 2005
[110] Powers R. Reinkarnation oder die Illusion der persönlichen Identität [Reincarnation, or the Illusion of Personal Identity]. Schliersee: Ch. Falk; 1989
[111] Qin J et al. "A human gut microbial gene catalogue established by metagenomic sequencing". Nature 2010; 464:59-65
[112] Raknes 0. Wilhelm Reich und die Orgonomie [Wilhelm Reich and Orgonomy]. Frankfurt: Fischer; 1973
[113] Reich W. Charakteranalyse [Character Analysis]. Frankfurt: Fischer; 1973
[114] Resch A. Psyche und Geist [Psyche and Spirit]. Innsbruck: Resch; 1986
[115] Riemann F. Grundformen der Angst [Basic Types of Fear]. Munich: Ernst Reinhard; 1968
[116] Rosenberg A. Die Seelenreise [The Soul's Journey]. Olten: Walter; 1952
[117] Rossaint A. Medizinische Kinesiologie, Physio-Energetik und Ganzheitliche Zahnheilkunde [Medical Kinesiology, Physioenergetics and Holistic Dentistry]. Kirchzarten: VAK; 2005
[118] Saint-Exupery A de. Wind, Sand und Sterne [Wind, Sand and Stars]. 3rd Ed. Düsseldorf: Karl Rauch; 2002
[119] Sanders L. Die Farben deiner Aura [The Colors of Your Aura]. Berlin: Goldmann; 1988
[120] Sartre J-P. Geschlossene Gesellschaft [No Exit]. Scene 5. Reinbek: Rowohlt; 1991
[121] Schimmel H. Bewährte Therapierichtlinien bei chronischen Erkrankungen [Proven Therapy Guidelines for Chronic Diseases]. Vols. 1-3. Gießen: Pascoe; 1990
[122] Schroeder B. Atemekstase – Rebirthing [Breath Ecstasy – Rebirthing]. Essen: Synthesis; o. J.
[123] Servan-Schreiber D. Das Antikrebs-Buch[The Anti-Cancer Book]. Berlin: Goldmann; 2012

[124] Shang C. "Prospective tests on biological models of acupuncture". Evid Based Complement Alternat Med 2009; 6(1): 31-39

[125] Sheldrake R. Das schöpferische Universum – Die Theorie des morphogenetischen Feldes [The Creative Universe – The Theory of the Morphogenetic Field]. Munich: Meyster; 1985

[126] Stein M. C.G. Jungs Landkarte der Seele [Jung's Map of the Soul: An Introduction]. Düsseldorf/Zurich: Walter; 2000

[127] Stevenson I. Concerns about Hypnotic Regression. Im Internet: www.medicine.virginia.edu/clinical/departments/psychiatry/sections/cspp/dops/regression-page

[128] Stevenson I. Wiedergeburt – Kinder erinnern sich an frühe Erdenleben [Rebirth – Children Recall Former Earthly Lives]. Frankfurt: Zweitausendeins; 1992

[129] Tansley D. Aura, Chakras und die Strahlen des Lebens [Aura, Chakras and the Radiations of Life]. Essen: Synthesis; 1984

[130] Tansley D. Energiekörper [Subtle Body: Essence and Shadow]. München: Kösel; 1985

[131] Tansley D. Radionik – energetische Diagnose und Behandlung [Radionics - Energetic Diagnosis and Treatment]. Essen: Synthesis; 1989

[132] Thie J. Gesund durch Berühren - Touch for Health. Munich: Irisiana/Hugendubel; 1995

[133] Tomatis A. Der Klang des Lebens [The Sound of Life]. Reinbek: Rowohlt; 1987

[134] Tompkins P. Das geheime Leben der Pflanzen [The Secret Life of Plants]. Frankfurt: Fischer; 1977

[135] Westlake A. Medizinische Neuorientierung [Medical Re-Orientation]. Zurich: Origo; 1963

[136] Wilber K. Wege zum Selbst [Ways to the Self: Eastern and Western Approaches to Personal Growth]. Munich: Kösel; 1984

[137] Woolger R. Die vielen Leben der Seele – Wiedererinnerung in der therapeutischen Arbeit [The Many Lives of the Soul – Re-Remembering in Therapy]. Munich: Hugendubel; 1992

[138] Zander H. Geschichte der Seelenwanderung in Europa - alternative religiöse Traditionen von der Antike bis heute [History of the Transmigration of Souls in Europe – Alternative Religious Traditions from Antiquity to the Present]. Darmstadt: Primus; 1999